Readers Loved

"Nothing else has worked in the past and I was more than a little skeptical that anything would work at this point. I have already lost about fourteen pounds in less than two months! It is amazing. I feel wonderful. . . . I almost don't feel like I'm doing anything that deprives me at all. Thank you, thank you, thank you, a million times. Thank you."

—*Carrie R.*

"*The Thyroid Diet* certainly was 'worth the weight!' Exactly nine weeks ago today I weighed in at 144 pounds. Today I weighed in at 121! Those twenty-three pounds have been with me for almost ten years and nothing was moving them. I had tried Atkins and after some weight loss I would stall on the scale, as soon as I ate again I would gain all the weight back and then some. I loved the diet plans and modified them to my benefit. I watched calories and found out carbs are my worst enemy. I eat healthy food and feel great. I just want to say thank you."

—*Linda W.*

"Mary Shomon has outdone herself again. In her easy-to-understand book [she] covers the details of how we digest our food, and the many herbs and minerals that can help thyroid disease sufferers lose weight, and what is just a waste of time or potentially dangerous. She doesn't just focus on hypothyroid patients, she discusses the whole spectrum of thyroid diseases, including thyroid cancer patients. There are also many valuable resources listed in the back of her book as well. Don't pass this book up—if you are suffering from thyroid disease and cannot seem to lose weight, this book will definitely give you hope and insight as to why."

—*Lea T.*

"I cannot believe that I have lived for three years without a thyroid, have been on a yo-yo medicine regimen, and am just now finding Mary! My doctor told me to just accept that I would never feel normal again! Now I know it doesn't have to be that way!" —*Cathy S.*

"I have taken Mary Shomon's suggestions on supplements and diet, and I have been impressed with her knowledge of what works and what doesn't. Mary, you are my hero! Thanks for saving so many of us from the pitfalls of trial and error in dealing with metabolism, diet, supplements, and prescriptions!" —*Shari D.*

"I had just been to one of my doctors and went on the scale, and it was just so depressing that no matter how hard I tried I couldn't get the weight off, even walking every day. Then I started the Thyroid Diet. When I went to my endocrinologist I had to get on the scales again. I had been on the diet for three weeks and I wasn't really expecting much. I was so surprised and happy to find out I had lost seventeen pounds. What really made me happy is that I don't feel hungry." —*Jackie B.*

"I have lost almost eighty-five pounds, found a new doctor who cares, and recommended *The Thyroid Diet* and Mary Shomon's website. Because of the information, I am now eighty-five pounds lighter, in less than one year!" —*Kathleen J.*

"I want to thank Mary Shomon for helping educate myself and others about thyroid disorders. Her frank, patient-centered manner has made me feel far more empowered and will allow me to start asking the right questions. I applaud Mary for turning the source of her pain into a blessing for others." —*Kelly Y.*

"I was about 140 for my life until I started to gain weight due to an undermedicated thyroid. I quickly went from 160 to 180 to 220 pounds. By following *The Thyroid Diet*, exercise, knowledge, and correct medicine, I am now maintaining my current weight of 135 pounds. I lost too many years of my life to being uninformed and passive about my thyroid condition. Now I am walking proof that you can live and be happy even with a thyroid condition!" –*Elissa C.*

"I used *The Thyroid Diet* to figure out how much I really should be eating and adjusted accordingly. Quite a scary feat for a gal who had gained steadily for four and a half years, despite constant exercise and diet, before being diagnosed as hypothyroid. I also use some supplements Mary recommended. I found an endocrinologist I love from Mary's Thyroid Top Doctors site—and after reading her research, I decided to switch medications (with my doctor's approval), and have never felt better. And so far I have dropped two dress sizes!"
                                                                    –*Natalie A.*

"I have had a hard several years trying to find ways to lower my weight, as nothing I tried seemed to work. With *The Thyroid Diet*, I was able to lose more than twenty-five pounds and am near a weight I am happy with. It's great to get help from someone who knows what I'm talking about."
                                                                    –*Sabrina P.*

"I really need to thank Mary Shomon for all of the useful information that has empowered me not to accept anything less than the best medical care. I have lost thirty pounds in about two years and feel fabulous. I am healthier and slimmer now at twenty-nine, than I was at my high school graduation. Thank you, Mary. What would my life be like without Mary's contribution to thyroid disease?"
                                                                    –*Rita H.*

"I ordered *The Thyroid Diet* a couple months ago and I would just like to say thank you. They gave me radioactive iodine, and then I quit smoking and gained weight. My doctor said no diet would help me. I have tried all the wrong things until I tried your book. I want to thank you for giving me hope and I feel so good about myself again. I have lost nineteen pounds in seventy-five days and dropped a few sizes already, and I have Mary to thank." —*Juanita S.*

"After dealing with hypothyroidism my entire life (diagnosed when I was about eighteen years old), I finally came across Mary's website and subsequently bought her book *The Thyroid Diet*. I literally thought myself crazy at times not understanding how slow my 'slow metabolism' could be! So finding other people who share my frustration, and someone who is an advocate for thyroid patients, literally brought tears to my eyes." —*Lauren W.*

"I started following Mary's diet in July, when I was about 146 pounds—the highest I've been since getting serious about exercise a few years ago. Today when I weighed myself I was at 124, about what I weighed twenty years ago when I was in grad school—and what I never expected to weigh again! It's been satisfying and really amazingly easy to give up my addiction to bread and pretzels, and I plan to keep following the plan for good." —*Anne M.*

"I feel like Mary Shomon is the only person who understands what I'm going through. I am a fitness instructor/personal trainer. I've been in the fitness industry for more than twenty-two years. For two years, doctors told me that my symptoms were due to depression over my mother's death, and the birth of a new baby, but I knew they were wrong and something was wrong with me. Over a few months, I gained twelve pounds, and I am someone who pays close attention to my nutrition, teaches group exercises classes every day of the week, strength training classes several times a week, and in addition to teaching, I also run three to five miles several times a week. Finally I was diagnosed with thyroid disease. Last week I picked up your book and read it—and found your advice helpful. I'm already down a few pounds. I feel like the weight should be melting off faster but I'm grateful that it is coming off."

—*Gina K.*

"I have just finished reading *The Thyroid Diet* and I am glad that I decided to read it. Not only did I come away from it with some great suggestions to make living with the condition easier, but it has also helped me realize that I am not alone in this—something I have felt since I was first diagnosed. I did not get more than four chapters into the book before I started crying. It was at this point that Mary's story, and the stories of several other women, resonated so deeply with me: from symptoms, diagnosis, treatment, and continual struggles. Breaking through the solitude I felt up until this point has given me new hope to improve my body and life."

—*Victoria G.*

THE
THYROID
DIET
REVOLUTION

THE
THYROID
DIET
REVOLUTION

Manage Your Master Gland

of Metabolism for Lasting

Weight Loss

MARY J. SHOMON

wm

WILLIAM MORROW
An Imprint of HarperCollins*Publishers*

This book contains advice and information relating to health care. It is not
intended to replace medical advice and should be used to supplement rather than
replace regular care by your doctor. It is recommended that you seek your physician's advice before embarking on any medical program or treatment. All efforts
have been made to assure the accuracy of the information contained in this book
as of the date of publication. The publisher and the author disclaim liability for
any medical outcomes that may occur as a result of applying the methods suggested in this book.

FIRST EDITION

Library of Congress Cataloging-in-Publication Data
    Shomon, Mary J.
        The thyroid diet revolution : manage your master gland of metabolism for
    lasting weight loss / Mary J. Shomon.
            p.   cm.
        Rev. ed. of: The thyroid diet.
        Includes bibliographical references and index.
        ISBN 978-0-06-198747-2 (pbk.)
        1. Hypothyroidism—Complications—Treatment. 2. Reducing
    diets. I. Shomon, Mary J. Thyroid diet. II. Title.
    RC657.S563   2011
    616.4'440654—dc22   2011005174

12 13 14 15 16   ov/RRD   10 9 8 7 6 5 4 3 2 1

For my precious children,
who are my joy and inspiration through thick and thin

Think with your whole body.
—Taisen Deshimaru

CONTENTS

ACKNOWLEDGMENTS

I'd like to thank my agent and friend, Carol Mann, as well as Jessica Deputato and her colleagues at HarperCollins for their wonderful guidance. Thanks to Jon, Julia, and Danny Mathis, and our fuzzy family members, who endured my long hours at the computer to help me make this book happen. Thank you to my dad, Dan Shomon, his fiancée, Gail Dana, and my brother, Dan Shomon, for their support, and to my mother, Pat, who, even though she is gone, is with me always in heart and spirit.

To my friends Jeannie Yamine, Jane Frank, Laura Horton, Kim Conley, Cynthia Wallentine, Gen Piturro, Viana Muller, Rebecca Elia, Julia Schopick, Lisa Moretti, Mohammed Antabli, Franca Fiabane, Michael Phillips, Nadia Krupnikova, Ric Blake, and Lisa Cook—thank you all for your support and friendship. And thanks to all the Momfriends!

Many thanks to my dear friend and colleague Teresa Tapp and the whole T-Tapp crew for their hard work and support. Ribs up, tuck butt, KLT everyone!

Thanks to Susan Osburn, Leslie Blumenberg, Lorena Veresh, Linda Souter, and Paige Waehner for research help on the current edition and the original book.

Continuing gratitude to Kate Lemmerman, MD; Scott Kwiat-kowski, DO; and Lauren Cafritz, who keep me running smoothly and breathing easily.

Special thanks to Katie Schwartz of DearThyroid, Geri Rybacki of the Coalition for Better Thyroid Care, Nicolet (Nikki) Hundt-Prohaska, Ali Jagger, Molly Shea Jester, Scott Rose, and Robert Chapman for your advocacy work and contributions to the thyroid cause.

To my unofficial news bureau, Rose Apter, Kim Carmichael-Cox, Sherri Leu, and Nicholas Bashour, among others, who have regularly sent me news reports, articles, and books that are right on target and always just what I need.

With thanks for their time and contributions to the book: David Clymer, Kat James, Jimmy Moore, Paige Waehner, and Daphne White.

Thanks to Kate Grossman, MD, Joy Victory, and all our colleagues at About.com, as well as my fellow guides, and to Aracely Brown and our colleagues at the New York Open Center.

Much gratitude to weight loss experts Marc David and Jena la Flamme, cofounders of the Weight Loss Pleasure Camp, for their time and for sharing their truly innovative thinking.

I must thank the many doctors, practitioners, and experts who provided information for the book, or who took time to brainstorm with me, shared their insights, or otherwise have contributed greatly to my thinking in the area of thyroid disease and nutrition. We are all fortunate to have these smart and caring people out there thinking about, researching, and caring for our health: Ken Blanchard, MD; David Brownstein, MD; Rob Carlson, MD; Hyla Cass, MD; Adrienne Clamp, MD; David Derry, MD; Rebecca Elia, MD; Udo Erasmus, PhD; Bruce Fife, ND, CN; Rick Ferris, PhD, ND; Ted Friedman, MD; Ann Louise Gittleman, PhD, CNS; Sara Gottfried, MD; Joy Gurgevich; Steven Gurgevich, PhD; Ron Hoffman, MD; Donna Hurlock, MD; Mark Hyman, MD; Dave Junno, PsyD; Karta Purkh Singh Khalsa, DN-C, RH ; Scott Kwiatkowski, DO; Stephen Langer, MD; Kate Lemmerman, MD; Scott Levine, MD; John Lowe,

DC; Ron Manzanero, MD; Viana Muller, PhD; Jan Nicholson, PhD; Richard Podell, MD; Byron Richards, CCN; Marie Savard, MD; Erika Schwartz, MD; Karilee Shames, PhD, RN; Richard Shames, MD; Robban Sica, MD; Mark Starr, MD; Jacob Teitelbaum, MD; Dirk van Lith, MD, MPH; and Ken Woliner, MD. A special thanks to Kent Holtorf, MD, for generously sharing so much of his innovative thinking about thyroid health.

And my heartfelt gratitude and commiseration to the thousands of people who have written to me to share their stories, pain, tears, laughter, joy, and sorrow as they go through this journey of thyroid disease and face the challenges of weight loss. I know exactly how you feel, and I can only hope that you find a glimmer of hope somewhere in this book, because you more than deserve hope, good health, happiness—and answers.

THE
THYROID
DIET
REVOLUTION

INTRODUCTION

Totie Fields once said, "I've been on a diet for two weeks and all I've lost is fourteen days."

If you're trying to lose weight, you may feel like Totie is talking about you.

You've probably tried diet after diet, joined Jenny Craig or Nutri-system, or tried whichever "lose twenty pounds in two weeks" diet program was being advertised the last time you watched late-night television. Maybe you sat through a few Weight Watchers meetings where everyone else lost weight that week . . . but not you. Maybe you tried herbal diet pills, or over-the-counter Alli, or overpriced açaí supplements. Maybe you've hitched your diet wagon to the likes of Valerie Bertinelli or Jennifer Hudson and the diet programs and products they promote. And I bet your bedside table is stacked high with diet books that tell you to eat only protein, eat like a caveman, smash your fat, flatten your belly, eat right for your blood type, and stay in the zone, right?

But whatever you're doing and whatever advice you're following, you're not losing weight. In fact, you may even be following one of these weight loss programs or diet gurus religiously, eating well, exercising regularly, and not only are you not losing, but you're actually gaining weight!

Mari, a personal trainer, found herself frustrated.

It just didn't make any sense. There I was advising my clients on fitness and nutrition, and somehow, I kept gaining weight, and couldn't drop a pound myself. I was eating a terrific, healthy diet—and believe me, in my business, I know about good sources of protein, organic fruits and veggies. I was working out with at least six clients a day—that's six hours of exercise on top of a low-calorie, low-fat, ultrahealthy diet. What else was I supposed to do, for goodness' sake, when I cut calories, cut fat, exercised more than ever before, and I still couldn't lose weight?

Maybe, like Mari, you never had a weight problem, but then suddenly the pounds started piling on. Many doctors say "calories in, calories out" and remind you that it takes 3,500 excess calories to gain a pound. But you—well, you seemingly defy the laws of physics! How it is humanly possible to eat the same things, in the same quantities, and do the same amount of exercise this month as you were doing last month, yet gain ten pounds? Logically, you would need to take in an extra 35,000 calories during the month—basically, the calories in sixty-five Big Macs—to gain ten pounds. And yet there it is, the extra weight . . . defying all logic and reason.

Andrea noticed that she had gained fifteen pounds unexpectedly, and to jump-start some weight loss, she did a three-week liquid cleansing fast—with no solid food, just drinking water and vegetable broth. At the end of the three weeks, she had *gained* two pounds.

I told my doctor that I was having trouble losing weight, even on the cleansing fast. My doctor laughed at me and said, "You won't lose weight unless you eat less." I looked at him and was thinking, "How much less could I possibly eat?"

When Corey first got married, she was a healthy 135 pounds.

Six months later, I was 175 pounds, miserable, and wondering how this had happened to me. At first, the doctor told me I was "clearly" eating too much and not exercising enough. I explained that my diet had actually *improved* after I got married and graduated from college. Before graduation, I ate fast food almost constantly. My new husband was a big fan of salad for dinner, so we primarily cooked at home and ate lots of salads.

When you're faced with this sort of unexplained weight gain or a total inability to lose weight on even the most rigorous diet and exercise program, what happens next? Well, most of us end up in a doctor's office, saying, "I think something is wrong with me."

Unfortunately, doctors often have little to offer, and you are likely to be sent home with one of the following:

- *An antidepressant.* "Depression makes you gain weight." Plus, it's easy and inexpensive to prescribe, because no blood tests are required.
- *A shrug of the shoulders.* The shrug is usually accompanied by one of those vague non-explanations like, "Well, you're getting older—it's to be expected" or "It must be your hormones" or "It's normal not to lose weight after having a baby" or "We all need more exercise," and so on.
- *A condescending look.* Often the look is delivered with patronizing advice along the lines of "Well, you clearly are eating too much!" or "Get off the couch and stop strapping on the feedbag!" And there's my personal favorite, the doctor who openly snickered at a woman and told her, "My diagnosis is that you have fork-in-mouth disease!"
- *A handout.* Usually this is a photocopy of the latest version of the USDA Food Pyramid, telling you to eat five servings of fruits and vegetables a day and . . . well, you know the rest. If your doctor is really fancy, maybe it'll be a color brochure of the food pyramid.

Gee, doctor, thanks for nothing.

You know something is not right. You are not overweight because you're sitting around lazily stuffing your face, but it seems like the doctor doesn't believe you. And you're not imagining that. The doctor *doesn't* believe you. One study showed that not only general practitioners—but even health professionals who specialize in treating obesity—have negative stereotypes about people who are overweight. They see someone who is overweight, and they associated that with being lazy or even unintelligent. Most doctors—and the people around you, to an even greater extent—have an automatic bias against people who are overweight.

You know something is wrong—but who believes you?

I believe you.

Because while your doctor is busy assuming that you're too lazy to exercise, that you're sneaking food when no one is looking, and that you don't have enough willpower to stop eating, what he or she is not doing is his or her job: to suspect that you could have a thyroid problem—a dysfunction in the small, butterfly-shaped gland in your neck—and run the proper tests to make a diagnosis.

A normal thyroid weighs just an ounce, but this little butterfly-shaped gland packs a punch, because it is your master gland of metabolism and energy. When your thyroid isn't functioning, your metabolism—and your ability to lose weight—can grind to a halt.

Unfortunately, some narrow-minded doctors dismiss thyroid disease as yet another "excuse" for being overweight. The reality, however, is that for millions of overweight people, undiagnosed, untreated, or improperly treated, thyroid disease is a very real reason for weight problems.

Learning about thyroid disease and its symptoms—beyond weight problems—and how to get properly diagnosed and treated are critical steps that can address an overlooked cause of your weight gain, help restore your hope, and finally allow healthy diet and exercise to work the way they should!

Recent studies have conservatively estimated that as many as 27 million people have a thyroid problem, *the majority of them undiagnosed*. Some experts believe that the actual number is substantially higher, more like 59 million people, and rapidly on the rise. At the same time, studies have shown that as many as two-thirds of all Americans—that's 200 million Americans—are overweight or obese.

Do you see the connection?

You may be one of the millions of people struggling to lose weight, sabotaged by your own thyroid! One study found that as many as 40 percent of overweight people had evidence of a dysfunctional thyroid.

That was the case for Mari, Andrea, Rick, and Corey. All were finally diagnosed with hypothyroidism, and after treatment, their weight normalized and their diet and exercise programs became successful again. This is what happens for some people who, struggling with undiagnosed thyroid issues, get diagnosed. It's as if a door opens. Weight doesn't magically fall off, but the diet and exercise programs that are no longer working begin to work again.

For some people, treating an undiagnosed, untreated thyroid condition can be the key to successful weight loss.

MY OWN JOURNEY

I wrote the first edition of *The Thyroid Diet* back in 2004, because it is a topic near and dear to my own heart.

I started inexplicably gaining weight at age thirty-three. After going through my twenties as a slender size 8, I quickly started packing on weight—so much so that I bought a size 12 wedding gown, and in the months before my wedding, I had to have my wedding dress let out two more sizes. (Is that a horrifying thing for a bride or what?) Even after I went on an intensive diet with daily exercise, I walked down the aisle as a size 16. After the honeymoon, the weight kept piling on. And it didn't make sense.

During that time before and after my wedding, I went to the doctor a number of times complaining about a variety of symptoms. I hadn't changed my diet and yet I was gaining weight rapidly. Even after I started an intensive diet and exercise program, the weight kept coming. I was exhausted. My hair was falling out. I felt moody and a bit blue. And I had muscle and joint pains and aches.

After a few visits, my doctor decided she should test my thyroid. I was surprised when she called and left a voice mail saying that I was hypothyroid and that she'd call in a prescription for me. I didn't even know what a thyroid was. Sure, I'd heard overweight people laughingly referred to as having "glandular problems," and I had an aunt who'd had a goiter once, but that was the extent of my knowledge about my master gland of metabolism.

My doctor put me on thyroid hormone replacement therapy. At that point, I assumed that all the symptoms, and particularly the pounds, would disappear as quickly as they had appeared, now that I was getting my thyroid back in order. But it wasn't so simple.

As we tweaked my medicine and dosage, I felt far better in some ways—less exhausted, less moody, my aches disappeared, and I felt clear-headed—and I lost a few pounds. But after that, the extra weight didn't budge.

Nothing I was doing moved the scale an ounce. I realized that it wasn't going to be so easy. So I set out on a mission to discover how best to optimize my thyroid treatment. To learn what and how much I could and couldn't eat in order to lose weight. To find out whether I needed to exercise, what type of exercise, and how much. To learn how to get back on track when my weight-loss efforts got stalled or even derailed.

So I started reading and learning. I interviewed hundreds of endocrinologists, internists, hormone experts, integrative physicians, nutritionists, weight-loss coaches, dietitians, herbalists, holistic health counselors, fitness experts, physiologists, and more.

Meanwhile, as I increasingly focused my time on thyroid advocacy, I also began to hear from other thyroid patients—in letters, in e-mails, in online forums, in calls to radio shows, in faxes, in telephone coaching sessions, and face-to-face at classes and events around the world. They would describe their symptoms, and ask if they too could have a thyroid problem. They would share their frustrations with inexplicable weight gain, the misery of not feeling well. They'd cry, telling me how being overweight made them feel ugly, old, worthless, and unattractive, and how nothing was working in their attempts to get the weight off. The ones who had figured out how to lose weight would share what was working and what wasn't.

I learned the most important fact of all: it doesn't have to be this way. There *are* answers.

And that's why I wrote *The Thyroid Diet*: to organize everything I'd learned about thyroid disease in one place, and to help others identify thyroid signs and symptoms, get properly diagnosed, navigate through the treatment options to get the best possible thyroid treatment, and tackle the issues of metabolism and hormonal imbalance that can make weight loss difficult even after proper treatment. I put together all the best ideas for thyroid patients who were trying to lose weight and not having success using the traditional "eat well and exercise" approach.

After *The Thyroid Diet* was published, I heard from thousands of people who were using the book to help transform their own health. *The Thyroid Diet* helped them recognize their own thyroid signs and symptoms and gave them the information and tools to find the right kind of practitioner, ask for the appropriate tests, and get treated. People were still coming up to me at conferences and sending me faxes and e-mails, saying: "I did it! I'm finally losing weight!" "My doctor can't believe it, even he wanted to know what I was doing!" And they cried . . . but this time tears of happiness!

Some thyroid patients—myself included—also discovered that the weight-loss journey for thyroid patients is an ongoing struggle. Certain people could optimize thyroid function, cut calories, reduce fat, cut starchy carbohydrates, and regularly exercise—and *still gain weight*. Again, seemingly defying the laws of physics!

What was going on?

Back to the medical journals, the literature, the endocrinologists, the hormone experts, the weight-loss coaches, the physiologists. Back to the patient community, to find out what was working and what wasn't. I realized that there was much more for us to know, and for some thyroid patients there were other hormonal issues that were getting in the way of weight loss.

And that's why I wrote *The Thyroid Diet Revolution*. Building on what we know from *The Thyroid Diet*, we are long overdue for a revolution in the way we think about the thyroid's impact on diet and weight loss, and a revolution in the way we help thyroid patients lose weight.

WHY DO WE NEED A REVOLUTION?

Some people think it should be obvious: you complain about fatigue and weight gain, and your doctor will run the right tests, interpret them correctly, and get you on the best thyroid treatments. Problem solved, right? Where's the issue? What's the controversy? Why do we need a revolution?

The truth is, it's rarely that easy. HMOs and insurers want to control costs, so they don't agree to pay for tests. Doctors don't agree on what tests to run or how to interpret them, creating a situation in which you can take the same blood test result and show it to two different doctors in the same practice, and one will say you have a thyroid condition and prescribe medication, while the other one will say you're fine.

But perhaps the biggest reason of all is that we are living with a tired, worn-out, and destructive stigma associated with the word *thyroid*.

If you say the word *thyroid* to someone who doesn't have or understand thyroid disease—and that means most people, including doctors, who don't personally have a thyroid condition—you're likely to hear laughter. These days, *thyroid* is code for "fat."

If you search for the term *thyroid* on Twitter, you'll see person after person tweeting a now famous "joke" from comedian Emo Phillips. The so-called joke goes like this: "I saw a woman wearing a sweatshirt with 'Guess' on it. I said, 'Thyroid problem?'"

It's no longer politically correct or acceptable in television shows or commercials to make fun of someone who is overweight. But the world loves to hate overweight people. So now they get around it by saying "thyroid problem."

Listen carefully—you'll hear it quite regularly in sitcoms, in conversation with friends and family, in celebrity interviews, in advertisements. Even major national companies such as Marriott and Dairy Queen have broadcast national advertising campaigns on television and radio that used references to "thyroid problems" to imply—in a failed attempt at humor—that someone was overweight.

Besides those who think it's just hilarious, you have the uninformed doctors, weight-loss experts, members of the media, and many of our own friends, family members, and colleagues who believe with all their hearts that thyroid problems are an excuse used by lazy, overweight people who want something to blame for being fat.

And, sad to say, there are even a few misguided, inept doctors who are out there yelling from the rafters that anyone who is overweight and asks the doctor for a thyroid test is just "drug-seeking"—as if the person were an addict looking to score a fix instead of a person with a hormonal imbalance looking for proper thyroid diagnosis and treatment!

Naturally, all of this laughter, prejudice, misinformation and mistreatment is coming from people who do *not* have thyroid conditions, so the bottom line is they have no idea what they're talking about. And that's clear when you start laying out real-life cases to them and they either quickly change the subject or argue that the person you're talking about "must be eating secretly"—even when I tell them about a lawyer I know named Rick, who was training for a marathon, running twenty to thirty miles a week, and eating a fastidiously healthy diet. Rick didn't know it yet, but he had become hypothyroid.

I was running regularly, subsisting on my usual diet of fish, chicken, and salads for the most part, I'd cut out the occasional glass of wine and had really tightened up my diet in preparation for the race. And the weight was piling on. I mean, every single week. Sometimes I felt like every day I got on the scale, it was up. In three months, I put on at least twenty pounds. It was if my body didn't belong to me. I asked the doctor if it could be a thyroid problem. But the doctor's answer? "Don't blame your thyroid. You just need more exercise!"

The stigma also extends to the celebrity world. When a high-profile celebrity announces that she is battling breast cancer, or he has had gastric bypass surgery for weight loss, there's no shame. In fact, they have their publicists announce it, they do interviews, and it's front-page news.

But what about when a celebrity has an underactive thyroid condition due to autoimmune Hashimoto's disease—the most common thyroid problem in America? Few celebrities seem inclined to publicly announce their hypothyroid conditions, and I can't think of anyone in recent years who has been willing to make it his or her own personal cause, or adopted it as an issue to promote.

For example, *Sex and the City* actress Kim Cattrall, NBC *Today* show host Meredith Vieira, singer Linda Ronstadt, and *My Big Fat Greek Wedding* star Nia Vardalos are all hypothyroid, and yet we rarely hear anything about their thyroid challenges. I even interviewed Nia Vardalos after she successfully lost forty pounds, and that was after she'd been diagnosed and treated for an underactive thyroid. She didn't want to talk about her thyroid problem, and implied that she didn't want to "blame" her thyroid for her weight gain, or attribute her ability to lose weight to getting properly diagnosed and treated. I have nothing but respect for Nia's amazing talent and intelligence, but, hello! When you get a thyroid condition properly diagnosed and treated, that is when many people find they *can* finally lose weight and keep it off!

(Of course it's okay to announce you have had thyroid cancer—like *JAG* and *Army Wives* actress Catherine Bell, singer Rod Stewart, Sofia Vergara of television's *Modern Family*, and comedian Joe Piscopo. For some reason, thyroid cancer does not have the same stigma.)

The truth is that many celebrities have thyroid problems, yet few of them have made it publicly known. The stigma surrounding thyroid problems ensures a celebrity code of silence.

There's another issue complicating the whole situation that we just can't overlook, and that's the Oprah factor.

I'll let you in on a secret—thyroid patients recognize each other. We look around us, and we see the puffiness around the eyes, the lack of hair on the outer edge of the eyebrows, the unexplained weight gain, the thinning hair, and we somehow just know. Since the late 1990s, I have had that feeling about Oprah Winfrey. And I was not alone. Other thyroid patients did too. Readers even wrote to me years ago, asking if I'd contacted Oprah. "Oprah looks hypothyroid to me," they'd write. "Please, Mary, get in touch with Oprah and tell her to get her thyroid checked!" And I did. Believe me, I did.

And I wrote not just to urge Oprah to get her own thyroid checked as she went up and down in her weight-loss struggles but also to urge her to cover thyroid disease on her program. For years, Oprah dedicated numerous episodes of her popular and influential talk show to important women's health concerns: menopause, low sex drive, weight loss, depression, infertility, PMS, and others. And time and again, she and her health experts listened to women complain of fatigue, weight gain or difficulty losing weight, depression, hair loss, muscle pain, lack of sex drive, erratic periods, and such, but thyroid disease was never mentioned! *Never!* Believe me, I was listening, not to mention writing to her and her producers, passionately encouraging them to bring up the issue of thyroid disease as an overlooked factor in all of these health concerns facing viewers. But Oprah continued on, and thyroid disease was not part of the discussion.

Meanwhile, Oprah seemed to successfully conquer her own weight-loss battle. Armed with her trainers, chefs, nutritionists, and staff, she had finally gotten to some sort of balance. She was at a healthy weight, she was exercising, and she seemed happy with herself.

But in 2006, she started to regain the weight that she'd lost. Again, I wrote to Oprah and her producers, and my readers wrote as well. The message: "Oprah, check your thyroid!"

No response.

In 2007, Oprah finally admitted what we had suspected along the way—she herself was hypothyroid. But instead of embracing it, doing a show on it, talking about the stealthy symptoms that can be difficult to identify and the issues around diagnosis and treatment, Oprah quickly backpedaled and claimed that she had "cured" her thyroid condition with a long Hawaiian vacation and a diet heavy in soy milk. She brought mind-body experts on her show to say that thyroid disease is due to women's inability to speak out, and that "finding your voice" is the solution. Oprah then came back and said that no, she wasn't actually cured, but that she'd decided *not* to take thyroid medication. Instead, she decided her problem was menopause, and she went on Suzanne Somers's controversial hormone regimen.

Meanwhile, she appeared to continue to gain weight, looking puffy around her eyes and in her face and neck. Was she still hypothyroid? Only her doctor knows, but she certainly fit the profile.

I'm not saying that Oprah's going public about her thyroid problem didn't have positive effects, because it did. There are some people who, listening to Oprah go back and forth about her thyroid issue, recognized the symptoms. Hearing about thyroid disease on Oprah was the wakeup call they needed to get properly diagnosed and treated.

But Oprah could have done so much more. She had it in her hands to help many millions of women around the world, women who look to her for advice and information and who follow Oprah's weight struggles because her struggles mirror their own.

Oprah had the opportunity to raise awareness of our epidemic of undiagnosed, untreated hypothyroidism. She had a chance to focus attention on the many challenges we face in getting properly diagnosed. Oprah could have explored the impact of an underactive and autoimmune thyroid on metabolism and weight. She was in a position to publicize the many issues surrounding proper thyroid treatment and restoring a metabolism that is affected by thyroid disease.

But Oprah did not do one of these things. Instead, she made it seem like having a thyroid problem was an embarrassment—something to be ashamed of, to brush away and ignore, and even to disown.

Oprah has also confused the weight-loss issue in particular for thyroid patients. By refusing thyroid treatment herself—a move that some of her followers will no doubt emulate—and by publicly advocating approaches that are known to be detrimental to some thyroid patients, she has made the weight-loss battle for thyroid patients more difficult.

She has publicly promoted a soy-heavy vegan diet, soy milk, vacations, bubble baths, and even blowing kisses at herself in the mirror as thyroid solutions. (I'm not saying that a nice soak in the tub and good self-esteem aren't great, but seriously—they are not treatments for thyroid problems.) And a diet heavy on certain raw vegetables and loaded with soy can actually slow the thyroid down further, making hypothyroidism worsen and causing further weight gain. So, thanks but no thanks, Oprah, for that advice.

The message women have taken away from Oprah is that thyroid problems really aren't worth focusing on, maybe you shouldn't even get treated for an underactive thyroid, and by the way, vegan diets, soy, self-love, and speaking out will help your thyroid—not exactly a road map to success for most people with thyroid conditions, and definitely *not* helpful for those thyroid patients who are having difficulty losing weight.

THE THYROID DIET REVOLUTION WILL HELP YOU GET OFF THE WEIGHT-LOSS MERRY-GO-ROUND

Not only is there a stigma attached to thyroid disease, but as we all know, it's not easy to be overweight. I know that you don't want to be overweight. Sure, there are some overweight people who feel entirely comfortable with themselves and don't have any body image issues. More power to them. But I'm not one of them, and if you're reading this book, neither are you.

And let's face it: in addition to the psychosocial burden—suffering emotionally or mentally because of the self-esteem and depression issues related to being overweight—there is also an increased risk of many serious health conditions, including:

- Insulin resistance and diabetes
- High blood pressure
- High cholesterol
- Cardiovascular disease
- Stroke
- Asthma
- Arthritis/degenerative joint disease
- Gallbladder disease
- Sleep apnea
- Fatigue
- Fertility problems and complications of pregnancy
- Stress incontinence

Being overweight or obese is also a risk factor for various cancers. A sixteen-year study by the American Cancer Society found that deaths from a wide variety of cancers—including those of the breast, endometrium, colon, rectum, esophagus, pancreas, kidney, gallbladder, ovary, cervix, liver, and prostate, as well as multiple myeloma and non-Hodgkin's lymphoma—are linked to excess weight and obesity. Only a few cancers—lung cancer, bladder cancer, brain cancer, and melanoma—were found to have no link to excess weight. All those health issues certainly provide enough incentive to lose weight.

But how?

If you read the newspapers and women's magazine articles, watch those middle-of-the-night infomercials, view morning television interviews, and talk to the staff at supplement stores, you'll hear from "experts" galore, and every one of them knows the magic answer, the key to weight-loss success. The key is . . .

   . . . detoxing the liver
   . . . regulating insulin
   . . . avoiding carbohydrates
   . . . avoiding fat
   . . . eating more good fat
   . . . staying away from the wrong carbohydrates
   . . . restricting calories
   . . . eating more calories
   . . . raw foods
   . . . juicing
   . . . being a vegetarian
   . . . being a vegan
   . . . going gluten- free
   . . . eating a high-protein diet
   . . . mini-meals and grazing all day
   . . . eating three meals a day and no snacks
   . . . eating Mediterranean style

. . . exercising
. . . taking supplements
. . . taking weight-loss drugs
. . . eating cabbage soup
. . . following a liquid diet
. . . having surgery
. . . managing your mind and emotions
. . . regulating brain chemistry
. . . drinking maple syrup and cayenne pepper

Blah blah blah! It's a weight-loss merry-go-round, and we need to get off.

That's hard for everyone, but it's even more so for people who have an undiagnosed—or even diagnosed and treated—thyroid problem.

Thyroid patients are generally not lazy or lacking willpower. And your weight problem is most likely not an emotional issue that can be shouted and bullied out of you by some anorexic television personality with abs of steel and a heart of stone. You know and I know that you're not downing an entire pizza or box of donuts every night when no one else is watching. Your eating habits are probably not very different from those of your friends or family members who are at a normal weight.

Your problem is that your body does not work the way it's supposed to, so a challenge that is already hard for most people is that much harder for you. And what you suspect about your body is probably true: you may gain weight more easily than others, and you probably won't lose weight as quickly as others.

In fact, if you are hypothyroid, your metabolism can become so inefficient—unable to burn fat, and capable of storing nearly every calorie you eat as fat—despite the most rigorous diet and exercise program. Your friend or spouse could go on the same diet as you, lose a pound or two a week, and you might stay the same or even gain weight. It's not fair!

Can we shout that together? *It's not fair!*

Okay, since we've established that it's not fair, it's time to move on. That's life—I've got a thyroid problem, maybe you've got a thyroid problem, and it's not likely to go away. This is something we'll probably both live with for the rest of our lives. The question is, are we going to live well with it, or it is going to define us and make us miserable? Is it going to stop us from feeling good about ourselves, fitting into clothes we like, feeling sexy, exercising or playing sports, having energy for work, family, and children?

It shouldn't, but it does.

But *The Thyroid Diet Revolution*—in a simple, understandable way—helps you get off the merry-go-round, offering you the support, encouragement, and information you need to lose weight, despite a thyroid condition.

ABOUT THE THYROID DIET REVOLUTION

The Thyroid Diet Revolution can be a weight-loss revolution for you in a number of ways.

First, if you don't yet know if a thyroid problem is sabotaging your efforts to lose weight, you'll learn about the signs and symptoms—including the subtle and less common symptoms—that can signal a potential thyroid condition. You'll get comprehensive guidelines on how to get properly diagnosed. And keep in mind that it's rarely as easy as asking your doctor to "test your thyroid." You'll find out which tests to ask for, and how to get them done—even if you have an HMO, insurance company, or practitioner who is interfering. You'll find out what the test results mean, and why "your thyroid results are normal" is not enough information and doesn't rule out the kind of thyroid problem that could make you gain weight—or stop you from losing weight. And if you are diagnosed with a thyroid condition, there's the issue of treatment. Some doctors believe that anyone with an underactive thyroid should just be put on the Synthroid brand of levothyroxine medication, and that's that. But there are actually many brands beyond Synthroid, and many other options beyond levothyroxine, that can be used to effectively treat your thyroid condition. The key is finding out which drug(s), at what dose(s), and in what combination(s) can safely and best resolve your symptoms. And, of particular interest to thyroid patients trying to lose weight, there is the issue of thyroid resistance—or, as Dr. Mark Starr calls it, type II hypothyroidism.

You'll also learn about hormonal imbalances and resistance issues, and how they can affect your ability to lose weight. First, some thyroid patients produce a particular kind of thyroid hormone that can make it especially difficult for you to lose weight. Few doctors test for it, and few doctors understand what it means and how to treat it. You'll learn about thyroid resistance in *The Thyroid Diet Revolution*. There are other types of hormonal resistance that are also more common in thyroid patients, including insulin resistance and leptin resistance. Again, there are very few physicians who are knowledgeable about the hormonal impact on weight gain and loss, but you'll find out the latest information on how these resistance syndromes can affect weight loss, and how they can be identified, tested, and, most important, treated. Other hormone imbalances can also affect your ability to lose weight, including estrogen dominance and deficiencies or excess levels of progesterone, adrenal hormone, DHEA, and testosterone. *The Thyroid Diet Revolution* will help you explore the interrelated balance of hormones and weight.

Nutrition is, of course, a critical component for thyroid patients who want to lose weight, and *The Thyroid Diet Revolution* has a comprehensive approach to help guide you. You'll learn about the challenges—nutritional and vitamin deficiencies, food allergies, food sensitivities, goitrogenic foods, phytoestrogens, and toxic exposures—that can get in the way of weight loss. You'll also learn about the importance of the glycemic index for thyroid patients who want to lose weight, as well as foods that help metabolism. And you'll get a number of structured recommendations that can get you started right away on the thyroid diet. You'll also get in-depth reviews of the most popular diet programs—everything from the South Beach Diet to Weight Watchers, Jenny Craig, and the Paleo Diet—from the perspective of thyroid patients. Is this a diet that is generally thyroid-friendly? Are thyroid patients losing weight on this diet plan? Should you avoid the diet entirely? Are there ways to customize it to make it more effective for thyroid patients? It's all here in *The Thyroid Diet Revolution.*

Movement is also an essential part of *The Thyroid Diet Revolution*'s approach to weight loss. But not just any exercise. Have no fear—I'm not going to suggest you start doing an hour of step aerobics six days a week, or start running five miles a day. Most of us aren't in shape to do that—plus it's not healthy for our adrenal system and may even prevent weight loss. The real key? Building muscle, detoxing the lymph system, and moving without exhausting ourselves. I have some recommendations regarding great ways to get into a regular exercise program, including a section created specifically for thyroid dieters by exercise physiologist Teresa Tapp, founder of the incredible T-Tapp exercise program. To whet your appetite: I lost twelve inches in two weeks, and I was doing three 45-minute sessions of T-Tapp a week.

And last but not least, there is the mind-body aspect of weight loss. What you think does affect what you eat, how you eat, how you digest, and whether or not you gain or lose weight. If you're inclined to dismiss that idea as "woo-woo," think again. Neuroendocrinology is the science of the relationship between our neurological and hormonal systems. And those two systems are indeed related. Think about how, if you watch a television commercial for something that looks delicious, you might start feeling hungry. You may even begin to salivate a little. Meanwhile, behind the scenes, a whole host of hormonal processes are beginning. What if you could tap into those hormonal processes and help guide them in the right direction? In *The Thyroid Diet Revolution*, you'll learn the skill of talking directly to your body in a language it can understand. You'll also learn why "loving your animal"—to borrow a phrase from weight-loss expert Jena la Flamme—is an essential part of weight loss. And how slowing down, savoring what we eat, and appreciating the experience can actually transform our relationship with food and help us lose weight.

The Thyroid Diet Revolution also includes a detailed resources section, to help you explore in even greater depth the many concepts, approaches, and techniques featured in the book, and so you can access all the skills, tools, experts, and resources you need to get started.

Isn't it time you started a revolution, your own *Thyroid Diet Revolution?*

Let's get started!

Mary J. Shomon
March 2011
Kensington, Maryland

PART 1

THE THYROID

CONNECTION

CHAPTER 1

Could You Have an Undiagnosed Thyroid Condition?

Knowledge is of two kinds: we know a subject ourselves,
or we know where we can find information about it.
—SAMUEL JOHNSON

The thyroid is a small butterfly-shaped gland located in your neck around the windpipe, behind and below your Adam's apple area. The thyroid produces several hormones, but two are absolutely essential: triiodothyronine (T3) and thyroxine (T4). These hormones help oxygen get into your cells and are critical to your body's ability to produce energy. This role in delivering oxygen and energy makes your thyroid the master gland of metabolism.

The thyroid has the only cells in the body capable of absorbing iodine. It takes in the iodine obtained through food, iodized salt, or supplements, and combines that iodine with the amino acid tyrosine. The thyroid then converts the iodine/tyrosine combination into the hormones T3 and T4. The 3 and the 4 refer to the number of iodine atoms in each thyroid hormone molecule.

Of all the hormones produced by your thyroid when it is functioning properly, approximately 80 percent will be T4 and 20 percent will be T3. Of the two, T4 is a storage hormone, and T3 is the biologically active hormone—the one that actually has an effect at the cellular level. So while the thyroid gland produces some T3, the rest of the T3 needed by the body is actually formed when the body converts stored T4 to T3. Once released by the thyroid, the T3 and T4 travel through the bloodstream. When it reaches cells, thyroid hormone helps convert oxygen and calories into energy to serve as the basic fuel for your metabolism.

As mentioned, the thyroid produces some T3. But the rest of the T3 needed by the body is actually formed by the conversion of the mostly inactive storage hormone T4. The process by which T4 becomes T3 is sometimes referred to as T4-to-T3 conversion. This conversion can take place in the thyroid, the liver, the brain, and other organs and tissues.

As T3 circulates through your bloodstream, it attaches to and enters your cells via receptor sites on the membrane of the cells. Once inside the cells, T3 increases cell metabolic rate, including body temperature, and stimulates the cells to produce a number of different hormones, enzymes, neurotransmitters, and muscle tissue. T3 also helps your cells use oxygen and release carbon dioxide, which assists metabolic function.

So how does the thyroid know how much T4 and T3 to produce? The release of hormones from the thyroid is part of a feedback process. The hypothalamus, a part of the brain, releases thyrotropin-releasing hormone (TRH). The release of TRH tells your pituitary gland to in turn produce thyroid-stimulating hormone (TSH). The TSH that circulates in your bloodstream is the messenger that tells your thyroid to make the thyroid hormones T4 and T3, sending them into your bloodstream. When the pituitary senses a sufficient amount of thyroid hormone circulating in the bloodstream, the pituitary makes less TSH. This reduction in TSH is a signal to the thyroid that it can slow down thyroid hormone production. When the pituitary senses that there is not enough thyroid hormone circulating, TSH goes up.

It's a smoothly functioning system when it works properly. But when the thyroid gland itself malfunctions, or when something interferes with the system and the feedback process doesn't work, thyroid symptoms develop.

PREVALENCE

At minimum, experts estimate, there are 27 million thyroid sufferers in the United States, and at least 13 million of them are undiagnosed. There are some scientists who suggest that the actual number is much higher, maybe as high as 59 million, which would mean that about one in five Americans has a thyroid problems. In the United States, the most prevalent thyroid disease is Hashimoto's disease, an autoimmune condition that causes hypothyroidism—an underactive thyroid. Thyroid problems are actually the most common autoimmune diseases in America today.

Women are seven to ten times more likely than men to develop thyroid problems. During their lifetime, women face as much as a one in five chance of developing a thyroid problem. For both men and women, the risk of thyroid disease increases with age, and by age seventy, the prevalence of subclinical hypothyroidism in men is nearly as high as in women.

In the United States, thyroid cancer is on the rise, with an estimated 45,000 new cases diagnosed in 2010. The incidence of thyroid cancer has increased substantially in the past decade, and experts believe it's in part due to exposure to radiation.

Thyroid problems are also common in many other countries, and autoimmune thyroid disease and thyroid cancer in particular are more prevalent in the areas around and downwind of the 1986

Chernobyl nuclear accident. Other areas that have a higher incidence of thyroid problems are those parts of the world that were
at one time covered by glaciers, where iodine is not present in the
soil and in foods. In many of these countries, an enlarged thyroid,
known as goiter, is seen in as many as one in five people and is usually due to iodine deficiency. Globally, an estimated 8 percent of
the population has goiter, most commonly women. Iodine deficiency
during pregnancy is also the leading preventable cause of mental
retardation around the world.

OVERVIEW OF CONDITIONS

The main conditions that can occur with the thyroid include:

- *Hypothyroidism:* when the thyroid is underactive and isn't producing sufficient thyroid hormone
- *Hyperthyroidism:* when the thyroid is overactive and is producing
  too much thyroid hormone
- *Goiter:* when the thyroid becomes enlarged, due to hypothyroidism
  or hyperthyroidism
- *Nodules:* when lumps, usually benign, grow in the thyroid, sometimes causing it to become hypothyroid or hyperthyroid
- *Thyroid cancer:* when lumps or nodules in the thyroid are ma-
  lignant
- *Postpartum thyroiditis:* when the thyroid is temporarily inflamed,
  in addition to hypothyroidism or hyperthyroidism triggered after
  pregnancy
- *Transient thyroiditis:* temporary inflammation or infection of the
  thyroid that can cause hypothyroid or hyperthyroid symptoms in
  some people

Causes and Risk Factors

The most common causes of thyroid conditions are autoimmune diseases, notably Hashimoto's thyroiditis and Graves' disease. In an autoimmune disease, the body's immune defenses inappropriately identify the thyroid as foreign to the body in some way. Hashimoto's disease may cause periods of hyperthyroidism, followed by permanent hypothyroidism as the antibodies produced by the immune system destroy the gland's ability to produce thyroid hormone. In Graves' disease, antibodies cause the thyroid to produce excessive amounts of thyroid hormone, a condition that is called hyperthyroidism and which can become life-threatening if not treated. If you have Graves' disease, you'll most likely receive antithyroid drugs, radioactive iodine, or surgery that will partially or entirely disable the thyroid's ability to produce thyroid hormone. Most people will become hypothyroid after treatment for Graves' disease.

The risk of developing thyroid disease is greatest if:

- You or a family member has a history of thyroid problems
- You or a family member has a history of autoimmune disease (e.g., rheumatoid arthritis, psoriasis, vitiligo, multiple sclerosis, lupus, or other conditions)
- You are or were a smoker
- You have had a stomach infection or food poisoning in the past, especially if the infection is diagnosed as being caused by the foodborne bacterium *Yersinia enterocolitica*
- You have allergies or a sensitivity to gluten, or have been diagnosed with celiac disease
- You've been exposed to radiation, by living near or downwind from a nuclear plant, or through particular medical treatments (e.g., treatment for Hodgkin's disease, nasal radium therapy, radiation to tonsils and neck area), have had numerous dental or neck X-rays

(without a thyroid collar), or were near or downwind of the Chernobyl nuclear disaster in 1986

- You've been treated with the medications lithium or amiodarone
- You have been taking supplemental iodine, kelp, bladder wrack, or bugleweed
- You live in an area (e.g., the midwestern "goiter belt") where there is low iodine in the soil, or you have cut down substantially on the iodized salt in your diet, leaving you iodine-deficient
- You've been exposed to excessive amounts of environmental estrogens, toxins, and other chemicals (e.g., perchlorate, fluoride, bisphenol A) via your water, food, or employment
- You've been excessively exposed to metals such as mercury
- You drink fluoridated water and use external fluoride (fluoridated toothpaste, fluoride treatments)
- You are a heavy consumer of soy products, especially soy powders or soy-based supplements
- You eat a substantial quantity of raw goitrogenic foods such as Brussels sprouts, rutabaga, turnips, kohlrabi, radishes, cauliflower, cassava, millet, cabbage, kale, and babassu (fruits from a type of palm tree native to the Amazon)
- You are over age sixty
- You are female
- You are in a period of hormonal variance such as perimenopause, menopause, pregnancy, or postpartum
- You have had serious trauma to the neck such as whiplash from a car accident or a broken neck
- You currently have or have in the past been diagnosed with any of the following diseases or conditions, known to occur more frequently in people with thyroid disease:
  - Other pituitary or endocrine disease (e.g., diabetes, a pituitary tumor, polycystic ovary syndrome [PCOS], endometriosis, premature menopause, adrenal disease)
  - Chronic fatigue syndrome
  - Fibromyalgia

- Carpal tunnel syndrome, tendonitis, plantar fasciitis
- Mitral valve prolapse syndrome (MVPS)
- Epstein-Barr virus (EBV)
- Mononucleosis
- Depression
- Infertility or recurrent miscarriage
- Celiac disease (gluten intolerance)

HYPOTHYROIDISM

The most common thyroid condition is hypothyroidism. It's estimated that the majority of people with thyroid conditions in the United States are hypothyroid. A concerning statistic: most experts believe that at least half of Americans with a thyroid disorder are undiagnosed.

If you have hypothyroidism, your thyroid fails to produce sufficient levels of the thyroid hormones needed by your body. This slows down a variety of bodily functions, as well as your metabolism. Hypothyroidism typically develops when:

- An autoimmune disease (Hashimoto's disease) has caused your immune system to attack and destroy your thyroid, making it unable to produce sufficient hormone amounts.
- You've had radioactive iodine (RAI) treatment for your overactive thyroid, which has made all or part of your thyroid unable to produce hormone.
- You have a goiter or thyroid nodule(s) that is interfering with your gland's ability to produce hormone.
- You've had surgery for goiter, thyroid nodules, Hashimoto's disease, or thyroid cancer, and all or part of your thyroid has been removed.

- You've been hypothyroid since birth. A small percentage of people experience this condition, known as congenital hypothyroidism, which results from a missing or malformed thyroid gland.
- You have an imbalance in your adrenal or reproductive hormones that is putting strain on the thyroid's ability to produce hormone.
- You have a significant excess or deficiency of iodine that is affecting the thyroid's ability to function properly.
- You are taking a medication, such as lithium, that is disabling the thyroid's ability to produce sufficient hormone.
- You are hyperthyroid and taking too much antithyroid medication.

Ultimately, however your thyroid problem started, if your thyroid is now unable to produce sufficient thyroid hormone, or if you don't have a thyroid at all, you are considered hypothyroid.

Symptoms

You may be hypothyroid if:

- You are extremely exhausted and fatigued
- You feel depressed, moody, or sad
- You're sensitive to cold, and you have cold hands or feet
- You're experiencing inappropriate weight gain, or having difficulty losing weight, despite changes in diet and exercise
- Your hair has become dry, easily tangled, or coarse
- You've lost hair, and in particular, hair from the outer part of the eyebrows
- You have dry or brittle nails
- You're feeling muscle and joint pains and aches
- You have carpal tunnel syndrome or tendonitis in the arms and legs
- The soles of your feet are painful, a condition known as plantar fasciitis
- Your face, eyes, arms, or legs are abnormally swollen or puffy

- You have an unusually low sex drive
- You have unexplained infertility, or recurrent miscarriages with no obvious explanation
- Your menstrual period is heavier than normal, or your period is longer than it used to be or comes more frequently
- You feel like your thinking is fuzzy (e.g., you have difficulty concentrating or remembering)
- You're constipated
- You have a full or sensitive feeling in the neck
- Your voice is raspy or hoarse
- Your heart rate or blood pressure is unusually low
- You have periodic heart palpitations
- Your total cholesterol and LDL ("bad") cholesterol levels are high and may not respond to diet and medication
- Your allergies have gotten worse, and you experience symptoms such as itching, prickly hot skin, rashes, and hives (urticaria)
- You regularly have infections, including yeast infections, thrush, or sinus infections
- You feel shortness of breath, sometimes have difficulty drawing a full breath, or often feel a need to yawn

Dana described how she determined that she needed to be tested for hypothyroidism:

I have a master's degree in nutrition and had worked for about eight years in health care at the time as a clinical dietitian. The crunch for me came when I put a woman on a weight-loss diet. I asked her to eat about 1,800 calories per day and try to do ten minutes on the treadmill daily. Meanwhile, I was doing eleven hours of step aerobics daily, and riding my bike to and from work, and eating a strict (and I mean strict!) 1,200-calorie diet. She lost eight pounds in one week, and I gained two!

Dana's doctor was astute enough to suspect hypothyroidism right away, and she was diagnosed and able to get on a treatment program.

Diagnosis

One possible sign of thyroid abnormality is a chronically low basal body temperature. To take a basal temperature, use a special basal thermometer, and take your temperature upon awakening before getting out of bed and moving around. Typically, basal body temperatures lower than 97.8 to 98.2 degrees Fahrenheit are thought to indicate hypothyroidism. This self-testing method was popularized by the late Dr. Broda Barnes. This test is not considered conclusive by many practitioners and does not definitively diagnose or rule out thyroid abnormalities.

To diagnose or rule out hypothyroidism, conventional doctors will typically start with a blood test that measures thyroid-stimulating hormone (TSH). As of the spring of 2003, laboratory guidelines and standards recommended that the reference range for the TSH test be revised to 0.3 to 3.0 mIU/L. Still, nearly a decade later, most American laboratories still use 0.5 to 5.5 as the normal reference range for the TSH test. When 5.5 is the top end of the normal reference range, a TSH above that level may be considered hypothyroid. With the newer guidelines, a TSH above 3.0 might be considered indicative of hypothyroidism.

Other blood tests that may be done to help diagnose hypothyroidism include:

- *Total T4 (total thyroxine).* A low level along with an elevated TSH may indicate hypothyroidism.
- *Free T4 (free thyroxine).* A low level along with an elevated TSH may indicate hypothyroidism. (Free levels refer to unbound, available thyroid hormone and are considered more accurate than total levels.)

- *Total T3*. A low level along with an elevated TSH may indicate hypothyroidism.
- *Free T3*. A low level along with an elevated TSH may indicate hypothyroidism.
- *Reverse T3*. A level above 150, or a ratio of free T3 to reverse T3 that exceeds 0.2 (when free T3 is measured in picograms per milliliter [pg/mL]), may indicate hypothyroidism.
- *Antithyroid antibodies (thyroglobulin and microsomal)*. The presence of these antibodies usually indicates thyroid autoimmunity and possibly Hashimoto's thyroiditis.
- *Antithyroid peroxidase (anti-TPO) antibodies*. The presence of these antibodies usually indicates autoimmunity and possibly Hashimoto's thyroiditis.

Hashimoto's thyroiditis is the most common cause of hypothyroidism. The characteristic Hashimoto's thyroiditis patient has high TSH values and usually low free T3 and T4 thyroid hormone levels. However, the greatest distinguishing feature for Hashimoto's is a high concentration of thyroid autoantibodies—anti-TPO antibodies in particular. Some patients have elevations in antibody levels for months or even years before elevation of the TSH level and a drop in the free T4 and free T3 levels.

Treating Hypothyroidism

The medical treatment for hypothyroidism is with prescription thyroid hormone replacement drugs, which are almost always taken daily.

Most commonly, conventional physicians prescribe a levothyroxine (T4-only) drug—i.e., Synthroid, Levoxyl, Levothroid—as this category of drug is considered the standard treatment for hypothyroidism. Generic levothyroxine is of good quality, but the problem is that you may wind up with generics from different makers—and thus with somewhat different potencies—with each prescription refill, making it more difficult to stabilize on a particular dose.

Integrative thyroid experts have shown through research and clinical practice that a subset of patients feel better with the addition of T3, so some practitioners are prescribing levothyroxine plus synthetic T3—known as liothyronine—in various forms.

Natural desiccated thyroid drugs—derived from the thyroid gland of pigs—are less commonly used but more popular with holistic and integrative physicians. These drugs, which contain natural forms of the T4 and T3 hormones, among other ingredients, are known by the brand names Armour Thyroid, Nature-Throid, Westhroid, and Erfa.

A more detailed discussion of hypothyroidism treatment and medications is featured in chapter 3.

HYPERTHYROIDISM

Hyperthyroidism occurs when the thyroid is overactive, producing more thyroid hormone than is necessary. Just as hypothyroidism slows down the body's functioning, hyperthyroidism speeds it up, causing accelerated heart rate, high blood pressure, and other concerns. Hyperthyroidism may be caused by:

- An autoimmune disease (Graves' disease) that has caused the immune system to attack the thyroid. Autoantibodies bind to the thyroid gland and cause the thyroid to overproduce thyroid hormone.
- Autoimmune Hashimoto's disease, which can include short spurts of overactivity and hyperthyroidism before the thyroid shifts into underactivity.
- A goiter, nodule, or nodules that have caused the thyroid to inappropriately produce too much thyroid hormone.
- Excessive exposure to iodine.

- Thyroiditis, an inflammation of the thyroid that makes the thyroid overactive.
- Being hypothyroid and taking too much thyroid medication.

Symptoms

Hyperthyroid patients often have an enlarged thyroid, which can be felt by a doctor upon examination. You may be hyperthyroid if:

- You're rapidly losing weight, or you are eating more and not gaining weight
- You're having a hard time falling asleep or staying asleep
- You're suffering from anxiety, irritability, nervousness, or even panic attacks
- You're finding it difficult to concentrate
- You're having palpitations, or your pulse and heartbeat are rapid, and blood pressure is elevated
- You're sweating more than usual, feeling hot when others are not
- You have tremors in your hands
- You're suffering from diarrhea
- You feel tired
- Your skin is dry, or you have a thickening of the skin on the shin area of your legs
- Your periods have stopped or are very light and infrequent
- You're having muscle pain and weakness, especially in the upper arms and thighs
- You're having eye problems, such as double vision or scratchy eyes, or you notice that your eyes are bulging or more of the white is showing than usual
- You're having trouble getting pregnant
- Your hair has become fine and brittle
- Your behavior is erratic

Diagnosis

A diagnosis is usually made by a thyroid-stimulating hormone (TSH) test. Levels lower than 0.3 to 0.5 are considered possibly indicative of hyperthyroidism.

Other blood tests that may be done to help diagnose hyperthyroidism include:

- *Total T4 (total thyroxine).* A high level along with a low TSH may indicate hyperthyroidism.
- *Free T4 (free thyroxine).* A high level along with a low TSH may indicate hyperthyroidism. (Again, note that free levels measure unbound, available T4 and T3, and are considered more accurate than total levels.)
- *Total T3.* A high level along with a low TSH may indicate hyperthyroidism.
- *Free T3.* A high level along with a low TSH may indicate hyperthyroidism.

Additionally, thyroid-stimulating immunoglobulin (TSI) or thyroid-stimulating antibodies (TSAb) in your blood may also be measured to diagnose Graves' disease, the autoimmune condition that frequently causes hyperthyroidism.

A radiographic picture of the thyroid that is taken after ingesting radioactive iodine by mouth may also be taken to see if the thyroid gland is overactive. This overactivity is a hallmark of Graves' disease. (*Note:* Because radioactivity can potentially damage the unborn or breast-feeding infant's thyroid gland, this procedure is not done during pregnancy or in nursing mothers.)

Treating Hyperthyroidism

Regardless of the method of treatment eventually used, as a first course of action a doctor may initially recommend that you take a beta-adrenergic blocking drug—also known as a beta-blocker—such as atenolol (Tenormin), nadolol (Corgard), metoprolol (Lopressor), or propranolol (Inderal) to block the action of circulating thyroid hormone in your tissue, slow your heart rate, and reduce nervousness. These drugs can be useful in rapidly reducing potentially dangerous symptoms until treatment has taken effect.

When the disease is mild, occurs in children or young adults, or needs to be promptly controlled (as with elderly patients whose heart disease puts them at risk from the increased heart rate associated with Graves' disease), the first treatment approach is often a course of antithyroid drugs such as methimazole (Tapazole). This drug make it more difficult for your thyroid to use the iodine it needs to produce thyroid hormone, resulting in a decrease in thyroid hormone production. Outside the United States, a similar drug, carbimazole, is frequently used. Another antithyroid drug, propylthiouracil (PTU), is still used by some patients and practitioners, but carries a slightly increased risk of side effects, and so increasingly doctors prefer methimazole.

Antithyroid drugs work well for about 20 percent to 30 percent of patients. In some patients, antithyroid drug treatment for twelve to eighteen months will result in prolonged remission of the disease, particularly if the disease is relatively mild when treatment is begun. These drugs can offer as much as a 40 percent chance of remission in some patients. This is another reason to see your doctor early if you suspect you have the disease.

In about 5 percent of cases, antithyroid drugs cause allergic reactions such as skin rashes, hives, and sometimes fever and joint pains. A rarer and even more serious potential side effect is a decrease in the white blood cells that are part of the immune system, thereby resulting in a decrease in resistance to infection. In very rare cases, these cells may disappear entirely (a condition called agranulocytosis), which can be potentially fatal if there is a serious infection.

If you experience an infection while taking these drugs, call your doctor immediately. The doctor will likely tell you to stop taking the drug right away and get a white blood count that same day. If the white count has been lowered and you continue taking the drug, the infection could become fatal. However, a lowered white count will return to normal once you have stopped taking the drug.

Despite the fact that patients treated with antithyroid drugs have a decent chance of permanent remission, radioactive iodine (RAI) is the treatment of choice in the United States. In RAI, a radioactive iodine pill is given. The iodine concentrates in the thyroid, making it partially or fully inactive, and reversing the hyperthyroidism. RAI is typically followed by an elevation in thyroid antibodies, which can further aggravate the autoimmune-related symptoms. According to experts, the majority of patients do become hypothyroid for life after RAI, and while this is sometimes due to radiation-induced follicular damage, there are suggestions that this promotion of antibodies worsens the underlying thyroiditis and causes hypothyroidism.

Some practitioners recommend a technique known as block replace therapy (BRT), which involves simultaneous use of antithyroid drugs to disable the overproduction and thyroid hormone replacement to suppress function and provide sufficient thyroid hormone.

In the United States, thyroidectomy is typically done only when the patient cannot tolerate antithyroid drugs or is not a good candidate for RAI (such as in a case of life-threatening hyperthyroidism during pregnancy). This surgery involves removal of all or part of the thyroid gland and typically can provide a permanent cure for hyperthyroidism. While the goal of surgery is to remove just enough of the gland so that thyroid production is normal, it's not often achieved. Determining how much of the gland to take is part science and part art. If too much is taken, then the patient becomes hypothyroid. If only part of the thyroid is surgically removed, hypothyroidism is still a strong possibility. There are several somewhat rare complications resulting from the surgery. One is vocal cord paralysis. Another is accidental damage to or removal of the parathyroid glands, which are located in the neck in back of the thyroid gland. Because the parathyroid glands regulate the amount of calcium in the body, their removal would result in low calcium levels.

Outside the United States, antithyroid drugs are the primary treatment, with surgery reserved for hyperthyroidism that does not respond to drug therapy.

GOITER

A goiter is an enlargement of the thyroid. The condition can be detected by ultrasound or X-ray, and may also be diagnosed visually, when the neck is visibly thicker due to the enlarged gland.

The thyroid can become enlarged due to hyperthyroidism, hypothyroidism, autoimmune thyroid disease, multiple nodules, or inflammation from thyroiditis. It can also become enlarged due to deficiency or overconsumption of iodine.

Symptoms

You may have goiter if:

- Your thyroid is enlarged, so your neck looks or feels swollen
- Your neck or thyroid area is tender to the touch
- You have a tight feeling in your throat
- You cough frequently
- Your voice is hoarse
- You have difficulty swallowing

- You have difficulty breathing and shortness of breath, especially at night
- You have a feeling that food is getting stuck in your throat

If not caused by an autoimmune condition that triggers an inflamed thyroid, a goiter can be due to the level of iodine in your body. If there's too much iodine (e.g., from heart medications such as amiodarone), excess thyroid hormone can be produced, and a hyperthyroid goiter can appear. If there is insufficient iodine in your diet, a hypothyroid goiter can develop. The use of iodized salt has wiped out the majority of goiters from iodine deficiency in the United States, but 10 percent to 20 percent of goiters in the United States are still due to iodine deficiency, and iodine-deficiency goiter outside the United States is still common.

Diagnosis

To self-test your thyroid, hold a mirror so that you can see the area of your neck just below the Adam's apple and right above the collarbone. This is the general location of your thyroid gland. Tip your head back while keeping this view of your neck and thyroid area in the mirror. Take a drink of water and swallow. As you swallow, look at your neck. Watch carefully for any bulges, enlargement, protrusions, or unusual appearances in this area. Repeat this process several times. If you see anything that appears unusual, contact your doctor right away. You may have an enlarged thyroid or a thyroid nodule, and your thyroid should be evaluated. Be sure you don't get your Adam's apple confused with your thyroid gland. The Adam's apple is at the front of your neck; the thyroid is farther down and closer to your collarbone. (Remember that this test is by no means conclusive and cannot rule out thyroid abnormalities. It's just helpful to identify a particularly enlarged thyroid or masses in the thyroid that warrant evaluation.)

These steps can be involved in diagnosing goiter:

- A doctor's examination to observe neck enlargement
- A blood test to determine if your thyroid is producing irregular amounts of thyroid hormone
- An antibody test to confirm an autoimmune disease, which may be the cause of your goiter
- An ultrasound test to evaluate the size of the enlargement
- A radioactive isotope thyroid scan to produce an image of the thyroid and provide visual information about the nature of the thyroid enlargement

Treating Goiter

Treatment for goiter depends on how enlarged the thyroid has become, as well as other symptoms. Treatments can include:

- Observation and monitoring, which is typically done if your goiter is not large and is not causing symptoms or thyroid dysfunction.
- Medications, including thyroid hormone replacement, which can help shrink your goiter, or aspirin or corticosteroid drugs to shrink thyroid inflammation.
- Surgery if the goiter is very large, if it continues to grow while on thyroid hormone, if symptoms continue, or if the goiter is in a dangerous location (e.g., impinging on the windpipe or esophagus) or is cosmetically unsightly. If the goiter contains suspicious nodules, this may also be reason for surgery.

THYROID NODULES

Sometimes your thyroid gland has lumps also known as nodules. These nodules, which can be solid or fluid-filled, can be overactive and produce far too much thyroid hormone—in which case they're called toxic nodules. When there are a lot of them, the condition is referred to as a toxic multinodular goiter. When nodules overproduce hormone, they can result in hyperthyroidism. Some nodules do not produce any hormone at all, or may impair the gland's ability to produce thyroid hormone, and contribute to hypothyroidism. Thyroid nodules are actually fairly common. An estimated 1 in 15 women and 1 in 50 men has a thyroid nodule. More than 90 percent of nodules are benign (except in pregnant women, in whom approximately 27 percent of nodules are typically cancerous). It's vital to have your doctor examine any nodule as soon as you notice it.

Symptoms

Symptoms of thyroid nodules include palpitations, insomnia, weight loss, anxiety, and tremors, which are all common in hyperthyroidism as well. Nodules can also trigger hypothyroidism, and symptoms might include weight gain, fatigue, and depression. Some people will cycle back and forth between hyperthyroid and hypothyroid symptoms. Others may have difficulty swallowing, feelings of fullness, pain or pressure in the neck, a hoarse voice, and neck tenderness. Many people have nodules with no obvious symptoms related to thyroid dysfunction at all.

Diagnosis

Nodules are usually evaluated by:

- A blood test to determine whether they are producing thyroid hormone
- A radioactive thyroid scan, which looks at the reaction of the nodule to small amounts of radioactive material

- An ultrasound of the thyroid to determine whether the nodule is solid or fluid-filled
- A fine-needle aspiration or needle biopsy of the nodules to determine whether they may be cancerous

Treating Thyroid Nodules

Depending on the results of the evaluation, nodules may be left alone and monitored periodically (assuming they aren't causing serious difficulty), treated with thyroid hormone replacement to help shrink them, or surgically removed if they are causing problems with breathing or if test results indicate a malignancy. Some endocrinologists are also treating some nodules with percutaneous ethanol injections (PEI) and ultrasound, to shrink the nodules without surgery.

THYROID CANCER

Thyroid cancer is not especially common and is considered very survivable, but according to the American Cancer Society, its incidence is rising rapidly. There were an estimated 45,000 new cases of thyroid cancer in the United States in 2010.

The treatment and prognosis for thyroid cancer depends on the type. Papillary and follicular thyroid cancer are the most common types; an estimated 80 percent to 90 percent of all thyroid cancers fall into this category. Most of these cancers can be treated successfully when discovered early. Medullary thyroid carcinoma (MTC) makes up 5 percent to 10 percent of all thyroid cancers. If discovered before it metastasizes to other parts of the body, it has a good cure rate. There are two types of medullary thyroid cancer: sporadic and familial. Anyone with a family history of MTC should have blood tests to measure calcitonin levels, which may indicate a strong possibility of a genetic predisposition. If found, a thyroidectomy may be performed as a preventive measure. Anaplastic thyroid carcinoma is quite rare, accounting for only 1 percent to 2 percent of all thyroid cancers. It tends to be quite aggressive and is the least likely to respond to typical methods of treatment, though new drug treatments are showing some promise with this most difficult form of thyroid cancer.

Symptoms

Although many patients are asymptomatic at first, possible symptoms of thyroid cancer include:

- A lump in your neck
- Changes in your voice
- Difficulty in breathing or swallowing
- Lymph node swelling

Diagnosis

The main diagnostic procedure for suspected thyroid cancer is a fine-needle aspiration (FNA) biopsy of the thyroid nodule. Using a needle, fluid and cells are removed from various parts of all nodules that can be felt, and these samples are evaluated. Frequently, FNA tests are done with an ultrasound machine to help guide the needle into nodules that are too small to be felt. Between 60 percent and 80 percent of FNA tests show that the nodule is benign. Only about one in twenty FNA tests reveals cancer. If a case is classified as suspicious, a surgical biopsy may be needed.

In everyone except pregnant women, a radioactive thyroid scan is frequently done in order to identify if the nodules are "cold," meaning they have a greater potential to be cancerous.

Treating Thyroid Cancer

There are three key treatments for patients with cancer of the thyroid. The following types are commonly used:

- Surgery (removal of the thyroid and the cancer)
- Radiation therapy (to kill remaining cancer cells)
- Hormone therapy (use of hormones to stop cancer cells from growing)

Surgery is the most common treatment of cancer for the thyroid. A doctor may remove the cancer using one of the following operations:

- *Lobectomy* removes only the side of the thyroid where the cancer is found. Lymph nodes in the area may be taken out (biopsied) to see if they contain cancer.
- *Near-total thyroidectomy* removes all of the thyroid except for a small part.
- *Total thyroidectomy* removes the entire thyroid.
- *Lymph node dissection* removes lymph nodes in the neck that contain cancer.

Radiation for cancer of the thyroid may come from a machine outside the body (external radiation therapy), but most commonly it is administered via a pill or liquid form of radioactive iodine (RAI). Because the thyroid takes up iodine, the radioactive iodine collects in any thyroid tissue remaining in the body and kills any remaining cancer cells.

After removal of the gland or radiation, patients typically end up hypothyroid for the rest of their lives, and must take thyroid replacement hormone. In some cases, suppression is also part of the thyroid cancer follow-up to help prevent a relapse of cancer; this means that the thyroid hormone replacement medication must be at a dosage to keep TSH levels low or even close to zero in some patients.

Overall, the prognosis for thyroid cancer is quite good. However, survivors need to be vigilant in case of a recurrence. Regular checkups and periodic scans by a physician are necessary to monitor for recurrence and ensure proper thyroid hormone replacement.

Thyroid Disease Risks and Symptoms Checklist

THYROID DISEASE RISK FACTORS

The following factors increase your risk of having a thyroid condition:

Age, Gender
____ Age over sixty
____ Female

Medical History
____ Past history of thyroid problems, radioactive iodine (RAI), thyroid surgery for goiter, nodules, Hashimoto's disease, or thyroid cancer
____ Family history of thyroid problems
____ Personal or family history of autoimmune disease
____ Currently or formerly a smoker
____ Allergies or sensitivity to gluten, wheat

Related Conditions: Currently or in the past diagnosed with the following diseases or conditions:
____ Other pituitary or endocrine disease (e.g., diabetes, pituitary tumor, polycystic ovary syndrome [PCOS], endometriosis, premature menopause)
____ Chronic fatigue syndrome
____ Fibromyalgia
____ Carpal tunnel syndrome, tendonitis, plantar fasciitis
____ Mitral valve prolapse syndrome (MVPS) (heart murmur, palpitations)
____ Epstein-Barr virus (EBV)
____ Mononucleosis
____ Depression

____ Infertility, recurrent miscarriage
____ Celiac disease (gluten intolerance)
____ Lyme disease
____ Elevated cholesterol (hypercholesterolemia)
____ Tinnitus (ringing in ears)

Radiation Exposure History
____ Work at a nuclear plant
____ Live near or downwind from a nuclear plant
____ Lived near or downwind from the Chernobyl nuclear disaster in 1986
____ Had radiation treatments to neck area (e.g., for Hodgkin's disease, nasal radium therapy, radiation to tonsils and neck area)

Medications, Supplements
____ Currently or formerly treated with lithium
____ Currently or formerly treated with amiodarone
____ Currently taking supplemental iodine, kelp, bladder wrack, or bugleweed
____ Currently taking supplemental estrogen—birth control pills or estrogen pills, patches, or creams

Dietary Factors
____ Live in midwestern "goiter belt"
____ Significantly cut back or eliminated iodized salt from diet
____ Heavy consumer of soy products
____ Heavy consumer of raw goitrogenic foods—Brussels sprouts, rutabaga, turnips, kohlrabi, radishes, cauliflower, cassava, millet, cabbage, kale, and babassu

Toxic Exposures
____ Work at a rocket fuel, fireworks, or explosives production plant
____ Live in an area where there is currently or formerly a rocket fuel, fireworks, or explosives production plant
____ Excessively exposed to mercury
____ High exposure to pesticides
____ Drink and use fluoridated water

Hormonal Status
____ Perimenopause (above age forty)
____ Menopause (no periods for a year)
____ Postmenopausal
____ Had a baby within the past year

Trauma, Injury
____ Have had serious trauma to the neck, such as whiplash from a car
accident or a broken neck

THYROID DISEASE SYMPTOMS

Energy, Mood, Thinking
____ Exhaustion, fatigue
____ Depressed, moody, sad
____ Difficulty concentrating
____ Thinking is fuzzy; difficulty remembering

Anxiety, Panic
____ Heart palpitations
____ Tremors in hands
____ Panic attacks
____ Erratic behavior
____ Anxiety, irritability, nervousness, or panic attacks

Temperature
____ Sensitive to cold, cold hands or feet
____ Sweating more than usual, feeling hot when others are not, hot
flashes

Weight
____ Inappropriate weight gain, or having difficulty losing weight
despite changes in diet and exercise
____ Rapid weight loss, inability to gain weight

Hair, Nails, Skin
____ Dry, easily tangled, or coarse hair
____ Fine and brittle hair
____ Hair loss, especially from the outer part of the eyebrows
____ Dry or brittle nails
____ Dry skin
____ Thickening of skin in shin area of legs
____ Itching, prickly hot skin, rashes, and hives (urticaria)

Muscles, Joints, Nerves
____ Muscle and joint pains and aches
____ Carpal tunnel syndrome, or tendonitis in arms and legs
____ Soles of the feet are painful

____ Muscle pain and weakness, especially in the upper arms and
thighs
____ Unusually slow or fast reflexes

Sex, Reproduction, Fertility, Menstruation
____ Low sex drive
____ Unexplained infertility, or recurrent miscarriages with no obvious
explanation
____ Recurrent donor egg or IVF failure
____ Menstrual period is heavier than normal, or period is longer than
it used to be or comes more frequently
____ Periods have stopped
____ Periods are very light and infrequent

Digestion
____ Constipation
____ Diarrhea

Neck, Throat
____ Full or sensitive feeling in the neck
____ Raspy, hoarse voice
____ Enlarged thyroid
____ Neck looks or feels swollen
____ Neck or thyroid area may be tender to the touch
____ Tight feeling in the throat
____ Frequent coughing
____ Difficulty swallowing
____ Difficulty breathing and shortness of breath, especially
at night
____ Feeling that food is stuck in throat

Vital Signs
____ Rapid pulse
____ Elevated blood pressure
____ Slow pulse
____ Low blood pressure

Eyes
____ Double vision
____ Scratchy eyes, dry eyes, sensitivity, glare
____ Eyes are bulging or more of the white is showing than usual

Other Symptoms
____ Lymph node swelling
____ Face, eyes, arms, or legs are abnormally swollen or puffy
____ Cholesterol levels are high and not responsive to diet and
medication
____ Allergies worsening
____ Frequent infections, including yeast infections, thrush, or sinus
infections
____ Shortness of breath, sometimes difficulty drawing a full breath, or
a need to yawn
____ Difficulty falling asleep or staying asleep
____ Antidepressant is not working
____ Estrogen therapy for menopausal symptoms is not working

CHAPTER 2

Thyroid Diagnosis and
Its Challenges

Don't defy the diagnosis, try to defy the verdict.
—NORMAN COUSINS

For some readers, just recognizing the symptoms of a thyroid problem will trigger a visit to your doctor, conventional tests will reveal your thyroid problem, the doctor will give you a thyroid prescription that works for you, and you'll be on your way to feeling better and normalizing your metabolism and weight. Yes, it truly may be as simple as that!

Unfortunately, for others, getting a doctor who will actually test, diagnose, and properly treat your thyroid condition may not be as smooth a process as you'd hope. Let's take a look at the diagnosis process and some of the inherent challenges.

THE DIAGNOSTIC EXAMINATION

A thorough diagnosis of thyroid problems should always include a clinical examination by a physician. The following is a recap of the components of a clinical thyroid exam.

Hands-on examination of the thyroid. The doctor should palpate (feel) your neck looking for a goiter, which is an enlargement of the thyroid, as well as nodules or lumps in your thyroid. Your doctor should also be feeling for increased blood flow in the thyroid (known as "thrill") on palpation.

Stethoscope examination of the thyroid. The doctor uses a stethoscope to listen for what is known as "bruit"—the sound of increased blood flow in the thyroid.

Reflex check. Hyperresponsive reflexes can be a sign of hyperthyroidism, and slow reflexes may point to hypothyroidism.

Heart and blood pressure check. Very high or very low blood pressure can be signs of thyroid problems. Other heart-related issues the doctor should look for include:

- *Abnormal heart rate:* fast but regular heartbeat (called atypical sinus rhythm or sinus tachycardia), over 100 beats per minute (normal heart rate is 70 to 80), or a very slow heart rate (bradycardia), under 60 in a nonathlete
- *Ventricular tachycardia:* rapid heartbeat, felt as palpitations and sometimes also pounding
- *Atrial fibrillation:* inconsistent rhythm in which the upper chambers of the heart (atria) beat faster than and the lower chambers (ventricles)
- *Mitral valve prolapse:* felt as palpitations or heart flutters

Skin and hair examination. Your skin and hair should be examined for visible signs of a thyroid condition, looking specifically for:

- Loss of outer edge of eyebrow hair
- Hair loss on the head or body
- Yellowish, jaundiced cast to the skin
- Warm, moist hands and palms
- Hives

- Lesions on the shins (pretibial myxedema, dermopathy)
- Blister-like bumps on the forehead and face (milaria bumps)
- Onycholysis (separation of nails from underlying nail bed; also called Plummer's nails)
- Swollen fingertips (acropachy)

Eye examination. Your eyes should be evaluated, and your doctor should be looking for the following possible signs of a thyroid problem:

- Bulging or protrusion of the eyes
- Red, inflamed, dry, watery, or bloodshot eyes
- Stare in the eyes, retraction of upper eyelids, infrequent blinking
- "Lid lag"—when the upper eyelid doesn't smoothly follow downward movements of the eyes when you look down
- Swelling or puffiness of eyelids
- Twitching in the eyes
- Uneven motion of upper eyelid
- Uneven pupil dilation in dim light
- Tremor of closed eyelids

Other clinical signs your practitioner should look for include:

- Tremors
- Shaky hands
- Hyperkinetic movements (table drumming, tapping feet, jerky movements)
- Enlarged lymph nodes
- Dull facial expression
- Slow movement
- Slow speech
- Hoarseness of voice
- Edema (swelling) of the hands or feet

THYROID BLOOD TESTS

Blood tests are an important part of the process of diagnosing thyroid disease, and a number of different blood tests are typically used to diagnose a thyroid condition.

(*An important note:* In some cases, I've included normal ranges and values associated with different tests, but keep in mind that normal ranges can vary from lab to lab, and may be expressed quite differently in various countries. So be sure to get a printout of your lab test rests, along with information from the lab and your practitioner on what the reference range is for each test—most lab reports will provide this along with the results—so that you can review where your tests fall according to your particular lab.)

Thyroid-Stimulating Hormone (TSH) Test

Most conventional doctors rely on the thyroid-stimulating hormone test to diagnose an overactive or underactive thyroid. The TSH test is a blood test that measures the amount of TSH in your bloodstream. (The test is sometimes also called the thyrotropin-stimulating hormone test.)

When the pituitary detects that there isn't enough circulating thyroid hormone, TSH is released. TSH is considered a messenger that tells the thyroid to produce more hormone. So TSH goes up when you don't have enough thyroid hormone. A higher TSH indicates low thyroid hormone production, or hypothyroidism. Conversely, with hyperthyroidism, where there is too much thyroid hormone circulating, TSH drops, and low TSH levels are indicative of hyperthyroidism.

The TSH level typically remains in what is called the normal reference range when the thyroid gland is healthy and functioning normally.

You'll need to know what the normal values are for the lab where your doctor sends your blood because what's considered normal varies from lab to lab. Thyroid normal ranges are in tremendous flux right now. Throughout the 1980s and 1990s in North America, the normal

TSH range was from 0.3–0.5 at the bottom end to 5.0–6.0 at the high end. At the lab where they sent my blood, for example, a TSH of over 5.5 was considered hypothyroid, and under 0.5 was hyperthyroid. Anywhere in between was considered normal, or euthyroid.

Values below the low end of the TSH normal range usually indicate hyperthyroidism. Values above the top of the normal range can indicate hypothyroidism, an underactive thyroid. The higher the number, the more underactive your thyroid is considered to be.

In November 2002, the National Academy of Clinical Biochemistry (NACB), part of the Academy of the American Association for Clinical Chemistry (AACC), issued revised laboratory medicine practice guidelines for the diagnosis and monitoring of thyroid disease. Of particular interest was the following statement in the guidelines:

> More than 95 percent of rigorously screened normal euthyroid volunteers have serum TSH values between 0.4 and 2.5 mIU/L. A serum TSH result between 0.5 and 2.0 mIU/L is generally considered the therapeutic target for a standard L-T4 replacement dose for primary hypothyroidism.

Based on these findings, in January 2003, the American Association of Clinical Endocrinologists (AACE) made an important announcement:

> Until November 2002, doctors had relied on a normal TSH level ranging from 0.5 to 5.0 to diagnose and treat patients with a thyroid disorder who tested outside the boundaries of that range. Now AACE encourages doctors to consider treatment for patients who test outside the boundaries of a narrower margin based on a target TSH level of 0.3 to 3.0. AACE believes the new range will result in proper diagnosis for millions of Americans who suffer from a mild thyroid disorder, but have gone untreated until now.

In the years since the original NACB guidelines were released, most laboratories have not yet adopted these new guidelines, and the medical world is still not in complete agreement about changing the guidelines.

This continuing debate between practitioners who are using the new range and labs and doctors using the older, wider range means that for patients who test below 0.5 or above 3.0, getting diagnosed and treated for a thyroid condition depends on how up-to-date your laboratory and practitioner are and whether they are using the new, narrower standards.

TSH LEVELS CHART			
	Hyperthyroid (overactive thyroid)	Normal (euthyroid), neither hyperthyroid nor hypothyroid	Hypothyroid (underactive thyroid)
Former guidelines*	Below 0.5	00.5 to 5.0–6.0	Above 5.0–6.0
New guidelines per NACB & AACE, as of 2003	Below 0.3	0.3 to 3.0	Above 3.0

*As of 2011, many laboratories and practitioners are still using these outdated guidelines, and all evidence indicates that this will continue.

Total Thyroxine (Total T4)

T4—known as thyroxine—is the storage hormone produced by the thyroid. Total T4 measures the total amount of circulating T4 in your blood. *Total* refers to a combination of both the T4 bound to protein and the T4 that is free, or unbound to protein. A high value can indicate hyperthyroidism, a low value hypothyroidism. Total T4 levels can be artificially high, however, because both pregnancy and estrogen (including the estrogen in hormone therapy or birth control pills) raise thyroid binding globulin (TBG), and TBG elevates total T4 even when the actual levels of T4 circulating in your bloodstream are normal. When bound, thyroid hormone is not available to the cells, so most practitioners prefer to use the free (unbound) T4 test.

Free Thyroxine (Free T4)

Free T4 measures the free, unbound thyroxine (T4) levels circulating in your bloodstream. Free T4 is typically lower than normal in hypothyroidism and higher than normal in hyperthyroidism. Free T4 is considered a more accurate and reliable test than total T4. Some practitioners consider optimal free T4 during hypothyroidism treatment to be in the top half of the normal reference range.

Total Triiodothyronine (Total T3)

Triiodothyronine, or T3, is the active thyroid hormone at the cellular level. Total T3 is a measure of the combined T3 bound to protein as well as the free (unbound) T3. The total T3 level will typically be lower than normal in hypothyroidism and higher than normal in hyperthyroidism.

Free Triiodothyronine (Free T3)

Free T3 measures free unbound triiodothyronine in your bloodstream. Again, the free levels are considered more accurate than the total levels in the case of T3. Some practitioners consider optimal free T3 during hypothyroidism treatment to be in the top 25th percentile of the normal reference range.

Thyroglobulin or Thyroid Binding Globulin (TBG)

Thyroglobulin, also known as thyroid binding globulin or TBG, is a protein produced by your thyroid primarily when it is injured or inflamed due to thyroiditis or cancer. The normal thyroid produces low or no thyroglobulin, and so undetectable thyroglobulin levels usually mean normal thyroid function. But when TBG is leaking into the bloodstream and becomes detectable, it indicates some sort of thyroid abnormality. Thyroglobulin is typically elevated in Graves' disease, thyroiditis, and thyroid cancer.

Thyrotropin-Releasing Hormone (TRH)

The TRH (thyrotropin-releasing hormone) test is a "stimulation" or "challenge" test rather than a measure of circulating hormones. It's much like a three-hour glucose tolerance test to diagnose diabetes versus a fasting glucose level. The TRH test is considered a particularly good blood test for detecting subtle underactive thyroid problems. The time and cost involved in the test and the difficulty of getting the drugs needed to perform the test, however, have made it hard to get from most physicians.

Reverse T3

When the body is under stress or there are nutritional deficiencies or other issues impairing the thyroid's ability to function, instead of converting T4 into T3—the active form of thyroid hormone that works at the cellular level—the body conserves energy by converting T3 into an inactive form of T3 known as reverse T3 (rT3). Elevated levels of reverse T3 can reflect a thyroid problem at the cellular level—a condition that Kent Holtorf, MD, calls "cellular hypothy-roidism"—even though TSH, free T4, and free T3 values may well be within the normal reference range. The value of measuring and treating reverse T3 is controversial among conventional physicians, but this test has become commonly used by integrative physicians who are looking to assess a person's full range of thyroid function.

Holistic gynecologist and hormone expert Sara Gottfried, MD, has integrated reverse T3 testing into her practice.

> I used to order reverse T3 in a patient if I'd optimized the TSH and free T3 but the patient still had hypothyroidism symptoms, but now I order it more often at the start, because I think it's in-formative in deciding about the formulation. For example, if a pa-tient has high reverse T3, I'm more likely to use the compounded, time-release T3 as part of their treatment.

Some practitioners feel that reverse T3 should be below 150 for optimal hypothyroidism treatment.

Thyroid Peroxidase Antibodies

One of the most common thyroid antibody blood tests is thyroid peroxidase or TPO antibodies (TPOAb; also known as antithyroid peroxidase antibodies, or anti-TPO). This test is often done as a first step in diagnosing autoimmune thyroid disease. Thyroid peroxidase antibodies attack thyroid peroxidase, an enzyme that plays a part in the conversion of T4 to T3. TPO antibodies can indicate that the thyroid tissue is being destroyed, such as in Hashimoto's disease and in some other types of thyroiditis such as postpartum thyroiditis, and TPO antibodies are detectable in approximately 95 percent of patients with Hashimoto's thyroiditis. It's thought that among pa-tients with Graves' disease, 50 to 85 percent will test positive for these antibodies.

Antithyroid Microsomal Antibodies or Antimicrosomal Antibodies

Antimicrosomal antibodies (also called antithyroid microsomal antibodies) are typically elevated when you have Hashimoto's thyroiditis, and it's thought that as many as 80 percent of Hashimoto's patients have elevated levels of these antibodies. However, measurement of antimicrosomal antibodies has been replaced, for the most part, by the more state-of-the-art TPO antibody test.

Thyroglobulin Antibodies

Testing for thyroglobulin antibodies (Tg antibodies; also called antithyroglobulin or anti-Tg antibodies) is common. Tg antibodies are found in about 60 percent of Hashimoto's patients and 30 percent of Graves' patients.

Thyroid-Stimulating Immunoglobulins

Thyroid-stimulating immunoglobulins (TSI) can be detected in the majority of people with Graves' disease—some say as many as 75 to 90 percent of patients. Their presence is considered diagnostic for Graves' disease. The higher the levels, the more active the Graves' disease is thought to be. The absence of these antibodies does not mean that you don't have Graves' disease, however. Some people with autoimmune hypothyroidism also have TSI, and this can cause periodic transient hyperthyroid episodes.

Thyroid Receptor Antibodies (TRAb)

TSH receptor antibodies (TRAb) are seen in most patients with a history of or who currently have Graves' disease. TRAb may be:

- Stimulatory, in which case they cause hyperthyroidism (TSH stimulating antibodies, TSAb)
- Blocking, in which case they prevent TSH from binding to the cell receptor, and cause hypothyroidism (TSH receptor blocking antibodies, TBAb or TSBAb)
- Binding, in which case they interfere with the activity of TSH at the cell receptor

Patients with Graves' disease tend to test positive for stimulatory TRAb, and patients with Hashimoto's disease tend to test positive for blocking TRAb.

Thyroid Imaging Tests

In addition to blood tests, a variety of imaging and evaluation tests are sometimes used to make a conclusive diagnosis of thyroid disease, including:

- *Nuclear scan (also called radioactive iodine uptake, RAI-U):* used to help differentiate between Graves' disease, toxic multinodular goiter, and thyroiditis.
- *Computed tomography (CT) scan:* a specialized type of X-ray that is used—not very frequently, however—to evaluate the thyroid, and frequently to diagnose a goiter or larger nodules.
- *Magnetic resonance imaging (MRI):* done when the size and shape of the thyroid needs to be evaluated.
- *Thyroid ultrasound:* done to evaluate nodules, lumps, and enlargement of the gland. Ultrasound can also determine whether a nodule is a fluid-filled cyst or a mass of solid tissue.
- *Needle biopsy (fine needle aspiration, FNA):* done to evaluate suspicious lumps or cold nodules and assess whether a nodule is cancerous.

DIAGNOSING A THYROID PROBLEM

Based on the results of the patient history, review of symptoms, clinical examination, and blood imaging tests, doctors should be able to make an accurate diagnosis.

Diagnosing Hypothyroidism

To diagnose hypothyroidism, in addition to the history, symptoms, and clinical examination, conventional doctors consider the TSH test results. A TSH level above the reference range is considered hypothyroid, and will be flagged as "high" on test results. Remember, however, that there is controversy over the reference range, with some groups recommending the new range of 0.3 to 3.0, and many labs and doctors still using the old range of 0.5 to around 5.5.

Other blood tests that are typically done to help diagnose a straightforward case of hypothyroidism include:

- *Free T4 (free thyroxine).* A low level along with an elevated TSH may indicate hypothyroidism.
- *Free T3 (free triiodothyronine).* A low level along with an elevated TSH may indicate hypothyroidism.

In some cases, additional tests can be helpful. Kate Lemmerman, MD, is my doctor, and she works with many thyroid patients. I asked her to describe some of the key tests she uses to diagnose hypothyroidism:

To begin with, I order a panel of labs, including TSH, free T4, and free T3. If these are normal but the patient has a number of symptoms pointing to thyroid disease, then I will add the more expensive tests for thyroid antibodies and reverse T3, as well as cortisol and DHEA-sulfate. But the most important part of the diagnosis is a thorough history: What is your family history of thyroid disease and autoimmune diseases? Did your symptoms begin at a time of other hormonal changes, such as childbirth or menopause? (These periods can affect the thyroid, as the whole endocrine system is interrelated.) Is there a history of radiation to the thyroid area? (I have seen women become hypothyroid after radiation for breast cancer, especially those cancers high on the chest wall). The physical exam is also very important. Dry skin, thinning hair, puffy eyes, fluid retention, overly slow or overly fast reflexes—the latter often shows up when people have a combination of hypothyroidism, low magnesium, and adrenal dysfunction.

Diagnosing Hashimoto's Thyroiditis

Hashimoto's thyroiditis is the autoimmune disease that is the most common cause of hypothyroidism. The characteristic Hashimoto's thyroiditis patient would have high or high-normal TSH values and low or low-normal free T3 and free T4 levels. The greatest distinguishing feature for Hashimoto's is a high concentration of thyroid autoantibodies—anti-TPO antibodies in particular. (Some patients have elevated antibody levels for months or even years before the TSH level changes. But elevated antibodies can cause symptoms. And there is some evidence that treating elevated antibodies with a low dose of thyroid hormone medication may help reduce antibodies and prevent progression to overt hypothyroidism.)

Occasionally, fine needle aspiration biopsy of thyroid nodules or lumps will reveal evidence of Hashimoto's disease, but FNA is not typically done just to diagnose Hashimoto's disease.

Diagnosing Hyperthyroidism

A diagnosis of hyperthyroidism is usually made by means of a thyroid-stimulating hormone (TSH) test. Levels below 0.3 may be considered hyperthyroid.

Other blood tests that may be done to help diagnose hyperthyroidism include:

- *Free T4*. A high level along with a low TSH may indicate hyperthyroidism.
- *Free T3*. A high level along with a low TSH may indicate hyperthyroidism.

Diagnosing Graves' Disease

In addition to hyperthyroid TSH levels (typically, a TSH level below 0.3) and high-normal or high free T4 and free T3, the thyroid-stimulating antibodies (TSAb) or thyroid-stimulating immunoglobulin (TSI) in your blood may be measured to diagnose Graves' disease, the autoimmune condition that frequently causes hyperthyroidism.

A radioactive picture of the thyroid, made by ingesting a small amount of radioactive iodine by mouth, may also be taken to see if the thyroid gland is overactive. This overactivity of the thyroid gland is a hallmark of Graves' disease.

Diagnosing Goiter

Several steps can be involved in diagnosing the enlarged thyroid known as goiter:

- Examining and observing your neck enlargement
- A blood test to determine if your thyroid is producing irregular amounts of thyroid hormone

- Antibody testing, to confirm that autoimmune disease may be the cause of your goiter
- An ultrasound test to evaluate the size of the enlarged thyroid
- A radioactive thyroid scan to produce an image of the thyroid and provide visual information about the nature of the thyroid enlargement

Diagnosing Thyroid Nodules

Nodules are usually evaluated by:

- A blood test, to determine whether your nodules are producing thyroid hormone
- A radioactive thyroid scan, which looks at the reaction of the nodule to small amounts of radioactive material
- An ultrasound of your thyroid, to determine whether the nodule is solid or fluid-filled
- A fine-needle aspiration or needle biopsy of your nodules, to evaluate whether the nodules may be cancerous

Diagnosing Thyroid Cancer

The main diagnostic procedure for suspected thyroid cancer is a fine-needle aspiration (FNA) of the thyroid nodule. In an FNA, a needle is inserted into various parts of the nodule, fluid and cells are removed, and these samples are then evaluated. Sometimes FNA tests are done with an ultrasound to help guide the needle into nodules that are too small to be felt. Between 60 percent and 80 percent of FNA tests show that the nodule is benign. Only about one in twenty FNA tests reveals cancer. The remainder of cases are classified as "suspicious," and frequently a surgical biopsy or thyroidectomy is needed in order to rule out or diagnose cancer.

CHALLENGES TO GETTING PROPERLY DIAGNOSED

While it's common for doctors to say, "Thyroid disease is easy to diagnose and easy to treat," the reality is that diagnosis can be complicated. Many doctors don't recognize thyroid symptoms, so patients who are struggling with weight are told to eat less and exercise more, instead of getting a thyroid test. Once thyroid problems are suspected, some doctors will perform only one test, the thyroid-stimulating hormone (TSH) test, and then base their diagnosis only on that result. This narrow approach misses patients who otherwise would be diagnosed by a thorough thyroid evaluation, such as one that takes into account clinical examination, review of symptoms, a thorough family and personal history, and other blood work and imaging tests as needed.

Uninformed Doctors

Surprisingly in this day and age, there are still practitioners who believe that they can simply look at a patient or feel her neck and rule out thyroid disease. Looking at the patient and feeling the thyroid gland for enlargement and lumps are only a small part of a clinical thyroid examination. As noted, a thorough clinical thyroid exam must also include a blood pressure and pulse check, weight check, evaluation of reflexes, and careful evaluation of clinical thyroid signs, such as loss of outer eyebrow hair, swelling in face and limbs, unusual skin patches, and other skin and hair disturbances. The doctor should then consider the findings, in addition to blood work and medical history, to make a diagnosis. If you are seeing a doctor who thinks he or she can rule out thyroid disease based on just looking at you or feeling your thyroid, get another doctor.

Ali Jagger, a thyroid patient, life coach, and weight-loss expert in the United Kingdom, explains her experience:

I intuitively knew something was wrong but my doctor had other ideas, accusing me of overeating and drinking too much. The most desperate time for me was when he said to me, "You know you're really not doing yourself any favors looking like that!" I was feeling very lethargic by this point and had almost given up. My doctor didn't recognize my classic symptoms and instead decided to focus on the fact that I had had a miscarriage six months earlier. He referred me to a private specialist, and I paid £500 to see a gynecologist who of course could find nothing wrong. The saddest thing for me was at the height of my illness I had absolutely no fight left in me, I was permanently exhausted and thought I was dying. I think that before I got ill—and I had never been sick previously—I had faith in the National Health Service and their staff . I now feel that there are many GPs practicing in the UK who are ignorant about this condition or just go by blood test results rather than listening to patients.

Over the course of two years, Kanya went to six different doctors complaining of weight gain.

I gained sixty pounds over two years, plus I had fatigue and depression. And every one of those six doctors said the same thing. "Yes, you have an enlarged thyroid, but the symptoms you are experiencing are a result of stress."

Nikki Hundt-Prohaska is a thyroid patient advocate who runs online thyroid support groups at MedHelp and hears hundreds of stories each week from fellow thyroid sufferers.

One of the most upsetting complaints I hear about is the initial visit that brought them in to see their doctors. They complain about not feeling well and can't quite put their finger on the cause or why. The discussion includes many things. Fatigue, foggy head, cold all the time, achy joints etc. Then the dreaded remark, nor-mally filled with tons of emotion: "I've been gaining unexplained weight!" What I hear is that frequently, after weight gain is men-tioned, it's as if the appointment is practically over, because far too often the physician concludes that this patient may not have a real clinical thyroid issue, but instead is a fat, lazy couch potato or an inactive or depressed housewife. Many patients leave the appointment with a limp pat on the back and prescriptions for antidepressants and a water pill as the doctor says, "Diet and go to the gym." Worst of all, sometimes the doctors say, "Well, you're not getting any younger, you know!"

Difficulty Getting Tested

You may find that your doctor isn't willing to test your thyroid. Sometimes it's because the test was your idea, which can be a threat to an insecure doctor's ego or sense of control. Or your doctor may be afraid that you are asking for a thyroid test because you think thy-roid drugs are glorified weight-loss pills. Some HMO doctors face re-strictions or financial disincentives to order laboratory tests. Finally, some doctors are simply not particularly aware of or informed about thyroid disease. I've even heard from patients that their doctors re-fused to perform thyroid tests, saying totally off-base things such as:

- "You're only in your twenties. Only older people get thyroid dis-ease."
- "You just had a baby, and if you had a thyroid problem, you wouldn't have been able to get pregnant."
- "You're a man, and men almost never get thyroid problems."
- "You're just looking for an excuse for being overweight."

You may also find that you describe thyroid symptoms but end up with another diagnosis. If you say "fatigue," "weight gain," and "depression" to many doctors, you'll leave the office not with a thyroid test but with a prescription for an antidepressant. Some researchers estimate that at least 15 percent of those diagnosed with depression are actually suffering from undiagnosed hypothyroidism.

Or you may be told that it's your hormones—which is essentially true, but they're talking about the wrong hormones here! Or you may be told you're experiencing the effects of getting older, that you're working too hard, that these are normal postpartum symptoms, or that it's the result of a lack of exercise. If you describe feelings of anxiety and weight loss, you may, as some young women with hyperthyroidism have experienced, even be diagnosed as anorexic or bulimic.

When faced with a doctor who is oblivious or resistant to what may be very obvious thyroid symptoms, or won't test when asked, the best option is to find another doctor, even if you have to pay for it yourself. But if you have no options, here are a few tips:

- Quantify your symptoms as much as possible. Many people go into the doctor saying, "I'm just so tired, and I can't stand it. I'm gaining weight!" The doctor's response is likely to be, "Get more sleep, get off the couch, exercise, and don't eat so much." Rather than saying, "I'm tired," explain that you need to sleep ten hours a night instead of eight hours, and you're still exhausted by dinnertime. Instead of saying, "I can't lose weight," say, "I'm eating 1,500 calories per day on a low-fat diet, doing four hours a week on the treadmill and two hours a week of muscle-building exercise, and I'm gaining two pounds a week."
- Be persistent but unemotional. You may want to bring your Thyroid Disease Risks and Symptoms Checklist to your doctor (see chapter 1) and go over the key points with the doctor.
- If your doctor reviews your checklist and refuses to order thyroid tests, ask that a copy of your checklist be included in your medical chart after the doctor signs and dates it, indicating that he or she

has read and discussed it. Keep a signed copy for yourself. Send a copy to the HMO or insurance company's consumer liaison, along with your request that testing be approved.

- Write a letter that states the various reasons you have requested thyroid testing and the fact that this doctor has refused. Insist that the doctor sign it, place a copy in your chart, and give you a copy. (You can then use this copy with the HMO to argue for a referral to another doctor if needed.)

In today's lawsuit-laden environment, doctors are especially concerned about officially documenting controversial medical decisions, so you'll probably get the tests you need. It may seem ridiculous that you have to struggle to get standard medical tests and treatment, but it's your health that is at stake, so keep fighting.

If you are unable to get your own physician to order the appropriate tests, then consider having your tests done through a patient-directed testing service. These services allow you to select the blood tests you want, pay for them out of pocket—usually at costs that are close to the wholesale rate and not the marked-up consumer rate—have the blood drawn at nationally certified laboratories, and the results sent back to you. You can then use this information as part of your criteria in choosing a new doctor, or you may find that the test results allow you to reopen the dialogue with your existing physician. There are a number of these services available—the one I have worked with for years is MyMedLab. More information is available in the Resources section.

TSH Is "Normal"

Frequently, even after being tested, patients are told, "Your thyroid tests were normal." This assessment is based on a misguided practice some doctors have of diagnosing hypothyroidism based only on the thyroid-stimulating hormone (TSH) test. These doctors believe

that if the TSH test result shows you as being within the TSH reference range for normal that they subscribe to, then you do not have
a thyroid dysfunction.

As noted earlier, there is disagreement as to the reference range
itself, and for almost a decade doctors have disagreed over the
guidelines. The upshot? While the so-called normal reference range
at many labs continues to be shown as from around 0.5 to 5.0, some
endocrinologists use the range of 0.3 to 3.0 in their practice, and a
subset of practitioners believe that the top end of the range actually
should be lowered even further, to 2.5.

Adrienne Clamp, a McLean, Virginia–based physician who now
works extensively with thyroid patients—and is a thyroid patient
herself—explains:

> I myself suffer from hypothyroidism and it was difficult for
> me to get help with it because my numbers were "normal," even
> though I did not feel well. There is nothing like personal expe-
> rience to teach one about an issue in a whole new way. I think
> that often patients are not taken seriously when they express
> how poorly they feel. In my experience, most thyroid patients
> have a very difficult time being taken seriously if their numbers
> are normal. They are often offered antidepressants and psycho-
> therapy when what they need is optimization of their thyroid
> hormone levels.

Any way you look at it, according to the narrower recommended
range, millions more people are considered hypothyroid and could
qualify for treatment.

Still, many doctors are operating according to the old normal
range and therefore will inaccurately rule out thyroid conditions.
Get a copy of the guidelines online at ThyroidDietRevolution.com
and share them with your doctor.

And if your TSH is borderline—or what some physicians refer

to as subclinical—your doctor may refuse to treat you, or suggest that you wait until the TSH goes up further before you get treatment. Don't accept a response of "wait and see." Ask for the actual number, and ask for the normal range for the lab where your blood was tested. Show your doctor your Thyroid Disease Risks and Symptoms Checklist and ask about a trial course of treatment to see if your symptoms improve. If your doctor is so number-obsessed that it's like talking to an accountant instead of a health care practitioner, start looking for a new doctor.

Fear of Osteoporosis

Some practitioners fear that diagnosing and treating mild or borderline hypothyroidism will increase the risk of osteoporosis. This fear is based on studies that have shown that extended periods of hyperthyroidism—and in particular, extremely low, suppressed TSH levels—can be a risk factor for osteoporosis. There are also several inconclusive studies that suggest that long-term treatment of hypothyroidism may increase the risk of osteoporosis. At the same time, there are many studies that show that thyroid treatment does not increase the risk of osteoporosis, and that treatment may in fact assist with bone growth and help halt or reverse osteoporosis. One important study looked at more than sixty studies of the thyroid-osteoporosis connection that were published throughout the 1990s. Ultimately, this meta-review found no association between the duration of thyroid treatment and an associated reduction of bone mineral density.

Some doctors, unfortunately, employ faulty logic and decide that if a very low TSH level poses a risk, treatment *might* pose a risk, so failing to diagnose hypothyroidism when TSH is at high-normal levels will avoid the risk.

Reliability of the TSH Test

There is also a question as to the reliability of the TSH test itself. Dr. Richard Shames, a noted thyroid practitioner and author of a number of books on thyroid disease, has found that the practice of allowing TSH blood samples to sit for hours before they are collected and shipped to a laboratory for analysis can result in degradation of the sample. Says Dr. Shames, "A TSH that might have been measured at a 6.0 or 7.0 can degrade so that by the time it's measured, it actually ends up in the normal range."

The time of day a TSH test is taken also affects the result. The highest TSH level is typically the level obtained from a fasting blood test first thing in the morning. TSH levels then start to drop significantly throughout the day. This results in as many as 6 percent of patients having a hypothyroid morning TSH but a normal reference range TSH later in the day.

Getting a proper diagnosis sometimes means you will need to be careful when and where you have your blood work done, and ask about whether the sample will be properly refrigerated and stored before it's sent to the lab for analysis. Given the significant questions about the TSH reliability overall, you may also need to see a physician who does not base his or her entire diagnosis on this test alone.

Overreliance on the TSH Test, and Failure to Test Free T4 and Free T3

Another challenge for patients who have a TSH that is normal—even if by the new standards—is that a normal TSH may not reflect what is actually going on in terms of the circulating levels of thyroid hormone in the body. To measure the thyroid hormone, the free T4 and free T3 tests are performed. (*Note:* The total T4 and total T3 are considered less useful by many practitioners, because they include bound thyroid hormone that is not usable by the body, while the free levels do not.)

Many practitioners and patients feel that the thyroid treatment is optimized when TSH is within the reference range but free T4 and free T3 are at the middle of the normal range or higher. Some practitioners feel it is especially important that the free T3, in particular, be in the upper end of the normal range for patients to feel well. In some cases, patients have been able to make a case to a physician for thyroid treatment even with a so-called normal TSH when free T4 and free T3 levels were on the low end of normal or below normal.

What this means is that if you have a normal TSH but your free T4, free T3, or both are in the lower half of the normal range, you may want to discuss treatment to help resolve this imbalance.

Failure to Test for Antibodies

Even though autoimmune problems are most frequently the cause of thyroid conditions, many physicians do not routinely conduct the antibody tests that diagnose autoimmune thyroid disease. This presents a problem because elevated thyroid antibodies, even in the presence of normal TSH levels, mean that you have autoimmune thyroid disease and that your thyroid is suffering from autoimmune dysfunction. The dysfunction may not be significant enough to register as an abnormal TSH level, but the presence of antibodies may generate symptoms and is predictive of thyroid problems down the road.

The practice of treating patients who have Hashimoto's thyroiditis but normal-range TSH levels is supported by studies that show that treatment for "euthyroid" Hashimoto's autoimmune thyroiditis—where TSH had not yet elevated beyond normal range—can actually reduce the chance and severity of autoimmune disease progression. The researchers speculated that such treatment might even be able to stop the progression of Hashimoto's disease or prevent the development of hypothyroidism.

Many doctors, however, will not treat patients who present clinical symptoms of hypothyroidism and test positive for Hashimoto's antibodies but have a normal TSH level. You may have to actively interview endocrinologists, as well as holistic doctors, osteopaths, and other practitioners, to find one who will treat you if you have a normal TSH level with thyroid antibodies and symptoms.

Failure to Test for Reverse T3

One of the most difficult situations is having an underlying thyroid problem that does not show up on standard thyroid blood tests. You may have a family history of thyroid disease or a number of thyroid symptoms—even a low basal body temperature—but you have TSH, free T4, free T3, and antibody levels that are normal. What you may be experiencing is thyroid hormone resistance, where your body is capable of producing thyroid hormone, but nutritional and metabolic dysfunctions have made your tissues unable to properly absorb and respond to it. This is similar to the better-known concept of insulin resistance, where your body produces enough insulin, but your cells become resistant to it, so your body loses its ability to respond to it.

You may also have thyroid hormone conversion problems, where you have enough T4 and T3 in the bloodstream, but the organs and tissues are not effectively converting the inactive T4 into the active T3 that you need at the cellular level. In both cases, you may show normal circulating levels, but you are hypothyroid at the level of your tissues, organs, and cells.

Thyroid hormone resistance and conversion problems are very difficult to diagnose with blood tests. The thyrotropin-releasing hormone (TRH) test—the one laboratory test typically able to detect this sort of dysfunction—is generally not being done anymore. Some practitioners perform a reverse T3 test, which measures the conversion of T4 to reverse T3—an inactive form of T3. This typically occurs when the body is under stress and is cause for treatment according to some practitioners. This test is considered irrelevant by many mainstream practitioners, however.

The bottom line is that if you suspect thyroid resistance or conversion problems, you will need a practitioner who is skilled in clinical, observational diagnosis and who, in the face of normal blood test values, will still be willing to try you on a course of thyroid treatment if you have observable signs of hypothyroidism. Typically, this would be a holistic or alternative medicine physician with expertise working with thyroid disease and other difficult-to-diagnose conditions.

CHAPTER 3

Hypothyroidism Treatment and Optimization

He who has health has hope, and he who has hope has everything.

—ARABIC PROVERB

Hypothyroidism is the thyroid issue most linked to weight-loss challenges. And, for most thyroid patients, hypothyroidism—an underactive thyroid condition that requires thyroid hormone replacement for life—is also the end result of the disease process or treatments.

There are occasionally people with an active case of Graves' disease who instead of losing weight—which is typical—will gain weight. But for the most part, as I sometimes say, "all roads lead to hypothyroidism." For Hashimoto's thyroiditis patients, the thyroid typically burns itself out over time, becoming less able to produce thyroid hormone, leaving most patients hypothyroid. With Graves' disease and hyperthyroidism, most doctors in the United States administer radioactive iodine (RAI), which leaves patients without a functional thyroid. So these patients end up hypothyroid, even if they started out with an overactive gland. With thyroid nodules and goiter, surgery may be performed to remove all or part of the thyroid. The end result is often hypothyroidism. And almost all thyroid cancer patients have their thyroid gland removed entirely, leaving them completely hypothyroid and reliant on outside thyroid hormone replacement.

So whatever the thyroid disease or condition, and particularly if you are a thyroid patient who is struggling to lose weight, it's likely that you are or will soon be hypothyroid, unable to produce sufficient thyroid hormone on your own, and taking thyroid hormone replacement medication. Getting proper treatment for your hypothyroidism may be the key to weight loss.

THYROID HORMONE REPLACEMENT MEDICATIONS

Conventional treatment of hypothyroidism typically involves replacing the missing thyroid hormone, using prescription thyroid hormone replacement drugs. The following summarizes the various drugs in this category:

PRESCRIPTION THYROID HORMONE REPLACEMENT DRUGS		
Generic Name	Brand Name	Description
Levothyroxine	Synthroid, Levoxyl, Levothroid, Unithroid, Eltroxin, generic levo-thyroxine	Tablet form of synthetic T4 treatment. Different brands may have different fillers, dyes, and potential allergens
Levothyroxine	Tirosint	A manufactured capsule for-mulation of levothyroxine
Liothyronine	Cytomel, generic	Synthetic T3, provides the ac-tive thyroid hormone
Liothyronine-SR/TR	Compounded	Synthetic T3 compounded in sustained-release or time-release form
Liotrix	Thyrolar	A combination of synthetic T4 and T3
Natural desiccated thyroid	Armour, Nature-throid, Westhroid, Erfa, Thyroid-S	Derived from thyroid gland of pigs; includes T4, T3, and other thyroid hormones including T1 and T2
Natural desiccated thyroid	Compounded	Natural desiccated thyroid specially compounded
Custom compounded thyroid medication	Compounded	Custom compounded formula-tions that may contain synthetic T4, T3, and/or natural desic-cated thyroid in various ratios

Levothyroxine

The most commonly prescribed thyroid hormone replacement drug is levothyroxine. Levothyroxine is the generic name for the synthetic form of thyroxine (T4). It is sometimes referred to as "l-thyroxine" or "L-T4." Some endocrinologists also incorrectly call it "thyroxine," which is actually the name of the hormone produced in the body.

Levothyroxine is considered by conventional doctors to be the standard treatment for hypothyroidism, and many doctors will only prescribe levothyroxine for thyroid hormone replacement. The rationale is that people only need the synthetic T4, and the body will convert the T4 in the medication into T3 (triiodothyronine)—the thyroid hormone active at the cellular level. Some people with hypothyroidism find that levothyroxine therapy is sufficient treatment for their hypothyroidism.

Many doctors do not recommend generic levothyroxine. They tend to prefer brand names because there are several manufacturers of generic levothyroxine, and with each refill you may end up getting medication from a different manufacturer. These medications can vary in some cases from 95 to 105 percent of the stated potency, causing symptoms and testing irregularities. (And, for thyroid cancer survivors, erratic dosing can jeopardize therapy to prevent cancer recurrence.).

The primary difference between brand names is that each brand has different fillers, binders, and dyes, and some patients may have allergies to those ingredients. The 50 (mcg) pills from the brand-name levothyroxine manufacturers typically are free of dyes and are more likely to be hypoallergenic.

Levothyroxine came on the market in the late 1950s, without approval from the Food and Drug Administration (FDA). It was grandfathered in under approval for natural thyroid (Armour Thyroid) that had been available since the early 1900s. In 1997, the

FDA required levothyroxine to go through the new drug application process and receive formal approval, given concerns over stability, potency, and reliability. The drugs were to be approved by 2000, but among the drugs on the market at the time, only Unithroid received approval within the FDA deadline. Levoxyl, Levothroid, and Synthroid were eventually approved.

There are several main brand names of levothyroxine on the market: These include

- Synthroid, the market leader, made by Abbott Laboratories. Synthroid is also one of the top-selling drugs in America.
- Levoxyl, the second highest-selling brand of levothyroxine.
- Levothroid, made by Forest Pharmaceuticals.
- The brand known as Unithroid, which was manufactured by Jerome Stevens, is now distributed as a generic by Lannett. This levothyroxine is considered to be of good quality.
- A newer, gelcap (instead of tablet) form of levothyroxine called Tirosint is also available. Tirosint has a liquid form of levothyroxine in its gelcaps, and a key benefit is that it is free of dyes, gluten, alcohol, lactose, and sugar.

As noted, a number of other manufacturers also make and distribute generic levothyroxine.

Synthroid, as a heavily marketed drug for more than three decades, enjoys a high degree of brand loyalty from physicians. Over the years, Synthroid's manufacturer has been a major financial supporter of medical meetings and physician education, and has taken many opportunities to get Synthroid's name in front of both new and established physicians. As a result, the name Synthroid is sometimes used by doctors to describe the whole category of thyroid hormone replacement drugs in general (in the same way that the brand name Kleenex has, for example, become synonymous with tissues or Xerox with photocopying).

Liothyronine

Liothyronine is the synthetic form of triiodothyronine (T3), the thyroid hormone active at the cellular level. Liothyronine is available in one manufactured drug, Cytomel, and as generic triiodothyronine.

Research has shown that some patients feel better with the addition of T3 in some form, and so practitioners prescribe a form of liothyronine along with a levothyroxine medication, or natural thyroid medication.

Francesca, who is perimenopausal with a thyroid problem, started going to a new nurse practitioner who put her on Cytomel.

My only side effect was a minor headache for two days, which went away with aspirin. The third day I realized I was awake. I woke up in the morning and was alert for the first time in years. It didn't take me a hour to drag myself out of bed. I was only taking 5 mcg of Cytomel, and had an immediate result. My body temperature has risen to 98.1 degrees, and I am noticing little things changing in my body and health.

Liothyronine is also available from compounding pharmacies, which can make it available in regular or time-release capsules.

Dr. Richard Shames has found that T3 can be a helpful addition to a patient's thyroid therapy.

When it comes to T3, some patients do well on T3, but it seems that some patients do better on time-release T3. It seems that the compounded, time-release form prevents that spike of T3 that you get with the manufactured T3 pills. For some patients, the time-release T3 provides the necessary gradient that helps to drive the T3 across the cell membrane barrier.

Sometimes thyroid cancer patients preparing for a scan are given T3 for several weeks, to help aid with hypothyroidism symptoms that result from the withdrawal from other thyroid medication that is needed for the scan's accuracy.

Increasingly, integrative physicians are also using slow-release compounded T3-only treatment as a treatment for reverse T3 dominance.

Liotrix (Thyrolar)

Thyrolar is the brand name for liotrix, a combination of synthetic T4 (levothyroxine) and synthetic T3 (liothyronine) that is made by Forest Pharmaceuticals. This drug is not very regularly prescribed, but it is preferred by some physicians who wish to provide both T4 and T3 but prefer a synthetic drug versus natural (desiccated) thyroid.

The primary benefit of Thyrolar was that, as a single pill, it simplified the taking of a T4/T3 synthetic combination, and because it is a manufactured drug, some doctors are more comfortable prescribing it than prescribing T3 as a separate treatment.

Thyrolar is rarely prescribed anymore, however, because long-term shortages of the drug have made it difficult to ensure a steady supply. The drug is also expensive and requires refrigeration in order to maintain potency. Many patients who took Thyrolar in the past have switched to synthetic T4 and T3 as individual pills.

Natural, Desiccated Thyroid (Armour, Nature-Throid)

Natural desiccated thyroid is the original form of thyroid hormone replacement that first came into use early in the 1900s. From the early 1900s to the 1950s, this was the only thyroid replacement drug available—namely, Armour Thyroid. The drug fell out of favor with some endocrinologists, as Synthroid's extensive marketing promoted synthetic thyroid drugs as a better, more modern option for thyroid treatment in the second half of the twentieth century. Marketing efforts aside, since the 1990s, the natural thyroid drugs have been enjoying a resurgence in popularity with some patients and practitioners.

Natural desiccated thyroid is derived from the thyroid gland of pigs and contains natural forms of the thyroid hormones T4 and T3, as well as other, lesser known thyroid hormones such as T2 and T1, the hormone calcitonin, and nutrients typically found in a natural thyroid gland. Some patients report improvement in symptoms using natural thyroid versus the synthetic medications. Decades ago, bovine (cow) thyroid was used, but prescription natural thyroid sold in the United States is currently porcine (from pigs).

The popularity of natural thyroid has grown with doctors, in particular osteopaths, naturopaths, integrative physicians, and holistic MDs, some of whom prefer to start their hypothyroid patients on a desiccated thyroid drug because they believe that since the drug contains a full spectrum of thyroid hormones as well as nutritional cofactors, it more closely mimics the action of human thyroid hormone, and their patients generally respond better.

The top-selling brand of natural thyroid is Armour Thyroid, made by Forest Pharmaceuticals.

RLC Laboratories also makes natural desiccated thyroid products Nature-Throid and Westhroid, which are hypoallergenic. The two RLC-manufactured natural desiccated thyroid drugs are identical except for the different names. Another brand of natural desiccated thyroid, from the manufacturer Erfa, is available in Canada, and some patients are importing this drug into the United States by prescription. A generic natural desiccated thyroid is available in the U.S. market, made by Acella.

Most endocrinologists and conventional practitioners tend to oppose use of natural thyroid on principle, primarily based on outdated concerns about potency, or because they are unfamiliar with the current manufacturing processes for desiccated thyroid or how to properly dose these medications.

Raw materials shortages, government-mandated manufacturing shutdowns, and other challenges to production have caused availability of natural desiccated thyroid drugs at times. It is also likely that the FDA will call for these drugs to go through a formal drug approval process—they have so far been able to bypass the formal approvals process because they were on the market and in safe use for decades before the FDA was created.

Compounded Thyroid Medications

Special pharmacies known as compounding pharmacies can create individualized combinations of thyroid medications at customized doses. Compounded thyroid medication, available only by prescription, can include:

- Combinations of synthetic T4 and T3 in regular or slow-release formulas
- Natural desiccated thyroid
- T4 only, in slow-release form
- T3 only, in slow-release form

WHAT THYROID MEDICATION SHOULD YOU TAKE?

You may wonder which thyroid medication you should take for hypothyroidism. The answer is not clear-cut.

In some cases, you may not have a choice. Your physician may make it standard practice to start everyone on a particular medication—often a levothyroxine drug such as Synthroid—although there are some holistic and integrative practitioners who start most of their patients on a natural desiccated thyroid drug. Your choice of medication or brand may also be dictated by cost, and you'll start out with a medication that is covered by your insurance or HMO.

Over time, and with careful monitoring of your thyroid levels and symptoms, you'll discover whether you might benefit from a different brand or a different medication.

There are some practitioners and patients who believe that one size fits all and suggest that everyone will and should feel perfectly fine on a particular thyroid drug. You'll hear this about Synthroid, but there are some equally strong voices arguing that natural desiccated thyroid is vastly superior to any synthetic combination drugs.

I disagree with them all.

The best thyroid medication is the one that safely works best for you. It's tempting to want to declare a particular drug the "winner"— but I've talked to too many thyroid patients in the past fifteen years to believe that any one treatment works for everyone. Patients want to keep in mind several important factors:

1. With any thyroid drug, one brand's fillers, dyes, and binders may affect you differently than another's, so you may want to try a different brand of medication.
2. Some patients seem to need additional T3; others are extremely sensitive to it and do well on T4-only treatment.
3. Some patients who are unable to relieve symptoms on synthetic treatments do better on natural desiccated thyroid.
4. Some patients who are unable to relieve symptoms on natural desiccated thyroid do better on synthetic treatments.

Some practitioners like to start with a T4 drug, add T3 if needed, and switch to a natural thyroid drug as a third option. Others may prefer to start with natural thyroid.

Hormone expert and holistic gynecologist Dr. Sara Gottfried explains her approach.

My tendency when I see someone from the start who is newly diagnosed as hypothyroid is to start them on a natural desiccated thyroid preparation, either Armour or Nature-Throid. I even use it with patients who have autoimmune thyroiditis, despite the old dogma not to use it with those patients. I find that clinically it's very effective. I frequently see patients who are already on Synthroid or Levoxyl, but the TSH not where it should be, and free T3 is low. With those patients, I'll often add T3—either Cytomel or a slow-release T3.

OPTIMIZING THYROID TREATMENT

If you are still suffering from thyroid symptoms and finding it difficult or impossible to lose weight, or if you're gaining weight even though you're on a healthy diet and exercise program, there's a good chance that your thyroid treatment is not optimized. Many integrative practitioners believe that the optimal TSH level for the majority of thyroid patients is between 1 and 2. Free T4 levels should be in the top half of the normal range, and free T3 in the top half—or in some cases the top 25 percent—of normal. Reverse T3 should not be substantially elevated. And many doctors, including thyroid and weight-loss expert Kent Holtorf, MD, like to see the ratio of free T3 to reverse T3 at 0.2 or above, with reverse T3 ideally below 150.

A number of situations can contribute to less-than-optimal thyroid treatment:

- Insufficient T4
- Insufficient T3
- Problems with conversion of T4 to T3
- Problems with the cells' ability to absorb the T3

Any of these problems can interfere with optimal thyroid function and disrupt metabolism. Here are some questions you can consider that address the various concerns relating to optimal thyroid function.

Are You at the Optimal TSH for You?

The first step, no matter what thyroid medication you are taking, is to make sure that you are on the right dose for you.

As noted earlier, while the normal reference range for TSH still typically shows up on lab reports as 0.5 to 5.0, many practitioners believe that levels above 2.5 to 3.0 are indicative of hypothyroidism. A study reported in the *Journal of Clinical Endocrinology and Metabolism* found that the mean TSH level for people who don't have a thyroid condition is actually 1.5.

So if your TSH is on the higher end of normal for you, it's no wonder that you may find it hard to lose weight. If you are on thyroid medication, check your most recent blood test results; if your TSH is above 2.0, consult with your physician about whether a slight increase in medication dosage would be better for your health.

Allie, age fifty, started having a weight problem around the time she hit forty. She also had a laundry list of symptoms, including dry skin, hot flashes, memory loss, and low sex drive. Her doctor decided it was menopause and depression. Allie kept insisting on a thyroid test. She was finally tested and diagnosed as hypothyroid at age forty-eight. Her symptoms continued, and she insisted on more blood work. Her TSH level was 5.2, which according to Allie's doctor was normal.

> I insisted that, knowing my body, it was too high for me. He was quite adamant that my problem was not my thyroid, but that I needed to admit that it was depression and that I had all the symptoms. When I told him that all of my symptoms were from a low thyroid problem and that the latest count just wasn't compatible with my body, and that I wasn't depressed, his answer was, "I'll bet 95 percent of the people in the psychiatric ward say the same thing."

Allie finally saw another physician, who said she was being undertreated and upped her dosage of thyroid hormone replacement. She's feeling dramatically better.

Do You Need a Seasonal Adjustment in Dosage?

One little-known issue for thyroid patients is the seasonal variation in thyroid function. A number of studies show that TSH naturally rises during colder months and drops to low-normal or even hyperthyroid levels in the warmest months. Some doctors adjust for this by prescribing slightly increased dosages during colder months and reducing dosage during warm periods. Most doctors and patients are not aware of this seasonal fluctuation, however, leaving patients suffering with worsening hypothyroidism symptoms during colder months, or going through warmer months suffering with hyperthyroidism symptoms due to slight overdosage. This seasonal fluctuation becomes more pronounced in older people and in particularly cold climates. Twice-yearly tests, at minimum during winter and summer months, can help assess fluctuations and guide any seasonal dosage modifications needed.

Are You on the Right Brand of Levothyroxine for You?

The reality is, most people start out taking a levothyroxine drug. But some people simply do not feel well on one brand of levothyroxine, and changing brands seems to help. Keep in mind that Synthroid is known to dissolve extremely slowly and may not get fully absorbed in someone with quick digestion. Synthroid also contains lactose and acacia as fillers, and these substances can make the medication less effective or problematic for people who have lactose intolerance or seasonal allergies to tree and grass pollen. The other leading brand name of levothyroxine, Levoxyl, does not contain these ingredients. Levoxyl is a very fast-dissolving formula—in fact, it should be taken with a big glass of water—and may be better suited for some thyroid patients. The new liquid capsule form of levothyroxine, Tirosint, has no fillers, dyes, binders, lactose, acacia, soy or gluten, and may be a better choice for some patients who are especially sensitive to any of these ingredients.

With several FDA-approved brands (Levoxyl, Synthroid, and Tirosint, among others) available, you may wish to discuss a change with your physician. Do stick with a brand name, however, and not a generic, to ensure consistency. (Unless you have a relationship with your pharmacist, who will ensure that you get the same manufacturer of generic each time. Otherwise, every time you refill a generic prescription, you are at risk of getting a different manufacturer's levothyroxine, and they can vary in potency from one maker to the next.)

Do You Need T3?

Some people do not feel their best and find it difficult to lose weight without the addition of a second thyroid hormone known as T3. T3 is the active thyroid hormone. Usually, the body converts T4 to T3, but nutritional deficiencies, toxins, and a variety of other physiological factors may prevent the body from accomplishing that conversion process properly, leaving you deficient in this most important thyroid hormone. In one research study, experts found that among a group of one hundred obese patients, more than 90 percent of those studied had T3 levels that were below the mean. So it's clear that low T3 or inability to convert T4 to T3 may contribute to weight gain or difficulty losing weight.

In late 2009, a Danish study, reported on in the prestigious *European Journal of Endocrinology*, studied the effects of a levothyroxine-only therapy versus levothyroxine plus T3 (in this case, a dosage of 20 mcg of T3 daily was used). Tests for quality of life and depression were performed at the start, and after twelve-week treatment periods where the study subjects were given levothyroxine plus T3, or levothyroxine plus placebo, and then switched for the next twelve-week period. Participants were "blind" in that they were not aware whether they were taking active T3 or placebo.

The quality of life and psychological factors evaluated included, among other factors: general health, social functioning, mental health, vitality, sensitivity, depression, and anxiety. The study showed that among the patients, most of whom were women, 49 percent of the patients preferred the combination treatment, and only 15 percent preferred levothyroxine-only treatment.

Researchers have been going back and forth for more than a decade about the value of T3, but based on their own practical experience with patients, and on the growing body of research evidence, integrative hormone experts are increasingly adding supplemental T3 as a solution to help optimize thyroid treatment for some patients. They add T3 in one of several ways:

- Adding T3 to levothyroxine treatment, via the addition of the prescription synthetic T3 drug Cytomel or generic synthetic T3
- Adding synthetic T3 via compounded sustained-release T3 in addition to levothyroxine
- Adding a dosage of a natural desiccated thyroid, such as the prescription drugs Armour Thyroid or Nature-Throid, to a levothyroxine treatment, or switching patients to a natural desiccated thyroid drug entirely
- Prescribing the combination synthetic drug Thyrolar, which includes both T4 and T3 (increasingly less common, as Thyrolar has gone through such extensive shortages, back orders, and manufacturing issues that it seems to be unavailable most of the time)

The key point? Check with your physician about whether supplemental T3 might be helpful for you.

It's important to keep in mind, however, that because T3 is the active hormone, it can have an overstimulatory effect on heart rate and pulse in some people, especially those with a history of heart disease, the elderly, and those with heart irregularities such as mitral valve prolapse. T3-savvy physicians evaluate the safety of T3 as compared to the potential benefits on a case-by-case basis.

Even in those patients who do not have any heart- or age-related issues that may make T3 problematic, some patients are simply more sensitive to T3. The heart is very sensitive to thyroid hormone in general, and for some people, even low doses of Cytomel or generic T3 can cause a rise in pulse, or heart palpitations.

For those patients, physicians often recommend a time-release form of T3 called sustained-release or slow-release T3, available by prescription from compounding pharmacies.

Many physicians, in fact, believe that the slow-release T3 is actually the optimal form for supplemental T3, as it more closely resembles the body's own conversion to and release of T3, and because the slow-release form is less likely to cause any side effects.

A 2008 Canadian study found that treating primary autoimmune hypothyroid patients who had persistent symptoms and signs of hypothyroidism with a combination of levothyroxine plus slow-release T3 (the dose in this study was approximately 13 mcg) resulted in a significant rise in the serum T3 level and a decrease in persistent hypothyroidism symptoms, without a change to the TSH.

Do keep in mind, however, that many conventional endocrinologists do not recognize the need for T3. Lou explains her situation:

After I had my thyroid removed due to nodules and went on Synthroid, I ballooned to over 200 pounds from 145 pounds over six months. My endocrinologist said I had "fork-in-mouth" disease and sent me to a psychiatrist for depression. The psychiatrist said he didn't think I was depressed, I just needed T3, and called the doctor and told him so. The endocrinologist was married to Synthroid and said no. In the meantime I continued to gain weight on a 900-calorie diet.

Eventually she found a new doctor, who added T3 to her treatment, and she was able to lose weight and shift to a healthier diet.

Kent Holtorf, MD, is finding that either a T4/T3 combination or, increasingly, a T3-only treatment is optimal for his thyroid patients who are struggling to lose weight. Says Dr. Holtorf:

> I find that T4 alone rarely works optimally for anyone. I've had a handful of patients who don't tolerate T3, but T4/T3 is so much better for most patients. I find, however, that the more symptomatic they are, the more T3 they often need.

Do You Need Natural Desiccated Thyroid?

Some practitioners believe that certain patients simply do best on natural desiccated thyroid. This drug—known as porcine thyroid, or sometimes as "natural thyroid" or "pig thyroid"—is manufactured from the dried thyroid gland of pigs. The drugs in this category include Armour Thyroid, Nature-throid, and Erfa Thyroid, and are prescription thyroid drugs that have been in use for more than a century. Integrative hormone experts believe that these drugs, which provide T4, T3, T2, T1, and other thyroid hormones and nutritional elements, more closely resemble human thyroid hormone than the synthetic drugs, and report that their patients feel better on them. Some patients find that they feel best on natural thyroid drugs, or on synthetic drugs plus some natural thyroid.

Keep in mind that the conventional view of natural thyroid drugs—and in particular, the view of many endocrinologists—is that these drugs are out of date and not "consistent," and many simply will not prescribe them. If you want this type of medication, you may have to find a holistic or alternative physician.

Margie describes her experience with natural thyroid:

At the age of forty-nine, I was diagnosed with hypothyroidism by my family practitioner. I had been gaining weight for about a year at that time, after having been thin to normal weight all through my adult life. She put me on Levoxyl. I continued to gain weight, along with all the other symptoms continuing unabated. I had horrible fatigue, no sex drive, mental fog, hair loss, brittle fingernails, irritability, fibroids and heavy bleeding (for which I ultimately had a hysterectomy), night sweats, sleep disturbances, and high blood pressure—you get the picture. My insurance company switched me to the generic levothyroxine, and I put on another quick seven pounds. We messed with the dose. Nothing happened. I consulted an endocrinologist, who switched me to Synthroid and changed my dose again. The symptoms and weight gain continued. She also told me that my weight gain was "the totally normal twelve to twenty-two pounds"! Over the course of six years, I was beginning to feel like I might have to spend the rest of my life dragging myself around feeling awful, and awful to be around. I decided I had to try Armour. I begged my endocrinologist to put me on a trial of Armour, as I sat crying in her office. She did, and immediately my life changed. Within days, the weight started coming off. My hair stopped falling out. My fingernails stopped breaking. I started to wake up in the morning rather than forcing myself out of bed, totally exhausted. I was less irritable, more productive at work, less overwhelmed. I did not change my diet, although I was less hungry for sugar and processed food, and did not require as much coffee to get me going in the morning, as I was sleeping through the night and the night sweats went away. I did not exercise more until I dropped the first fifteen pounds. In fact, I was not exercising at all! All in all, I lost thirty pounds. My only regret is that I didn't do this much, much sooner. It has taught me many lessons about being proactive with health professionals and my own health care needs, lessons that I will use the rest of my life.

At first, Alex struggled to get diagnosed:

My TSH was never above 4.9 and I have Hashimoto's antibodies. With this TSH, however, my doctor never treated me, however,
telling me my thyroid tests were perfect. Over time, after my TSH
went up, I finally was treated, but meanwhile, I had gone from a
slim person with small bones to this really quite fat person for my
bone structure. Even at 112 mcg of Synthroid, I was getting worse
every day. I left my GP and my endocrinologist and went to a doctor
who put me on desiccated thyroid. My weight gain stopped within
two weeks. So far, on the natural thyroid, I have lost thirty-one
pounds. I actually didn't diet. What happened was that my switch
from my brain changed back to telling me, I had eaten enough.
When I was not treated and on Synthroid, this turnoff switch in my
brain was gone and my brain never told me I was full. I was eating
quite a lot and I think it was because I was so tired all the time, but
more than that, my disease made me into a binge eater. Now I am
a new person. It is magic to not be eating so much, not because I
have to try and diet, but because my brain is getting what it needs
to stop the binging. My taste in food has altered totally too, and I
don't crave carbs day and night; I crave good food now.

Should You Take Your Thyroid Medication More than Once a Day?

If you are taking a levothyroxine drug, there is no benefit to splitting
or staggering your dose and taking it multiple times a day because
the drug such a long half-life in your body.

For drugs that contain T3, including Cytomel, Thyrolar, Armour
and the other desiccated thyroid drugs, and compounded drugs that
contain T3, you may in fact want to stagger your dosage throughout
the day, to help maintain a steady level and offer the best possible
relief of symptoms. T3 is faster-acting and has a shorter half-life in the

body, and some people report better results when they take their thyroid medications two or three times a day. Some patients take a dose in the morning and at bedtime; others take a morning, lunchtime, and bedtime dose. Time-release compounded drugs eliminate the need for split dosages by gradually releasing T3 throughout the day.

Note: You should always discuss any change in the way you take your medication with your physician.

Are You Being Deliberately Underdosed?

Some practitioners make it a practice to underdose thyroid medication. This means that they will give you just enough thyroid medication to get your TSH level into the top end of whichever normal range they follow—even though many practitioners and patients recognize that the majority of patients feel best at a level more like the general population's average TSH of 1.0 to 2.0.

The main reason for this policy of underdosing is the fear of osteoporosis, which was discussed earlier in the chapter. Practitioners are mistakenly concerned that maintaining a woman's TSH level at a level of, say, 1.0 to 2.0, rather than above 4.0, is a risk factor for osteoporosis. Meanwhile, if you're being treated but your TSH is still in the high-normal range—and I consider that to be 3.0 and above—then you may not feel well.

If you have a doctor who has this philosophy, you may be able to get the doctor to work with you on increasing dosage by agreeing to have periodic bone densitometry testing. This will assure your doctor that the medication is not having an adverse effect.

Are You Taking Your Medication Properly?

There are a number of guidelines on how to properly take thyroid hormone to ensure that you are absorbing the drug and receiving the maximum possible benefit.

- Don't take your thyroid hormone replacement drug within four hours of taking calcium supplements or calcium-fortified juice. This includes antacids such as Tums or Mylanta in liquid or tablet form, which also contain calcium. Calcium can delay or reduce the absorption of your thyroid hormone.
- Don't take thyroid hormone replacement drugs within four hours of taking any supplements that contain iron, including prenatal vitamins, which are usually high in iron.
- Don't take your thyroid medication until at least an hour after you have had coffee. Coffee can block absorption of your thyroid pill.
- Try to take your thyroid hormone around the same time each day. For best results, maximum absorption, and minimum interference from food, fiber, and supplements, doctors recommend taking it in the morning on an empty stomach, about an hour before eating.
- If you need to take your thyroid hormone with food, be consistent and always take it with food.
- If you start or stop a high-fiber diet while you are on thyroid hormone, have your thyroid function retested around six to eight weeks after your dietary change. High-fiber diets can change the speed of thyroid drug absorption, and you may require a dosage adjustment. You should also be consistent about your daily fiber intake. Don't have 10 grams one day, 30 grams the next day, and so on, or you're risking erratic absorption.
- If you start or stop an antidepressant medication, or a medication that contains estrogen, have your thyroid function retested around six to eight weeks later to see if you need a adjustment to your medication, as these drugs can affect thyroid absorption or effectiveness.
- If you are taking the Levoxyl brand of levothyroxine, take the drug with a lot of water and swallow the pill quickly. The pill dissolves rapidly, and if it dissolves in your mouth before swallowing it, you risk not absorbing all of the active ingredients.

Are Other Medications Interfering with or Interacting with Your Thyroid Medication?

Use of tricyclic antidepressants such as doxepin (Adapin), amitriptyline (Elavil), desipramine (Norpramin), and imipramine (Tofranil) at the same time as thyroid hormones may increase the effects of both drugs and may accelerate the effects of the antidepressant. Be sure your doctor knows you are on one before prescribing the other.

Also, researchers have found that taking thyroid hormone replacement while taking the popular antidepressant sertraline (Zoloft) can cause a decrease in the effectiveness of the thyroid hormone replacement. This same effect has also been seen in patients receiving other selective serotonin reuptake inhibitors (SSRIs) such as paroxetine (Paxil) and fluoxetine (Prozac).

If you are taking an antidepressant and your doctor prescribes thyroid medication (or vice versa), be sure get your thyroid retested six to eight weeks after starting your new medication to evaluate any possible interactions.

A number of other drugs interact with thyroid hormone or affect thyroid function:

- *Insulin.* Thyroid hormone can reduce the effectiveness of insulin and the similar drugs for diabetes. Be sure your doctor knows you are on one before prescribing the other.
- *Cholestyramine (Questran) or colestipol (Colestid).* These cholesterol-lowering drugs bind thyroid hormones. A minimum of *four to five hours* should elapse between taking these drugs and thyroid hormones.
- *Anticoagulants (blood thinners).* Anticoagulant drugs such as warfarin (Coumadin) or heparin can sometimes become stronger in the system when thyroid hormone is added to the mix. Mention it to your doctor if you are on one or the other.

- *Corticosteroids, adrenocorticosteroids.* Steroid drugs like prednisone can suppress TSH and can block conversion of T4 to T3 in some people.
- *Amiodarone (Cordarone).* This heart drug can cause hypothyroidism or hyperthyroidism and interfere with T4 metabolism. People taking amiodarone should be monitored periodically for thyroid changes.
- *Ketamine.* Some patients using ketamine, a drug used as an anesthetic (and illegally as a recreational hallucinogen known as "K" or "Special K"), experience elevated blood pressure and a racing heartbeat when taking levothyroxine sodium and ketamine at the same time.
- *Maprotiline.* This antidepressant can increase a risk of cardiac arrhythmias when taken with thyroid hormone products.
- *Theophylline.* This drug for asthma and respiratory diseases may not clear out of the body as quickly when someone is hypothyroid, but usually clears normally when the thyroid is in the normal range.
- *Lithium.* Lithium, used to treat bipolar disease and some forms of depression, is known to actually create hypothyroidism by blocking secretion of T4 and T3. People taking lithium should be monitored periodically for thyroid changes.
- *Phenytoin (Dilantin).* This anticonvulsant may accelerate levothyroxine metabolism, and tests may show decreased total T4 levels.
- *Carbamazepine (Tegretol).* This anticonvulsant pain medicine may accelerate levothyroxine metabolism, and tests may show decreased total T4 levels.
- *Rifampin.* This antituberculosis agent may accelerate levothyroxine metabolism, and tests may show decreased total T4 levels.

Are You Forgetting to Take Your Medication?

Surprisingly, one of the key reasons patients don't feel well on thyroid treatment is that they are failing to take their medications regularly, as prescribed. When you are taking thyroid hormone replacement, it's critical that you take it every day as prescribed. Even a day or two's failure to take thyroid medications can throw off your treatment regimen and have a dramatic effect on your overall health. Here are some tips on how to remember to take your thyroid medication.

- *Write it in your datebook.* Write it in a special color that is hard to miss.
- *Schedule a reminder.* If you use a computer, cell phone, or personal digital assistant (PDA) such as a BlackBerry or iPhone, consider putting a reminder in your scheduling program. Some programs allow you to set a regular daily "appointment" at a particular time. Some even have an alarm function you can set to remind you.
- *Use a screen saver.* You may be able to put a message on your computer's screen saver.
- *Keep your pill container right on top of your alarm clock.* This can help you remember to take your medicine first thing in the morning. (But be careful to keep your medications away from children.)
- *Link taking your medicine with key daily events.* One example might be brushing your teeth in the morning.
- *Put a note wherever you'll notice it every day.* Try on the refrigerator, on your coffeemaker, on your toothbrush, or on your bathroom mirror.
- *Take your medicine the same time every day.* This will help it become a habit.
- *Hire a calling service to give you a daily wake-up call to remind you to take your pill.* If you have a home voice mail answering system, you may be able to program a daily reminder call at the same time each day. You can even sign up online for free services

such as those at Wakerupper.com, which will make free reminder calls to you.

- *Use a pill sorter.* This device, also known as a dosette, has compartments for different days, or even different times of the day.
- *Get a special device to remind you to take your pill.* You can get medication computers, vibrating watches, automatic dispensers, beepers, and other alarms that can help keep you on schedule for taking your medication.
- *Enlist the aid of a family member or friend.* Sometimes just a few weeks of friendly reminders can help you get into the habit of taking your medicine at the right time every day.

RELATED IMBALANCES

For thyroid patients, several other imbalances should be tested for.

Ferritin

Ferritin is a protein that stores and releases iron, and it has a relationship to hormone balance, energy, and hair. Dr. Sara Gottfried explains:

> My opinion is that we need ferritin to be between 50 and 80 ng/mL (nanograms per milliliter) to feel our best and for hormones to operate properly. I find that to be especially true for menstruating women. If I find a low ferritin, my preference is for a patient to get it from food. If someone is not vegan, I'd recommend grass-fed beef, organic lamb. Leafy greens are also good, especially kale, chard, and watercress. For iron supplements, sometimes I will use glandulars like Integrative Therapeutics Iron Complex. Because people can have trouble absorbing iron, I also sometimes recommend Floradix liquid, which is a ferrous gluconate form that is better absorbed, but more expensive.

According to Jacob Teitelbaum, MD:

> If ferritin comes back under 50 (normal is anything over 12), taking iron is helpful. If it is over 50, you likely don't need iron unless you have hair loss, in which case supplement with iron until your ferritin is over 100.

Adrenals

For some thyroid patients, an important factor that must be addressed simultaneously in order to treat hypothyroidism is an adrenal dysfunction, or a condition known as adrenal fatigue. Thyroid and hormone expert Dr. Richard Shames explains the different levels of adrenal fatigue:

> A failing adrenal gland goes through a hyper phase before it becomes totally exhausted. In the 1950s, the famous researcher Hans Selye divided the physiology of fight-or-flight into three phases. In the first phase, adaptation, a person intermittently secretes slightly higher levels of the fight-or-flight hormones in response to a slightly higher level of stress. The second phase, called alarm, begins when the stress is constant enough, or great enough, to cause sustained excessive levels of certain adrenal hormones. This can be the very earliest glimmer of what later can become stress-induced illness. The third phase is called exhaustion, wherein the body's ability to cope with the stress is now depleted. At this point, adrenal hormones plummet from excessively high to excessively low. It is this latter phase of adrenal exhaustion that sometimes accompanies, or is confused with, low thyroid. Where do low thyroid and adrenal stress intersect? If you find yourself in the alarm phase of adrenal stress (high levels of ACTH and high levels of cortisol), one result might be altered conversion of T4 into T3, or thyronine. Thus, your adrenal

situation might profoundly affect the availability of biologically active thyroid hormone.

In addition to the continuation of thyroid symptoms after treatment and feeling "tired but wired," some common signs of adrenal fatigue include:

- Excessive fatigue
- Unrefreshing sleep (you get sufficient hours of sleep, but wake fatigued)
- Feeling overwhelmed by or unable to cope with stress
- Feeling especially run down or exhausted after stressful physical or emotional experiences
- Exhaustion or slow recovery after exercise
- Poor resistance to respiratory infections
- Difficulty recuperating from illness
- Slow to recover from injury
- Difficulty recuperating from jet lag or time changes
- Generally feeling run-down or overwhelmed
- Cravings for salty foods
- Excess mood responses after eating carbohydrates
- Feeling exhausted in the morning, or at highest energy in the evening
- Difficulty concentrating; brain fog
- Low sex drive
- Dark circles under the eyes
- Particularly low blood pressure
- Momentary light-headedness after standing up
- Extreme sensitivity to cold
- Chronic food or environmental allergies
- Cystic breasts
- A history of mononucleosis or Epstein-Barr virus reactivation
- A history of chronic fatigue syndrome

According to Richard Shames, MD:

If low-thyroid people with these symptoms are put on thyroid hormone alone, they sometimes respond negatively. These people may have coexistent, but hidden, low adrenal. If they take thyroid hormone by itself, the resultant increased metabolism may accelerate the low adrenal problem. The addition of thyroid hormone in this situation unmasks the low adrenal situation.

Many integrative physicians use the twenty-four-hour saliva cortisol test to evaluate adrenal function, looking at the levels of cortisol at four or six points during the daily cycle. Other hormones measured to evaluate adrenal function include pregnenolone and dehydroepiandrosterone (DHEA). Pregnenolone, which is synthesized from cholesterol, is a precursor for three hormones: the adrenal hormone cortisol and reproductive hormones DHEA and progesterone. Because it is the precursor for all the other reproductive hormones, pregnenolone is sometimes called a "parent hormone." Pregnenolone has roles in helping to elevate mood and energy, relieve joint pain, and improve concentration, and it is thought to help with brain function. DHEA is a steroid hormone produced by the adrenal glands as well as by the brain and the skin. DHEA levels peak around age twenty-five to thirty and steadily decline after that, so that by age eighty, the DHEA level is typically only about 15 percent of the peak level. DHEA is derived from pregnenolone and broken down into estrogen and testosterone. DHEA helps with memory, the immune system, reduction of fatigue, strength, and building muscle.

Dr. Adrienne Clamp incorporates adrenal analysis into her overall hormone balancing approach. According to Dr. Clamp:

The role of suboptimal adrenal function is not very well addressed or recognized. It can wreak havoc and undermine health and wellness if not addressed. When thyroid function appears to be normal and still someone suffers with all the symptoms of hy-pothyroidism, often adrenal hypofunction is to blame. Diagnosis can be suggested by the history of recent or prolonged stress, or recurrent bouts of serious illness. It is best confirmed by mea-surement of saliva cortisol levels throughout the day and evening. Measurement of the other hormones made by the adrenal gland such as DHEA sulfate and aldosterone is also helpful.

Treatment of the adrenal gland dysfunction depends on the pattern. I usually turn to herbal adaptogens first, as well as rec-ommending work on stress reduction by means such as medi-tation, relaxation, learning different coping mechanisms and psychological counseling, among others. Sometimes hormone re-placement is needed and, in extreme cases of hypofunction, even low doses of cortisol, though this is typically recommended only after trying the other approaches.

If evidence of adrenal imbalance or fatigue is found, some practi-tioners recommend adaptogenic supplements, such as ashwagandha. If adrenal fatigue is evident, a variety of herbal and vitamin ap-proaches may be tried. In some cases, a combination glandular adre-nal/herbal support formula is recommended. One that I have found helpful for me is Enzymatic Therapy's Fatigued to Fantastic: Adre-nal Stress End, formulated by Jacob Teitelbaum, MD, or Adreset, by Metagenics. In some cases where adrenal insufficiency may be more severe, some practitioners prescribe low doses of hydrocortisone, a bioidentical form of the hormone cortisol.

Keep in mind that traditional endocrinologists do not typically rec-ognize the existence of low-level adrenal dysfunction. Much as it took several decades for endocrinology to recognize the concept of predia-betes or insulin resistance, the endocrinology community is slow to recognize that imbalance or mild insufficiency of adrenal hormone rep-resents a diagnosable, treatable hormonal imbalance in some patients.

NUTRITION AND SUPPLEMENTS FOR THYROID FUNCTION

You'll also want to make sure that you are getting proper nutritional supplements to help support your thyroid. The following are the basics that many physicians recommend.

Multivitamins

A high-potency multivitamin is essential for thyroid patients. Look for one that has high amounts of vitamins B, C, and E and a good range of minerals. One that I particularly like is Dr. Jacob Teitelbaum's formulation, known as Daily Energy Revitalization (see Resources). The vitamin comes as a flavorful powdered drink and this replaces more than 30 vitamins and supplement pills each day. The formulation includes only a trace amount of calcium, so it's suitable for thyroid patients to take with their thyroid medication. The formula includes a low dose of iodine that Dr. Teitelbaum feels is a healthy maintenance level to help support the thyroid. You may want to slightly reduce your daily dosage if you are iodine sensitive. Says Dr. Teitelbaum: "I also added vitamin K, strontium, lipoic acid, and increased vitamin D levels to make it even more optimized for people with thyroid problems and the general public."

A good option if you want an iodine- and iron-free antioxidant multivitamin is the Advanced Nutritional System line of vitamins from Rainbow Light. They have a SafeGuard Iron-Free, Complete Nutritional System Iron-Free, and Just Once Iron-Free SafeGuard multivitamins.

Specifically, you want to make sure you are getting:

- *Vitamin A*. A deficiency in vitamin A may limit the ability to produce thyroid hormone.

- *Vitamin B$_2$ (riboflavin)*. A shortage of vitamin B$_2$ can depress endocrine function, especially the thyroid and adrenals.
- *Vitamin B$_3$ (niacin)*. Vitamin B$_3$ helps keep cells working by aiding in respiration and delivery of energy to cells.
- *Vitamin B$_6$ (pyridoxine)*. Vitamin B$_6$ helps the body convert iodine to thyroid hormone.
- *Vitamin B$_{12}$ (cyanocobalamin, methylcobalamin)*. Hypothyroidism makes us less able to absorb sufficient B$_{12}$ from diets. Some experts believe we should be getting 1,000 to 5,000 micrograms (mcg) a day, even via injection when possible. Sublingual B$_{12}$ is a more effective form of delivery than other B$_{12}$ supplements.
- *Vitamin E*. Vitamin E is an essential antioxidant, and also can help with immune function.

Vitamin C

Many experts recommend that you add 2 to 3 grams—that is, 2,000 to 3,000 mg—of vitamin C each day. You can use capsules, tablets, or powdered forms of vitamin C.

Some research has also shown better absorption of thyroid medication when it's taken along with vitamin C.

One particular favorite of mine is Emergen-C drink mix. It's very low in calories and sugar but very flavorful (I particularly like the raspberry, cranberry, and tangerine flavors). Each envelope makes one drink, and the drink has a bit of fizz to it, so it functions like a soda. But it's packed with 1,000 mg (1 gram) of vitamin C, as well as B$_6$, B$_{12}$, potassium, and a variety of other useful nutrients.

Vitamin D

Vitamin D is a vitamin, but it also functions as a hormone. It is necessary in order for the pituitary gland to produce thyroid hormone, and it may play a role in T3 binding to its receptor. Vitamin D is part of the necessary supporting apparatus that enables the enzyme deiodinase to convert T4 (inactive thyroid hormone) into T3 (the active type). It is also thought that vitamin D is necessary for healthy immune system functioning.

Cardiologist and hormone expert Dr. Rob Carlson believes that vitamin D is especially important for thyroid patients:

> I feel that screening for vitamin D deficiency should be strongly recommended for all thyroid patients. Vitamin D is required for thyroid hormone production in the pituitary gland, and is involved in the early stages of triiodothyronine or T3 binding to its receptor and initiating receptor activity. In the presence of low levels of circulating vitamin D_3, our body's ability to produce and regulate thyroid hormones may be hindered. And low levels are common, especially between September and May, in areas above 35 degrees latitude (the border between North Carolina and Georgia), and in those who avoid the sun or use sunscreen. I recommend using vitamin D_3 gelcaps, which are very inexpensive and easy to take.

Vitamin D deficiency is so rampant that this is one vitamin level that you should have tested. Dr. Sara Gottfried likes to see vitamin D levels in the 50 to 80 ng/mL range, and Dr. Kent Holtorf feels that a level of at least 80 is optimal for immune health and weight loss.

Probiotics

Probiotics are supplements that contain the "good" bacteria found in fermented foods such as miso and dairy products such as yogurt and some cheeses. We are meant to have these bacteria in sufficient quantities in our intestinal system. One of the more well-known probiotic bacterium is acidophilus, the live cultures found in yogurt. According to a report in the *European Journal of Clinical Nutri-*

tion, the probiotic bacteria known as *Bifidobacterium lactis* HN019 boosts the activity of various disease-killing immune system cells in healthy adults. Probiotics help proper digestive functioning, which enhances the immune system. They also promote a healthy balance of bacteria in the digestive system.

You can eat yogurt, but the concentration of live cultures in many brands of yogurt is not typically high enough to get a substantial effect—plus many people are sensitive to dairy. So a daily probiotic supplement is your best option. Some probiotic supplements can be expensive and require refrigeration, but I recommend a patented formula from Enzymatic Therapies, the Probiotic Pearls. This tiny pearl-shaped supplement contains a guaranteed level of live bacteria in the millions and requires no refrigeration.

Another reason to take probiotics is that they can help prevent absorption of some xenoestrogens—toxic substances that have estrogen-like effects, such as bisphenol A (BPA).

(*Note:* If you have a history of mitral valve prolapse or heart valve irregularities, check with your practitioner before starting any probiotics. There are a small number of cases of heart infection linked to probiotic intake in people with preexisting heart conditions.)

Zinc

Zinc is important for thyroid hormone production and conversion, and 15 to 25 mg of zinc a day can help ensure optimum zinc delivery to the thyroid. Zinc, along with selenium, can also help prevent the decline of T3 when you are on a lower-calorie diet. (Before you supplement with zinc, check to see if it's already included in your multivitamin.)

Selenium

Research has shown that selenium is an important mineral for thyroid function. It activates an enzyme responsible for controlling thyroid function by the conversion of T4 to T3. Stress and injury appear to make the body more prone to selenium-deficiency. Supplemental selenium appears to offset the potentially damaging effect of high iodine intake on thyroid function, according to one study. Also, selenium supplementation has been shown to reduce inflammation in patients with autoimmune thyroiditis. Too much selenium can be dangerous, so multivitamin and additional supplementation should never exceed a total of 400 mcg per day. (Before you supplement with selenium, check to see if it's already included in other supplements you are taking.)

L-tyrosine

L-tyrosine is an amino acid that contributes to the process of creating and releasing thyroid hormone, and low levels can make it difficult for the thyroid to function properly. It is a common component of many thyroid support supplements that combine several nutrients in one capsule. Tyrosine supplements at the level of 85 to 170 mg a day may be helpful to the thyroid.

Guggul

Guggul (*Commiphora mukul*) is a plant that has been used in Ayurvedic medicine as an anti-inflammatory, antiobesity, thyroid-stimulating, and cholesterol-lowering agent. Its active ingredient is Z-guggulsterone. Guggul is considered particularly important for prevention of a sluggish metabolism, and studies have shown that Z-guggulsterone may increase the thyroid's ability to take up the enzymes it needs for effective hormone conversion. It also increases the oxygen uptake in muscles. Some people find that guggul is over-stimulating, so you need to be careful with this supplement.

Iron

Iron is critical to thyroid function, and if the body is low in iron, the thyroid gets shortchanged. Iron is used to support the production of T4 and T3 and the conversion of T4 to T3. When iron is in short supply, however, iron will forgo supporting the thyroid in favor of its role in red blood cells.

To determine if you have a sufficient iron level, the best test is for ferritin, a protein that stores iron and releases it in a controlled fashion.

Sara Gottfried, MD, prefers that patients get their iron from food:

> If someone is not vegan, I'd recommend grass-fed beef and organic lamb. Leafy greens, especially kale, chard, and watercress, are also good sources of iron. For iron supplementation, sometimes I will use glandulars like Integrative Therapeutics Iron Complex. Because people can have trouble absorbing iron, I also sometimes recommend Floradix liquid, which is a ferrous gluconate form that is better absorbed, but somewhat more costly.

Some experts suggest that you eat a diet rich in vitamin C, because it helps the body absorb iron more effectively.

It's important to remember that if you take an iron supplement, you need to take it at least three to four hours apart from your thyroid hormone replacement medication, because the iron can interfere with thyroid drug absorption.

Essential Fatty Acids

Essential fatty acids (EFAs) cannot be produced in the body, so you must get them through diet or supplements. The key essential fatty acids are:

- *Omega-3s.* These include alpha-linolenic acid (ALA), eicosapentaenoic acid (EPA), and docosahexaenoic acid (DHA). They are found in fish from cold, deep oceans. Some popular fish in this category include mackerel, tuna, herring, flounder, sardines, and salmon. Other sources include linseed oil, flaxseeds and flaxseed oil, black currant and pumpkin seeds, cod liver oil, shrimp, oysters, leafy greens, soybeans, walnuts, wheat germ, fresh sea vegetables such as seaweed, and fish oil. Usually your body can convert ALA into EPA, then into DHA.
- *Omega-6.* These include linoleic acid and gamma-linolenic acid (GLA). They are found in breast milk, sesame seeds and sesame oil, safflower seeds and safflower oil, cottonseed and cottonseed oil, sunflower seeds and sunflower oil, corn and corn oil, soybeans, raw nuts, legumes, leafy greens, black currant seeds, evening primrose oil, borage oil, spirulina, and lecithin. Linoleic acid can be converted into GLA.

According to Dr. Udo Erasmus, author of *Fats That Heal, Fats That Kill*, imbalances and deficiencies in essential fatty acids are the cause of, a trigger for, or a contributing factor to many diseases and conditions, and addressing those deficiencies through proper foods or use of healthy oils can have huge implications for health. He believes that essential fatty acids are critical to thyroid function because (1) they are required for the structural integrity of the membrane of every cell, (2) they increase energy levels in the cell, and (3) there is some evidence that essential fatty acids, especially omega-3s, improve the body's ability to detect and respond to thyroid hormone effectively.

Erasmus also points to the role that EFAs play in preventing and reducing inflammation. In particular, essential fatty acids make hormone-like eicosanoids, substances that regulate immune and inflammatory responses, and omega-3s in particular have anti-inflammatory effects that can slow autoimmune damage. Inflammation of the thyroid is central to many cases of autoimmune thyroid disease, and inflammation is generally seen in almost all autoimmune diseases. Erasmus believes that if protein reactions lead to inflammation, allergies, and autoimmune disease, essential fatty acids seem to help prevent the proteins from becoming hyperactive and triggering these various immune reactions.

Nutritionist and naturopath Dr. Ann Louise Gittleman, author of *Eat Fat, Lose Weight* and the bestselling *Fat Flush* series of books, believes that good fats are essential to good health and weight loss, and that today's low-fat diets are counterproductive. Dr. Gittleman says, "Even as we have cut back on fat in the last decade, weight has steadily increased, an average of eight pounds per person. We may be eating less fat, but we are eating more calories." Ultimately, Dr. Gittleman, like many other nutritional experts, believes that if you include good fats in the diet, you rev up the body's fat-burning potential and you stay full longer, so you eat fewer calories without feeling hungry.

Overall, EFA supplements appear to be an important part of any weight-loss effort for the following reasons:

- EFAs help your body metabolize stored fat more efficiently.
- EFAs help reduce the output of inflammatory markers from fat tissue and reduce inflammation in joints and muscles.
- EFAs can help reduce insulin resistance.
- EFAs can help balance blood sugar.
- EFAs can help reduce appetite.
- EFAs can improve cholesterol levels.
- EFAs can help reduce blood pressure.
- EFAs help keep hair, skin, and nails healthy.

In addition to adding more of the foods that contain these essential fatty acids, some of the ways you can add EFAs to your diet include:

- *Fish oil supplements* are a popular choice for adding omega-3s to your diet. Go for a toxin-free, decent-tasting oil or a "burpless" capsule. Carlson's, Barlean's, and Enzymatic Therapies are known for their high-quality, pure oils and supplements. Enzymatic has my favorite burpless capsules—called Eskimo Oil—and Barlean's has a liquid fish oil with a lemon flavor that tastes surprisingly like lemon pudding. (Even my children will take it!)
- *Flaxseeds and flaxseed oil* are another choice for omega-3s. You can add flaxseed to meals, either in the oil form or as freshly ground seeds. Flaxseed oil is also available in capsules. Some people like to make salad dressing out of the oil or add it to soups or smoothies. Taking flaxseed oil with each meal helps slow down digestion and modulate blood sugar fluctuations (which helps with insulin levels).
- *Evening primrose oil* and *borage oil* are good sources of omega-6s. These are usually taken as supplements. GLA is thought to help and activate brown fat, a kind of fat that helps generate heat and burn calories.

OTHER THYROID ISSUES

Watch Goitrogens

Goitrogens are products and foods that promote goiter formation and can act like antithyroid drugs in disabling the thyroid and causing hypothyroidism. Specifically, goitrogens inhibit the body's ability to use iodine, block the process by which iodine is used to produce the thyroid hormones T4 and T3, inhibit the actual secretion of thyroid hormone, and disrupt the peripheral conversion of T4 to T3.

If you are hypothyroid due to thyroidectomy—such as for thyroid cancer, a goiter, or nodules—don't be concerned about goitrogens. If you still have a thyroid, however, you need to be careful not to eat raw goitrogens in large quantities. The enzymes involved in the formation of goitrogenic materials in plants can be partially destroyed by cooking. Eating cooked goitrogenic foods is probably not a problem for most people, though if you are a heavy consumer of cooked goitrogens and have a difficult time balancing your thyroid, you may want to consider some dietary changes.

The following list contains some of the more common and potent goitrogens (particularly when consumed raw):

- Cassava
- Broccoli
- Cabbage
- Kale
- Millet
- Radishes
- Rutabaga
- Babassu (fruits from a type of palm tree native to the Amazon)

- Turnips
- Brussels sprouts
- Cauliflower
- Kohlrabi
- Mustard
- Watercress

Understand Soy

Experts can't seem to agree on the subject of soy, a goitrogen, and there is heated debate about the potentially harmful effects of over-consumption of isoflavone-intensive soy products. Soy contains isoflavones, which have some structural similarities to estrogens and in large enough quantities function in the human body like a weak estrogen. Soy also acts as an antithyroid agent, working against the thyroid by inhibiting thyroid peroxidase (TPO), which disturbs proper thyroid function.

There are concerns about adult consumption of soy products. Inhibition of thyroid peroxidase can be expected to generate thyroid abnormalities, including goiter and autoimmune thyroiditis. One U.K. study involving premenopausal women gave participants 60 grams of soy protein per day for one month. This was found to disrupt the menstrual cycle, with the effects of the isoflavones continuing for a full three months after the soy was stopped. Another study found that intake of soy over a long period causes enlargement of the thyroid and suppresses thyroid function. Isoflavones are also known to negatively affect fertility and sex hormones, and in some animal studies have been shown to produce serious health effects including infertility, thyroid disease, and liver disease.

Soy is also a common allergen, and concerns are growing about the impact of genetically modified (GM) soy on health and hormones.

If you don't have a thyroid, as is the case for thyroid cancer patients and others who have had the thyroid surgically removed, some soy food is probably fine for you. Avoid processed soy foods like bars, shakes, and soy-based snack foods, along with genetically modified soy. Do be careful about consuming high levels of soy, however, because even in the absence of a thyroid gland, soy binds to thyroid hormone and can reduce the effectiveness of your medication.

If you still have a thyroid gland, you'll want to be more careful about using too much soy, especially soy pills, powders, and supplements. Daily overconsumption of soy foods may contribute to the worsening of your thyroid problem, and the high concentration of isoflavones found in some soy products transforms them from a food into something more like a drug.

If you want to eat some soy, again, avoid highly processed and genetically modified soy, and stick to tempeh, soy sauce, miso and other fermented forms of soy foods that are least likely to affect you negatively.

Reduce Toxic Exposures

In the past, fluoride was used as a treatment for hyperthyroidism, because it has the ability to suppress thyroid function. In one study, it was shown that 2.3 to 4.5 mg of fluoride per day was a successful treatment for hyperthyroidism. In areas where water is fluoridated, typical fluoride intake ranges from 1.6 to 6.6 mg/day, which in some cases exceeds the dosage used for medical treatment of hyperthyroidism. This means that for some of you, ingested fluoride is slowing down your thyroid gland.

What can you do? Drink water that is not fluoridated. A reverse osmosis filter can remove fluoride from tap water. Use a fluoride-free toothpaste. And consider refusing fluoride treatments at the dentist. (These treatments have not been clearly demonstrated to be helpful in adults for reducing or preventing cavities anyway.)

Perchlorate, a chemical by-product of the manufacture of rocket fuel and explosives, is known to disrupt thyroid function and cause other health problems, is increasingly the focus of public, media, and government attention. Perchlorate has contaminated areas of the U.S. water supply, most commonly in the western part of the country. Eating lettuce or other vegetables and fruits irrigated with perchlorate-contaminated water may expose some consumers to high levels of the toxin; this produce is sold around the country. Perchlorate is also a component of fertilizers and can contaminate foods grown with them. There's not much you can do to avoid eating perchlorate-contaminated foods, except to grow your own produce and water it with water that you've had tested for perchlorate contamination. If you drink well water, you should also have that water tested, and if you live in an area near a current or former production facility for rockets, explosives, or fireworks, consider having your water independently tested. Most important, become aware of the issue, and monitor the status of perchlorate legislation through the comprehensive site www.perchlorate.org.

Bisphenol A (abbreviated as BPA) is a compound used to make plastic and resins. Some of the most common sources of exposure to BPA include the lining of cans used for foods and soft drinks; poly-carbonate plastics used in eating or drinking; and infants drinking from polycarbonate plastic bottles. Besides avoiding canned foods and using BPA-free water bottles, for example, toxicology experts also recommend avoiding microwaving food in plastic containers, putting plastics in the dishwasher, or using harsh detergents on plas-tics, to avoid leaching of BPA into food. Dr. Ann Louise Gittleman recommends choosing glass jars instead of cans. As noted, some studies have shown reduced absorption of BPA in people who take probiotic supplements.

Mercury exposure comes through amalgam (silver-colored) dental fillings and through some larger fish that concentrate high levels of mercury. Mercury levels can be tested by a holistic physi-cian or nutritionist using hair analysis. If you have excessive levels of mercury, some experts recommend chelation—the process of help-ing the body excrete excess metals and minerals. This can be done through intravenous infusion or herbal supplements. In some cases, practitioners recommend removing amalgam fillings and replacing them with composite materials that contain no mercury. This is con-troversial, because it can be very expensive. Some patients have re-ported that their thyroid problems and other symptoms were greatly relieved with removal of amalgam fillings.

Naturopath Dr. Ann Louise Gittleman explains the health impact of chronic overexposure to electromagnetic frequencies (EMF), elec-trical pollution, and radiation in her groundbreaking book *Zapped*. In the book, Dr. Gittleman says to think back to your grandparents' house and count up the total number of major electrical and elec-tronic appliances in each room. Often a home might have contained a television, clock radio, stereo, oven, dishwasher, and phonograph. Now, we have large-screen televisions, wireless Internet systems, cordless telephones, game systems, computers, laptops, BlackBerry devices, iPads, cell phones, and a whole host of other gadgets and appliances. According to Dr. Gittleman, there is evidence that EMF exposure can be a chronic stress to the body, which can then suppress both adrenal and thyroid function. Her book provides detailed guidelines on how to minimize and protect against EMF exposure in daily life.

Radiation is also a definite danger to your thyroid. New research is now linking an increased risk of thyroid disease to multiple X-rays without adequate protection. Some experts are suggesting that you ask your dentist to avoid regularly scheduled X-rays unless there is a medical reason to perform the X-ray, and when dental X-rays or mammograms are necessary, ask for a thyroid collar—a small lead collar placed around your neck—that protects the thyroid gland against radiation.

Treat Infections

Infection is also thought to be a trigger for some thyroid problems. The food-borne bacteria *Yersinia enterocolitica*, for example, has been associated with elevated levels of thyroid antibodies, a sign of autoimmune thyroid disease.

A laboratory analysis by Genova Laboratories (see Resources) can help detect intestinal bacterial overgrowth that could be contributing to underlying immune system problems that may be fueling your thyroid condition. Harmful bacteria are typically treated with antibiotics; a holistic practitioner may suggest a special diet, nutritional supplements, and herbs that function in an antibiotic-like capacity.

Deal with Iodine Excess or Deficiency

Iodine supplementation is a controversial topic for thyroid patients. Too little iodine can cause a variety of thyroid problems. But the opposite problem—too much iodine—is also a risk factor for trigger-ing or worsening thyroid problems. The key is in knowing if you need iodine supplementation, and if so, how best to take it.

Holistic or nutritional practitioners sometimes assume that every thyroid patient needs iodine, or an iodine-containing herb such as bladder wrack, seaweed, or kelp. But there is controversy over the amount of iodine deficiency in the United States. On one hand, statis-tics show that one-fourth to one-third of Americans may have some degree of iodine deficiency. On the other hand, some practitioners, such as Michigan's Dr. David Brownstein, one of the pioneers in iodine testing and therapy, says that the vast majority of his thyroid patients test positive for iodine deficiency. According to Dr. Brownstein, his thyroid patients who show suboptimal iodine levels and receive iodine supplementation treatment usually find that their symptoms improve.

Should you take iodine? Answering that question requires that you be tested and, if you are deficient, carefully trying iodine supple-mentation under the direction of a practitioner.

The key way to evaluate your iodine levels is the urinary iodine clearance test. Dr. Brownstein does iodine testing with his patients, and he has those who are iodine-deficient follow a protocol for iodine supplementation that uses a specialized combination of iodine and iodide designed to ensure maximum use of the nutrient. The com-bination is found in a pill format, known as Iodoral, and in a liquid, called Lugol's solution.

Dr. Brownstein has outlined an entire program for iodine testing and supplementation in his book *Iodine: Why You Need It, Why You Can't Live Without It*, and I highly recommend that anyone inter-ested in iodine testing and supplementation read this book to learn how to get properly tested and safely supplement with iodine.

Some practitioners and patients have found that even if a mild iodine deficiency is documented, iodine-containing supplements and herbal products aggravate hypothyroid symptoms. In my own case, I have a mild iodine deficiency according to the tests, and I have tried iodine on numerous occasions. Within a day or two, however, I always feel exhausted, with a swollen, irritated neck, and after a week, I am barely functional. I have found, however, that I respond well to iodine-rich sea vegetables and iodine-rich foods such as shellfish, so perhaps the obstacle is a sensitivity to processed iodine rather than iodine in food.

Iodization of salt and foods has helped eliminate epidemic goiter and cretinism in areas that are iodine-deficient, but excess inorganic iodine may contribute to thyroid imbalances in other areas where there is sufficient iodine. One gram of salt contains 76 mcg of iodine, and we need approximately 100 mcg of iodine per day. The average person in the United States, however, actually consumes as much as 3 grams of salt, so some of us may be overdosing on iodine. If you have an excess of iodine, one way to cut back on iodine intake is to stop buying commercially iodized salt (salt that has potassium iodide) and use sea salt instead. An added plus is that sea salt tastes better!

Consider Coconut Oil

If you search the topic "thyroid" on the Internet or read some of the women's magazines, you'll find ads touting coconut oil as a cure for thyroid disease and a weight-loss miracle food and supplement. Coconut oil is controversial, however.

Nutritionist Bruce Fife, author of *The Healing Miracles of Coconut Oil*, is a firm believer in coconut oil for thyroid patients. He says, "Coconut oil by itself is not a thyroid cure. But when used as part of a thyroid-enhancing program it can be invaluable in improving some forms of hypothyroidism and even bring about complete recovery." Fife believes that coconut oil can rev up the metabolism, and he suggests replacing all refined vegetable oils with it, including margarine, shortening, and hydrogenated oils. He also recommends using coconut products and foods such as coconut milk as much as possible in cooking.

Coconut oil contains medium-chain triglycerides (MCTs), which are a special type of saturated fat. It's theorized that MCTs may promote weight loss by increasing the burning of calories.

Research on the topic is contradictory. One Canadian study found that medium-chain fatty acids (MCFAs) such as those found in coconut oil are quickly oxidized in the liver, and this speed of oxidation leads to greater energy expenditure. No weight loss, however, was associated with the demonstrated increase in energy expenditure. Another study put a group of women on a very low-carbohydrate diet for four weeks. Half received a regular fat supplement; the other half received an MCT supplement. Those on the MCT supplement had increased fat burning and less loss of muscle mass during the first two weeks, but these benefits declined during the last two weeks of the trial. Other trials showed that MCTs and coconut oil failed to enhance weight loss.

You can see if it works for you. And remember that the way to use coconut oil is not to add a few tablespoons to your diet on top of your regular foods, including fats. If you want to see if it's going to help, you need to cut out most of your other fats and oils and substitute coconut oil.

PART 2

METABOLISM,

WEIGHT LOSS,

AND HORMONES

CHAPTER 4

Thyroid Dysfunction and Metabolism

Our own physical body possesses a wisdom which we who
inhabit the body lack. We give it orders which make no sense.
— HENRY MILLER

You may think that if you have an undiagnosed thyroid condition, once you get treated, your weight problems will be over. And they can be. Some people, once diagnosed and treated, find that they will lose weight and eventually stabilize at a normal weight, without major changes to diet or exercise.

Unfortunately, that happy ending is for the minority of patients.

Many thyroid patients, even after getting diagnosed and treated, continue to struggle with a variety of symptoms, including fatigue, mood swings, and, of course, weight gain or difficulty losing weight.

This is where the issue becomes particularly challenging, because there is a fear among some physicians to even connect thyroid and weight problems. The fear borders on paranoia—some doctors refuse to acknowledge that thyroid disease is connected to weight gain, and openly disdain anyone who claims that there is a connection. Those doctors have suggested that an overweight person asking for a thyroid test is someone looking for an excuse, and inappropriately seeking drugs to cure a weight problem. Others claim that thyroid disease causes only a few pounds of weight gain at most.

Where do this misinformation and hostility come from? Well, for one thing, in the past, just as amphetamines were abused by doctors and patients for weight loss, thyroid drugs were also used by a small number of doctors in a similar way. The so-called diet doctors—doctors who were known to dispense amphetamines (aka "speed" or "uppers") and other drugs to help with weight loss—had a bad reputation. In fact, the stigma was so bad that today's doctors specializing in weight loss call themselves bariatric physicians, and they are more likely to be handing out antidepressants and suggesting gastric bypass than ever testing for an underactive thyroid. Today's doctors fear being lumped into the old category of the diet doctors handing out diet pills to the *Valley of the Dolls* or *Peyton Place* housewives who want to lose weight.

Some doctors also seem to think that if they connect your weight with your thyroid, even if you don't have a thyroid problem, you will get the idea that thyroid medication can help you lose weight. And that means you could become what they call a "drug seeker"—someone who looks for prescription drugs inappropriately.

Another reason doctors actively don't want to connect thyroid disease with weight gain is that they don't want to admit how little they actually understand nutrition, metabolism, and the thyroid. They know the basic thyroid symptom list, they know how to do a thyroid-stimulating hormone (TSH) test, and they know how to write out a prescription for levothyroxine. But they don't know about nutrition or the hormonal effect on metabolism. You've heard the old bromide that most doctors spend about an hour on nutrition in medical school. Well, in addition to that hour, they spend a couple of hours on thyroid disease, and that completes their education on nutrition, the thyroid, and metabolism. The complexities of the endocrine system and the delicate interplay that goes on between hormones, the brain, the stomach, the appetite, and the ability to store and burn fat are topics few doctors have studied and even fewer understand.

Dr. Rob Carlson explains an aspect of the issue:

There has been some movement among endocrinologists to be critical of too "aggressive management" of thyroid disease in patients. I see so many patients who started out complaining to their physicians about weight gain issues (or an inability to lose weight despite eating very little and working out diligently), as well as fatigue and low energy. Being afraid to check labs in these patients, or ridiculing these patients because they aren't "telling the truth" about what they are eating or about how much they are exercising, seems counterintuitive. The logical approach, since they are coming to a physician for help, is to realize that something metabolically must be going on, and to search it out, not ridicule or dismiss the patient.

Katie Schwartz, a thyroid patient advocate and founder of the DearThyroid.org website, struggled for years to get a diagnosis of Graves' disease but was discouraged to discover that even after RAI treatment, her health battle continued:

Atypical of Graves' disease, I was gaining weight at the speed of light. The more weight I gained and the more misdiagnoses I received, the more doctors blamed everything but my thyroid. Even before I was properly diagnosed, I racked up a long list of unforgettable advice, including "Katie, stop eating whole pies," "Katie, you really need bariatric surgery," and "If you stopped eating, you'd be able to live off of your own body fat for at least six months!" After diagnosis, the fat slams were equally offensive. I was told, "You blame your thyroid, but your thyroid doesn't make you fat. What you put into your mouth makes you fat," "At best, a thyroid disorder will cause ten to fifteen pounds of weight gain," "You need to join Overeaters Anonymous," And "Why do you lie about the food you eat? You're obviously consuming thousands of calories a day or you wouldn't keep gaining weight."

Katarina gained more than sixty-five pounds after she developed hypothyroidism. In desperation to get some of the weight off, she did a three-week fast:

I ate no real food, just water and a very light vegetable soup. But instead of losing weight, I gained more than two pounds. Apparently I am a medical miracle! So I went to the doctor and explained everything for him. He just laughed at me and sent me home saying, "To lose weight, you just have to eat less!" Just one of many doctors who don't listen to their patients and do not believe in what patients tell them.

Lauren is a fitness trainer, with a degree in biochemistry and nutrition:

I know all about the 3,500-calories-equals-one-pound stuff and a ton of other things that should work—which I think made the whole process even more frustrating. I just couldn't understand why it was so hard for me to lose weight. Right now, I have a maintenance calorie intake of 1,000 calories per day. I count everything that I put in my mouth, from the lettuce in my salad to the crust of my daughter's bread from her sandwich at lunch if I eat it. If I go to 1,200 calories, I gain. Also, let me add that I am an aerobics and studio cycling instructor. I teach five classes a week, plus I manage to take one other spin class and run one day a week too. All this exercise, and still, I can only eat 1,000 calories to maintain my weight. It's not fair! It is very hard in my profession to be doing all the right things, and not be able to drop the three to five pounds I want with all the exercise and eating as little as I do.

The truth is, the thyroid is intricately connected to metabolism and weight. Interestingly, research published in the *Journal of Clinical Endocrinology and Metabolism* demonstrated that even slight hypothyroidism can cause weight gain. The study looked at almost four thousand people and found there was definitely a link between body mass index (BMI)—a measure of obesity—and the TSH level. BMI rose as TSH rose. They also found a negative association between BMI and free T4, meaning that as free T4—a measure of circulating thyroid hormone in the bloodstream—rises, BMI tends to drop. Even among people who had a so-called normal TSH level, those at the high end of normal TSH levels (with a median TSH of 4.5) weighed approximately twelve pounds more than those who had a TSH on the low end of normal (with a median TSH of 0.28).

The researchers concluded:

> We suggest that differences in thyroid function, within what is considered the normal range, are associated with differences in BMI, caused by longstanding minor alterations in energy expenditure. This is more pronounced when mild hypo- or hyperthyroidism is present. The prevalence of such abnormalities in thyroid function is high and may be influenced by environmental factors. Because small abnormalities in thyroid function are common, thyroid function may importantly influence the prevalence of obesity in a population.

I can guarantee you, however, that most doctors—including most endocrinologists—have never read that particular journal article, just as most doctors really don't know what to advise about losing weight. The majority of Americans are overweight, and doctors don't have much more advice than telling people to get off the couch, get more exercise, and eat less. Even for those who don't have a thyroid problem, this advice obviously isn't working, given that two-thirds of Americans are overweight. And when you add in the difficulties of a thyroid problem, doctors have even less to offer.

What you will hear from endocrinologists, other physicians, and even patients, however, are supposed facts about thyroid disease and weight gain that are spread around without question, but should actually be looked at quite critically.

FACTS VERSUS MYTHS

There is a variety of myths about thyroid disease and weight gain, and I don't need to repeat any of them here, because you can find them everywhere—in magazine articles, drug company literature, and perhaps even firsthand from your doctors. So instead, here are the facts.

Fact: When You Are Hypothyroid, You May Lose Weight

There is a small percentage of hypothyroid patients who have difficulty gaining weight, or who maintain a normal weight throughout diagnosis and treatment. Also, some hypothyroid people do not have weight gain right away but find that over time it slowly creeps up on them.

Fact: When You Are Hypothyroid, Your Weight Gain May Be Significant

If you talk to some physicians, they will suggest to you that hypothyroidism can't cause more than a few pounds of weight gain. Another myth. Just ask the thousands upon thousands of thyroid patients who were at a perfectly normal weight—myself included—until they started to pile on weight faster than seemingly physically possible, only to get diagnosed with hypothyroidism shortly afterward. Of course, there are always some patients who gain only a few pounds and who lose them fairly easily once treated, but they appear to be in the minority.

Laura, an active fifty-one-year-old mother of two children, knew something was wrong when she started to gain weight and feel tired, moody, and achy.

I went from a vibrant, in-shape woman to a totally out-of-control, overweight couch potato! I wanted to scream but could not, since I also lost my voice! I did not want to leave my house and was too tired to do anything. I felt so sick I thought I would die! I gained about forty pounds in a period of about three months. That alone was pretty scary.

Elizabeth is sixty-one and describes herself as at least seventy pounds overweight. In the past, the heaviest she had been was 190 after two pregnancies.

In 1999, I was told I had nodes on my thyroid and had a biopsy, which showed all was well. I had a severe case of vertigo in 2000, and the doctor I was taken to found out that my heart rate was out of control and my thyroid readings were bad. I was seriously hyperthyroid. Diagnosis: multitoxic nodular thyroid. I went to an endocrinologist and he had me take RAI (a high dose), and then I was put on Synthroid. He never told me that I was going to gain this much weight. I ballooned up to 230 pounds. That is my current weight! So I went from 190 to 230! What I find most frightening is the way my body has changed shape. Also my neck, which used to be long and graceful, is now squat and short, and I have these fat bulges in the indentations of my collarbones. I kept crying to the endocrinologist about how big I was getting. He said nothing and did nothing. I then went to a woman endocrinologist—she looked at me and pooh-poohed everything I said. She said I was fat from eating! At this point my regular internist takes care of me. But I must say that not a day goes by that I do not cry in the privacy of my home. I am so heavy my back is killing me. I barely have enough breath or energy to do things like I used to. It seems the doctors are unwilling to see the pain we are in. In plain English, I am not the same person I was before I had RAI. I am so miserably unhappy. I must try to get a grip on my weight before it does me in altogether.

Fact: If You Are Hyperthyroid, You May Gain Weight

While the majority of people lose weight when actively hyperthyroid, a percentage actually gain weight. Why they do is not clear. It may be they are simply so hungry that they are taking in more calories than even their revved-up metabolism can burn. Or it may be that their impaired endocrine system sets into motion a variety of the problems discussed in the last chapter, such as poor digestion, insulin resistance, and adrenaline resistance.

Fact: After Hyperthyroidism Treatment with Antithyroid Drugs, You Are Likely to Gain Weight

Doctors will tell patients, "You won't gain weight after RAI if you exercise and eat right," but they are not accurately representing the true situation. Patients who are hyperthyroid frequently lose a great deal of weight before their diagnosis. It's expected that after treatment, they will regain the weight that was lost. But many patients continue to put on weight even after they've regained the weight and thyroid levels are normalized. One study found that even after thyroid levels return to a normal range in patients treated with antithyroid drugs, many individuals continue to gain weight at three, six, and nine months, with the weight gain at three months being around five pounds or more.

Fact: After Hyperthyroidism Treatment with Radioactive Iodine (RAI), You Will Most Likely Become Hypothyroid, and You Will in All Likelihood Gain Weight

Doctors who tell you that they can somehow calculate just the right amount of RAI are living in fantasyland, because most patients post-RAI become hypothyroid, and many complain of weight gain. In fact, one research study found that more than 85 percent of patients receiving RAI became hypothyroid, and despite being treated with levothyroxine, their median weight gain was eleven pounds after six months, twenty pounds after twelve months, and twenty-five pounds after two years. Before the therapy, 27.5 percent were considered underweight by body mass index calculations, and 19.3 percent were obese, with a BMI above 30. Two years after treatment, only 8.7 percent of patients were underweight and 51.3 percent were obese. Overall, the researchers found that there was a 32 percent increase in obesity in previously hyperthyroid patients following RAI therapy, with the main weight gain coming in the first two years.

Miya had this experience:

I used to be chronically underweight. In high school I wore a size 4 and I'm five foot nine! My mom was convinced I had an eating disorder. I always felt light-headed and would get dizzy spells. When my thyroid was hyper, I was literally eating four to seven meals a day. I ate Dairy Queen on a regular basis and was outeating my six-foot-two boyfriend. I gained maybe five pounds the whole time (months and months) I was hyper. Once I went on Tapazole, I started to gain. I guess I began to be a weight that my body was supposed to be. I went up to a size 8, then a 10. When I was diagnosed, I was about 130 pounds. When I had RAI, after a year of Tapazole, I think I was about 150. After RAI, there was a two-week period where I literally gained ten or fifteen pounds. It was insane. My weight went up to 175.

Fact: Some Thyroid Cancer Patients Can Have Weight Problems

Some doctors will suggest that thyroid cancer, either in its early stages or after treatment when the thyroid cancer patient no longer has a thyroid gland, doesn't ever cause weight problems. Not true. The reality is that when you do not have a thyroid gland, you are hypothyroid for life, and reliant on outside thyroid hormone medication to help regulate your metabolism. This can be a problem for some patients.

It's not guaranteed that you'll gain weight in this situation, however, because when you have been treated for thyroid cancer, doctors do not typically wait for months until you become hypothyroid and your TSH levels elevate before they start thyroid hormone replacement. It's usually started right away, and levels of thyroid hormone replacement are high enough to suppress thyroid hormone production, which means that your TSH level will be in the hyperthyroid range. Even so, you may find weight piling on or impossible to lose.

Jody was diagnosed with thyroid cancer at age twenty-one and had a complete thyroidectomy followed by one radiation treatment.

During the time period that my thyroid was all out of whack when I was going through all the ultrasounds and biopsies to determine cancer or not, I gained forty pounds. Yes, I went from a very healthy and in-shape size 3/4 to a tired, miserable, and flabby size 13/14. I hated what had happened to my body as well as my mental well-being. I felt disgusting and that I had lost control of the one thing that I used to be very in control of. After the surgery, I could only thank God for getting me through it all and I could call myself a cancer survivor.

Fact: If All or Part of Your Thyroid Is Removed, You May Gain Weight

Some people who have had a full or partial thyroidectomy—surgery to remove the thyroid—gain weight. Someone who has a full thyroidectomy to remove a thyroid that is enlarged or filled with nodules is typically started on thyroid hormone replacement medication soon after surgery. Even then, however, over time, relying on external thyroid hormone replacement may destabilize metabolism and contribute to weight gain or difficulty losing weight. For those patients who have a partial thyroidectomy, the situation may be further complicated, because some practitioners wait until a patient has visible, physical symptoms of hypothyroidism and blood tests show significant hypothyroidism before providing thyroid hormone replacement. Their theory is that because they have removed only part of the thyroid, the remaining part should be able to provide sufficient hormone. The truth is that most patients who have even part of the thyroid removed do eventually need some thyroid medication in order to avoid hypothyroidism. Even with thyroid treatment, however, some of these patients will gain weight inappropriately, or find it impossible to lose weight.

Fact: The Weight Will Probably Not Just Melt Off After You Start Thyroid Hormone Replacement

There is always the story of the thyroid patient who started taking levothyroxine or natural thyroid and lost twenty pounds in a month. And I have heard doctors say to patients, "Once you're on thyroid hormone, the weight will drop off." But actual occurrences of this are few and far between. More likely is that after starting thyroid medication, you'll lose a few pounds, usually water weight, as the water retention of hypothyroidism starts to abate, then . . . nothing.

There are a number of reasons why thyroid patients have a more difficult time losing weight. These hormonal issues are discussed in the next section.

THYROID-RELATED CHALLENGES TO WEIGHT LOSS FOR THYROID PATIENTS

Another important fact is that thyroid patients frequently have a more difficult time losing weight than people who do not have a thyroid dysfunction.

There are a number of physiological factors that make weight loss more challenging for some thyroid patients.

Cellular Hypothyroidism, Thyroid Resistance, and Reverse T3 Dominance

In some thyroid patients, there appears to be a dysfunction in thyroid hormone transport—the ability of thyroid hormone to actually cross over the cell wall and into cells.

The transport of thyroid hormones into the cell is dependent on energy. Says Kent Holtorf, MD:

> Any condition associated with reduced production of the cellular energy (mitochondrial dysfunction) will also be associated with reduced transport of thyroid into the cell, resulting in cellular hypothyroidism despite having standard blood tests in the "normal" range. Conditions associated with reduced mitochondrial function and impaired thyroid transport include: insulin resistance, diabetes and obesity; chronic and acute dieting; diabetes; depression; anxiety . . . ; chronic infections; physiologic stress and anxiety [among others].

Dr. Holtorf has also identified chronic emotional or physiologic stress as factors that can cause a substantial reduction of transport of T4 into the cells. The pituitary gland, which produces TSH, is typically unaffected by stressors. This means that TSH levels may appear to be normal, yet cells remain deficient in thyroid hormone, resulting in cellular hypothyroidism. According to Dr. Holtorf, some studies have shown that significant physiological stress can reduce the tissue levels of T4 and T3 by as much as 79 percent, without any corresponding increase in TSH.

A variation of this problem, says Dr. Holtorf, is chronic over-production of reverse T3:

> A high reverse T3 demonstrates that there is either an inhibition of reverse T3 uptake into the cell and/or there is increased T4 to reverse T3 formation. . . . Reverse T3 is an excellent marker for reduced cellular T4 and T3 levels not detected by TSH or serum T4 and T3 levels. . . . high or high normal rT3 is not only an indicator of tissue hypothyroidism but also that T4 only replacement would not be considered optimal in such cases and would be expected to have inadequate or sub-optimal results.

Thyroid expert Richard Shames, MD, coauthor of the books *Thyroid Power, Thyroid Mind Power,* and *Fat, Fuzzy and Frazzled,* says that while every hormone can have resistance, physicians are less likely to understand the idea of thyroid resistance.

> They have heard of the condition known as "resistance to thyroid hormone"—and that is a rare genetic condition. But there are many people who have normal circulating thyroid levels, but they are not normal in terms of the thyroid function in the brain and cells, where so much is actually taking place.
>
> So, you—and your metabolism—could be literally starving for thyroid hormone, and yet a so-called normal TSH means that you may not get the proper treatment to address hypothyroidism due to transport problems or reverse T3 dominance.

The answer? According to integrative practitioners, one of the key ways to overcome reverse T3 dominance and help reset proper thyroid function is in thyroid treatment with time-release T3. In some cases, the T3 is added to a T4 or natural desiccated thyroid treatment, but in other cases, the T3 may be prescribed as a stand-alone thyroid treatment.

Metabolic Impact of Yo-Yo Dieting

Many thyroid patients are recurrent or repeat dieters, losing and then regaining weight on a regular basis. This pattern is especially harmful to ongoing thyroid function and, in particular, can sabotage thyroid patients who are trying to lose weight.

One study showed that after repeated cycles of dieting, weight loss occurs at half the rate compared to controls eating the same calorie level. And when weight gain occurred, it occurred *three times faster* than in the controls. No longer is the adage "Yo-yo diets wreck your metabolism" an old wives' tale.

Kent Holtorf, MD, explains:

> People on chronic diets—or those who lose significant amounts of weight—will have a lower metabolism than a person with the same weight and muscle mass who had not lost significant weight or drastically dieted in the past. This was demonstrated in a study by Leibel published in the journal *Metabolism* . . . [that] compared the basal metabolic rate in individuals who had lost significant weight to those of the same weight who had not lost significant weight in the past. The authors found that those who had dieted and lost weight in the past had, on average, a 25 percent lower metabolism than the control patients who had not lost significant weight.

Metabolic Impact of Starvation Dieting

Some thyroid patients, in frustration, have turned to very low-calorie diets—sometimes called "starvation dieting." This can also have a negative effect on metabolism.

According to Dr. Holtorf:

One study found that dieting obese individuals had a 50 percent reduction of T4 into the cell and a 25 percent reduction of T3 into the cell due to the reduced cellular energy stores. This demonstrates that in such patients, standard thyroid blood tests are not accurate indicators of intracellular thyroid levels. This also demonstrates why it is very difficult for obese patients to lose weight; as calories are decreased, thyroid utilization is reduced and metabolism drops. These thyroid changes are not, however, detected by standard TSH, T4, and T3 testing.

Free T3 and reverse T3 levels can aid in the diagnosis; if low free T3 or elevated reverse T3 is found, treatment with a T3 medication may help increase the thyroid utilization and metabolism.

OTHER CHALLENGES TO WEIGHT LOSS FOR THYROID PATIENTS

Even if your thyroid treatment is optimized, as described in chapter 2, as a thyroid patient, you may still face a variety of challenges that make it more difficult to lose weight than it is for the typical person. Again, I'm focusing primarily on hypothyroidism because it is the end result for almost all thyroid conditions, whether you have your thyroid surgically removed or radioactively ablated or you have an otherwise underactive or nonfunctioning thyroid gland.

Diagnosis Delay

For many people who become hypothyroid, it can be months or even years from the time their thyroid condition develops to when it is diagnosed and treated. During this period, a variety of symptoms can appear, even before TSH elevates enough to officially qualify for a conventional diagnosis of hypothyroidism. Even a slight decrease in metabolism mean fewer calories burned every day, so if you ate the same amount and kept up your same level of activity over time, you would see weight gain due to the reduction in metabolism. Unfortunately, many people who are becoming hypothyroid also experience fatigue, low energy, and muscle pain, which makes them less likely to exercise and incorporate physical activity into their daily lives. So you have another factor that can further reduce metabolism. Finally, as you become more tired, you may eat more in an unconscious attempt to generate energy. So it's a triple whammy to your metabolism: you're eating more food, burning off even less of it because of a lowered basal resting metabolism, and doing less physical activity.

If this resulted in a metabolism that was, for example, even 350 calories a day less efficient, you could gain a pound or more every ten days, or three pounds a month. Go undiagnosed for a year, and that's thirty-six pounds. It can be even more, because the more weight you gain, the more efficient your body becomes at fat storage and the less active you typically become. All the more reason to become your own best advocate and push for diagnosis and treatment as early as possible.

Hypothyroidism After a Period of Hyperthyroidism

As hyperthyroidism develops, some people actually enjoy the ability to eat anything they want without weight gain or even with weight loss. Excess energy in some hyperthyroid people may also result in their doing a great deal of exercise. So during this period, there's an increase in resting metabolism and often an increase in activity level that may outweigh increased appetite. Or, if appetite remains the same, some people enjoy desirable weight loss that occurs because of improved metabolic efficiency.

The problem is that hyperthyroidism needs to be treated. It can cause rapid pulse and high blood pressure, and untreated hyperthyroidism puts you at risk for thyroid storm, an episode of uncontrollably high blood pressure and heart rate that can result in heart attack, stroke, or even death. So at a minimum, your doctor will give you antithyroid drugs, and perhaps beta-blockers, to help slow things down temporarily and see if you respond. Or you may get RAI treatment or surgery to permanently make you hypothyroid.

The problem is that you may continue to eat as you did before. If you were eating at higher calorie levels and all of a sudden you go on antithyroid drugs to slow down your thyroid and beta-blockers to slow down your heart rate, it's like taking your metabolism from 60 mph to zero. You're going to be burning up fewer calories, and you can start gaining weight quickly at your former calorie level. The double whammy comes when you find yourself feeling tired, so you cut back on activity and burn even less.

Even if you did not increase your food intake, you may have been eating at a level that maintained your weight. But after you are diagnosed and your metabolism adjusts to antithyroid medication and beta-blockers, you may find yourself gaining weight if you don't cut calories and/or increase physical activity.

Erich was a cross-country runner, five feet ten inches tall, who kept himself at a trim 145 pounds for most of his life, until he developed hyperthyroidism, went on antithyroid drugs, and then had a thyroidectomy.

My weight just prior to surgery had climbed to an astounding 195 pounds, fully thirty pounds more than I weighed for the majority of my life. Following surgery, I was placed on a minimal dosage of Levothroid, which failed to provide me with the necessary supplement for my removed thyroid gland. Gradually, the dosage was increased (sometimes by my taking two pills on my own) until the point where I was taking 500 mcg per day. Unfortunately, the higher dosage failed to alleviate many of the symptoms of hypothyroidism such as cold hands, lethargy, weight gain, etc. By the time I switched doctors, my weight had climbed to approximately 236 pounds.

Another problem for people who start out with hyperthyroidism is the delay in getting on thyroid hormone replacement after RAI. Honestly, I have no idea what motivates some of the doctors who are treating thyroid patients, but if you are hyperthyroid and are going to have RAI, your doctor should sit down and tell you these things:

1. It's likely that you will become hypothyroid.
2. This can happen quickly, maybe several weeks after RAI, or it may take months.
3. Be aware of and on the lookout for hypothyroidism symptoms. If you have any of these symptoms, make a doctor's appointment immediately so that your thyroid levels can be checked.
4. As soon as symptoms appear or you have an elevation in TSH above a certain level, you will need to start thyroid hormone replacement drugs.

Most of you will not have this discussion with your doctor. Unfortunately, the longer you go with your TSH elevating and without thyroid hormone replacement treatment, the more likely it is that you will gain excess weight.

Once you've had RAI, forget about being hyperthyroid and start considering yourself hypothyroid. Familiarize yourself with hypothyroidism symptoms and treatments (my book *Living Well with Hypothyroidism* can help), and take control of your own health. Monitor your symptoms. If you have to, order your own thyroid blood work, and push for proper treatment for your now hypothyroid condition.

Slowed Digestion and Elimination

Many physicians don't tell you that thyroid disease causes water retention and bloating—especially hypothyroidism, which can cause
puffiness and bloating in the face (and especially the eye area), arms,
hands, legs, and feet. You also may not know that the body will hold
on to water fiercely unless you are taking in enough water. Because
you feel or look bloated or swollen, you may not drink enough water,
but that is counterproductive. Dehydration can interfere with proper
metabolism.

Hypothyroidism also slows down digestion and elimination. In
fact, constipation is one of the most common symptoms, even for
people who are optimally treated. Slower and less efficient digestion
and elimination means that toxins spend more time in the intestines, where they can do damage and pass into your body. Allergens spend more time in contact with your intestinal lining, where
they can cause irritation and inflammation. All of these factors can
impede weight loss.

Other Related Issues

A number of other factors may make it more difficult for thyroid
patients to lose weight.

- *Inflammation from autoimmune disease.* Most thyroid disease is
  due to autoimmune conditions, such as Hashimoto's disease and
  Graves' disease. Autoimmune diseases are conditions where there
  is internal inflammation. And, as noted in the previous chapter,
  inflammation can be a factor that impedes weight loss.
- *Lowered body temperature.* The reduction in body temperature associated with an underactive thyroid can communicate to your
  brain that you are facing a period of starvation. This sends out a

variety of signals that increase appetite, encourage fat storage, and discourage fat burning—all as a means of ensuring survival.

- *Less fitness, less muscle.* When you have a thyroid dysfunction, even with optimal treatment you may feel more fatigued than normal. This level of fatigue may mean that you exercise less and move around less, which reduces the amount of energy you expend and reduces your muscle mass. Thyroid disease also commonly causes joint and muscle aches and pains, carpal tunnel syndrome, tarsal tunnel syndrome, and tendonitis, all of which make exercise and movement harder and may discourage you from physical activity, which means you expend less energy. In both cases, the less you move, the more likely you are to lose muscle mass. And reduced muscle mass also reduces metabolism.

- *Fatigue and increased food intake.* Many people with thyroid problems experience ongoing fatigue. When you are tired, one of the body's ways to try to generate energy is to increase your appetite, encouraging you to eat more for energy.

- *Carbohydrate cravings.* Dutch researchers studying the energy and nutrient intake of thyroid patients found that thyroid disease and hyperthyroidism in particular may be linked to increased appetite for carbohydrates. This increased craving for and intake of carbohydrates appears to stem from various changes in brain chemistry and sympathetic nervous system activity due to the thyroid condition.

- *Depression.* Thyroid disease can trigger or worsen depression. Depression is known to trigger eating in some people and especially increase carbohydrate cravings. Depression can also make you less likely to exercise and disrupt your ability to get restorative sleep.

- *Sleep disruptions.* Thyroid patients may have difficulty getting sufficient levels of restorative sleep. A lack of restorative sleep affects fat burning, serotonin levels, and hormone levels, all of which can make weight loss more difficult.

DRUGS THAT MAY PROMOTE WEIGHT GAIN

There are a number of drugs that can actually cause weight gain. It's important to read through the complete list of side effects for all drugs prescribed for you. If weight gain is listed as a possible side effect, discuss with your physician whether there are any options that are more diet-friendly.

Some of the drugs that may contribute to weight gain include:

- Steroidal anti-inflammatories (e.g., prednisone)
- Propylthiouracil (PTU)
- Lithium
- Estrogen and progesterone independently, or together in birth control pills
- Antidiabetic drugs, such as insulin
- Various antidepressants, especially Prozac, Paxil, and Zoloft
- Mood-stabilizing and anticonvulsant drugs such as those given for bipolar disorder, including lithium, valproate (Depakote), and carbamazepine (Tegretol)
- Beta-blockers
- Sedatives
- Tranquilizers

Remember, don't stop taking any prescribed medications without discussing it in advance with your physician or practitioner. Some medications are less likely to cause weight gain than others, however, and a conversation with your doctor may help you choose a better course for your medication.

CHAPTER 5

Metabolism, Hormones, and Sensitivities

Metabolism is not a thing. It's a journey.
— MARC DAVID

I have to admit that I went through numerous versions of this chapter. It started out as a sixty-page dissertation on the entire process of metabolism—from the intake of food to the expenditure of energy, along with the intricate hormonal interactions that affect appetite, fat burning, and blood sugar. When I realized that I was starting to talk medicalese—after all, do I need to use the term *gluconeogenesis* ten times in one chapter?—I knew it was time to go back to square one and answer the really important question: how can metabolism be an obstacle to losing weight?

So if you want a comprehensive understanding of the physiology, I'd suggest a textbook on nutrition or endocrinology, where you can learn everything you'd ever want to know about gluconeogenesis (starting with how to pronounce it). In the meantime, here are the key points that affect your ability to lose weight.

HOW FOOD BECOMES ENERGY

To understand how metabolism can be an obstacle to weight loss, you first have to understand how food becomes energy in your body. Food is converted into energy by the processes of digestion and metabolism. Let's use a typical lunch as an example: a turkey sandwich on white bread with mayo, sweetened soda, and spinach salad. Where you see common foods such as bread, turkey, mayonnaise, soda, and spinach, your body sees carbohydrates (bread, spinach, and soda), protein (turkey), and fat (mayonnaise). Each type of food is digested and metabolized into energy in different ways.

Digestion starts in the mouth. Saliva contains enzymes that start to break down food, which means that the act of chewing works together with your saliva to moisten and start dissolving food. The food heads down the esophagus into your stomach, where enzymes and acids are released from the stomach lining. The food is chemically broken down, with each type of food headed for a different objective.

- Carbohydrates become glucose, the energy source for cells.
- Proteins such as meat, poultry, and dairy products become amino acids.
- Fats, such as those found in oils, nuts, fats, meat, and dairy products, become triglycerides and fatty acids.

Not all foods are digested at the same rate. Carbohydrates (which include everything from bread, rice, and sugar to potatoes, green vegetables, and fruits) are usually digested more quickly than proteins and fats. But how quickly you digest carbohydrates also depends on the type of carbohydrate. For example:

- The sugars in simple carbohydrates in liquid form, such as in a sweetened soft drink, are already so small that they require almost no digestion before they can be absorbed into the stomach lining. Their small size enables them to pass quickly—usually in less than thirty minutes—into the small intestine, then the blood. So the transit period from ingestion to hitting your bloodstream is very quick.

- Plain white bread is another refined, simple carbohydrate that has little to no fiber. With its easily dissolvable molecules, it will be digested fairly quickly. (Contrast this with high-fiber bread, which is a complex carbohydrate, meaning that it is less easily broken down and therefore is digested more slowly.)

- The carbohydrate that will be digested most slowly is the spinach, because like all fruits and vegetables, it is a complex unrefined carbohydrate (meaning that it has to go through more digestive processes, which take longer, before it becomes glucose). The fiber in the spinach also slows down its digestion.

- The turkey and mayonnaise will require more time to digest because it takes longer for protein and fat to go through the first round of digestion by the stomach enzymes. Proteins and fats are more complicated molecules than carbohydrates and may take as long as three and a half hours to digest. This is why meals that contain sufficient protein and fat make you feel full longer.

After digestion in the stomach, food moves quickly through your small intestine, where all absorption of nutrients occurs.

- The carbohydrates in bread have been broken down into glucose, which transfers easily across the lining (mucosa) of the small intestine into your blood.

- The indigestible carbohydrates (fiber) in spinach move through your system unconverted into energy, since humans (unlike cows) do not have the enzymes to digest fiber.

- Turkey, partially digested by enzymes in the stomach, is met by more enzymes from your pancreas, helping to complete the breakdown of protein into amino acids.

- Once in the small intestine, the fat in mayonnaise is turned into a watery substance of fatty acids and cholesterols with the help of bile acids from the gallbladder. Inside the mucosa, fatty acids and cholesterols are rebuilt into fats called triglycerides and released into the blood.

Meanwhile, there is another process going on in your bloodstream. Glucose, amino acids, and triglycerides start surging through the bloodstream to be used as energy, to aid in cellular repair, or to be stored as fat.

When faced with high amounts of glucose, your pancreas secretes a hormone known as insulin. Insulin's role is to keep blood glucose levels from rising too high. When insulin is present, glucose—your body's favorite and easiest-to-use energy source—is more rapidly absorbed by cells, especially the important area known as the mitochondria. The mitochondria are sometimes called the powerhouse of the cell, since this is where the largest production of energy occurs.

What happens to the amino acids and triglycerides? Usually, triglycerides end up stored in fat tissue. They can be converted into glucose by your liver, but usually only as a last resort when glucose is not readily available, because it costs the body more energy to metabolize these stored fats into energy. In case of a brief starvation, the liver holds a twelve-hour supply of glycogen, which it can convert into glucose to help fuel the body. Otherwise, the body is very stubborn about letting go of its fat and amino acid reserves. This is one reason why it can be hard to lose weight: the body readily and quite efficiently uses all the glucose it gets directly from food.

When you haven't eaten for hours and blood glucose levels are low, the pancreas releases not insulin but another hormone, glucagon. Glucagon acts in a way opposite to insulin and actually pulls sugar out of storage from the liver; if more is needed, it converts fatty tissue into glucose. The release of glucagon is also typically triggered by protein-heavy meals and exercise. Glucagon does not come into play, however, when a high-carbohydrate meal has been eaten and insulin levels are high.

Once you have finished digesting all the carbohydrates you last ate, release of glucagon causes the liver to convert its stored glycogen back into glucose to help maintain blood sugar. When the liver runs out of glycogen and in the absence of new carbohydrates or glucose sources, the liver shifts to a process called gluconeogenesis (there's that word!)—which means that it starts converting amino acids into glucose.

There's another important hormone in the picture: ghrelin. Ghrelin is sometimes referred to as the hunger hormone, and is produced by your stomach to signal that it's time to eat—now! Ghrelin rises sharply before you eat and falls quickly afterward. The ghrelin signal itself has a short-term effect, lasting up to an hour. If you don't eat when the signal presents itself, it goes away fairly quickly, and appetite disappears. When you lose weight, however, baseline ghrelin levels can go up. One study found ghrelin levels rose an average of 24 percent in dieters. In this way, it's thought, ghrelin may be part of the body's efforts to avoid starvation and maintain a particular weight range.

As you can see, your metabolism is designed to do everything it can to:

- Make sure you get every glucose molecule out of the food you eat
- Store sufficient fat so that you have energy sources during periods of "starvation"

Primal Blueprint author and nutritional expert Mark Sisson summed it all up best: "Carbohydrate controls insulin; insulin controls fat storage."

UNDERSTANDING METABOLISM

Now that you know about the process by which food is converted into energy and some of the various hormones and processes involved, it's time to look at the factors that affect the efficiency of that process.

Metabolism actually refers to the way in which your body processes and uses the food you eat each day, not the speed of the process. The idea of a faster or slower metabolism is not really as accurate as the idea of an efficient or inefficient metabolism.

Metabolism itself is made up of several components:

- *Basal metabolism.* From 60 percent to 65 percent of calories you eat each day are spent just keeping you alive and giving you energy for basic life support. If you were to lie in bed all day, you would still need these calories to support basic body functions.
- *Physical activity.* Optimally, about 25 percent of your calories go to movement and physical activity.
- *Thermic effect of food.* Normally, about 10 percent of calories taken in are spent processing the food you eat. For example, if you are eating 2,000 calories a day, optimally you would be burning 10 percent that, 200 calories a day, simply eating and digesting your food.

The essential formula is that input should equal output.

INPUT	OUTPUT
Calories from food =	Calories expended from basal metabolism + Calories expended by activity + Calories expended digesting food (thermic effect)

Many overweight people do not eat any more than people of average weight. Let me repeat that, because it's something that is counterintuitive to many readers, and to some doctors as well: *many overweight people do not eat any more than people of average weight.*

The problem for those people is on the output side of the equation. Basal metabolism is lower, activity is less, activity burns less fat than normal, and the thermic effect of food is blunted. Bottom line: many overweight people just don't burn as many calories or as much fat as people who have normal weight and an efficient metabolism.

METABOLIC EFFICIENCY

The efficiency of your metabolism is affected by a number of factors.

Body Composition: Muscle Versus Fat

Muscle cells are as much as eight times more metabolically active than fat cells. So the greater the proportion of muscle to fat, the more efficient your metabolism is at burning fat. It's estimated that a pound of muscle costs around 50 calories a day to maintain, and a pound of fat costs just 2 calories. One study actually found that lifting weights boosted resting metabolic rate by 9 percent over a four-month period by adding four pounds of muscle mass.

Building muscle mass usually requires some sort of weight-bearing or resistance work such as lifting weights, using exercise bands or hand weights, using the body as a weight, and other similar forms of exercise.

Brown Fat

According to Stephen Langer, MD, an expert on weight loss and thyroid function, one less well-known aspect of metabolism is brown fat, also known as brown adipose tissue. Brown fat is a special kind of fat that collects below the neck and extends down the back. It helps convert deposits of body fat into heat. The hypothalamus helps your nervous system trigger the action of brown fat, whose specialized mitochondria are particularly effective at generating heat and energy. People who are overweight may have lost the assistance of brown fat, and their excess calories go into fat storage.

Aerobic Exercise

Aerobic exercise, which increases heart rate, will also raise metabolism while you're exercising. And some experts believe that aerobic exercise boosts resting metabolism for several hours afterward, as your muscles burn calories to recover and repair themselves.

Food Intake

Metabolism is affected by how much you eat. When you are eating an insufficient amount of calories, your body perceives itself to be in starvation mode and may start to cannibalize your own muscle, burning it off for fuel. It will hold on to fat as protection. In his book *Turn Up the Heat*, Philip L. Goglia talks about the impact of a diet too low in calories on weight problems:

> I have found that most of the people who come to me with weight and health problems are usually already ingesting far fewer calories than they should in order to efficiently fuel their bodies. Therefore, their metabolism, the body's calorie-burning furnace, is already running 25 percent to 60 percent below its ideal metabolic-efficiency level. In turn, the body is storing much of the limited amounts of food these individuals eat as fat and wasting muscle tissue as an adaptive mechanism to create an alternative energy source.

At the same time, eating more food increases metabolism. One study found that as calorie intake increases, there is a corresponding increase in metabolic efficiency that is designed to maintain you around a particular body weight. However, if your caloric intake exceeds your body's ability to burn up those calories over time, the excess calories are converted into fat and glucose.

Your Age

The body typically starts to lose muscle after age thirty, so everything else being equal—activity level, calorie intake—you can gain weight due to this loss of muscle.

Genetics

Some people simply have a naturally more efficient metabolism than others.

Nutritional Status

Metabolism requires the smooth running of many complex physiological processes. When there are nutritional deficiencies, particularly in B vitamins and vitamin C, metabolism can become less efficient.

Water Intake

When the body has taken in sufficient water, body temperature can be maintained for optimal metabolism. Dehydration can make the body temperature drop slightly, and with a reduction in temperature, the body will attempt to help raise temperature by storing fat to act as an insulator. So drinking too little water can contribute to an inefficient metabolism and hoarding of fat.

INSULIN AND INSULIN RESISTANCE

When you eat carbohydrates, insulin is generated by the pancreas. Insulin's job is to take glucose (sugar) out of the bloodstream and store it—first as glycogen in the liver, and then, after the glycogen reaches sufficient levels, as saturated fat.

When you have eaten a normal-size meal that is low in simple carbohydrates and includes fats, proteins, and fiber in addition to complex carbohydrates, the up-and-down pattern of insulin and glucose is balanced. The processes of digestion and absorption are slow, glucose and insulin levels do not get exaggerated or substantially drop.

When you have eaten an especially large meal, however, or you've eaten many simple carbohydrates—a candy bar or a soda, for example—the body generates a stronger insulin response, in order to prevent a high level of blood glucose or blood sugar. This large insulin response in turn can trigger a more substantial drop in blood sugar—sometimes to levels that are even too low—in the three to five hours after the simple carbohydrate was eaten.

When someone chronically overeats in terms of volume, or regularly eats a diet high in simple carbohydrates, the circulating levels of insulin stay at a high level consistently, in response to the elevated glucose levels. The brain and cells don't always react to the insulin in the bloodstream, and elevated glucose continues to circulate. Over time, the cells can become less and less responsive to insulin, and glucose levels remain high—a situation that is referred to as insulin resistance. Dr. Ron Rosedale, author of *The Rosedale Diet*, explains:

> Cells become insulin resistant because they are trying to protect themselves from the toxic effects of high insulin. They down regulate their receptor activity and number of receptors.

The continued high levels of glucose cause the pancreas to continue to pump out even more insulin, in an attempt to store the glucose left in the blood. Over time, the overworked pancreas can tire and may lose its ability to produce any insulin at all, leading to type 2 diabetes. Insulin resistance is, in fact, sometimes called prediabetes.

The high levels of insulin circulating through the bloodstream also stimulate the storage of fat and amino acids and prevent the breakdown of fat and protein. In addition, they prevent the release of glucagon.

The fat cells in your abdomen are particularly sensitive to high insulin levels and are very effective at storing energy—far more so than fat cells you'd find in other areas such as the lower body (i.e., hips, rear end, thighs). Because abdominal fat cells are so close to your digestive organs and there is an extensive network of blood vessels circulating in the abdominal area, it's even easier for fat cells to store excess glucose there.

Recent studies have shown that thyroid hormones appear to have a role in insulin resistance, and low free T4 and higher TSH levels appear to have some connection to greater insulin resistance.

Testing for Insulin Resistance

A fasting glucose test measures your blood glucose after you have gone overnight without eating. This test is most reliable when done in the morning. After an overnight fast, the normal level is below 100 mg/dL. Fasting glucose levels of 100 to 125 mg/dL are above normal but not high enough to be called diabetes. This condition is called prediabetes or impaired fasting glucose, and it suggests that you have probably had insulin resistance for some time. Insulin resistance is considered a prediabetic state, meaning that you are more likely to develop diabetes but do not have it yet. A result of 126 or higher, if confirmed on a repeat test, typically indicates type 2 diabetes.

A glucose tolerance test measures your blood glucose after an overnight fast and two hours after you drink a sweet liquid provided by the doctor or laboratory. Your blood glucose level will elevate after drinking a sugar solution, but it should still be below 140 mg/ dL two hours after the drink. If your blood glucose falls between 140 and 199 mg/dL two hours after drinking the liquid, your glucose tolerance is above normal but not high enough for diabetes. This condition, also a form of prediabetes, is called impaired glucose tolerance and, like insulin resistance, it points toward a history of insulin resistance and a risk for developing diabetes. A level of 200 or higher, if confirmed, can mean diabetes.

Anyone with a thyroid condition who is struggling to lose weight— and, frankly, anyone who is overweight—should consider being evaluated for insulin resistance and metabolic syndrome (discussed later in this chapter). Other risk factors that warrant testing:

- A personal or family history of diabetes
- Low HDL cholesterol and high triglycerides
- High blood pressure
- A history of gestational diabetes (diabetes during pregnancy) or having given birth to a baby weighing more than nine pounds
- Ethnic background (African American, American Indian, Hispanic/Latino, or Asian American/Pacific Islander)

Treatment of Insulin Resistance

Before it has progressed to full type 2 diabetes, insulin resistance is considered a condition that is reversible with lifestyle changes. The National Institutes of Health's Diabetes Prevention Program study actually found that lifestyle changes alone reduced the risk of developing diabetes by 58 percent.

Specifically:

- *Eat fewer simple carbohydrates.* Cutting back—or, better yet, cutting out—processed and simple carbohydrates can reduce the overall circulating blood glucose levels.

- *Avoid overeating.* This prevents excess calories from all sources from being released into the bloodstream as glucose. The less glucose, the less insulin; when insulin levels are low, the body turns to fat reserves for energy and starts to break down large fat molecules into fatty acids for easy energy production.
- *Exercise.* Getting healthy exercise can help cells respond more effectively to insulin, which then helps reduce the excess glucose in the bloodstream before it is stored as fat.
- *Sleep.* Sufficient sleep is essential, and researchers have found that a lack of sleep—typically, less than eight hours a night for most people—can markedly reduce glucose tolerance and increase the risk of insulin resistance.
- *Reduce stress.* Stress reduction is important, because chronic stress contributes to excess cortisol, which makes cells less responsive to insulin.
- *Stop smoking.* Smoking contributes to insulin resistance.

Some experts are also recommending a reduction in processed foods and meats, refined grains, diet sodas, and artificial sweeteners. Diet soda in particular is strongly associated with an increased risk for metabolic syndrome.

Amy was able to use lifestyle changes to deal with insulin resistance:

I have Hashimoto's and I was feeling worse than ever, not losing any weight. I switched doctors and found out that I also had insulin resistance. Now I had two things working against me. My new doctor, a naturopath, suggested going grain-free to reverse the insulin resistance. I was already on a gluten-free diet, so this was fairly easy for me to do. I immediately started losing weight and feeling much better. In three months I lost twenty pounds. I did this by cutting way back on sugar, eating no grains at all and no processed foods, and walking. Some people see this as a really restrictive diet, but to me it is very basic and easy. It has reversed my insulin resistance and has been good for my thyroid as well.

Several type 2 diabetes medications are sometimes also used to treat insulin resistance, and some studies have shown that use of these medications may prevent progression of some patients from insulin resistance or metabolic syndrome to full diabetes. The medications typically used include metformin (Glucophage), taken as a pill, and injectable medications including pramlintide (Symlin), exenatide (Byetta), and liraglutide (Victoza). These medications are discussed at greater length in chapter 10. However, the only way to truly reverse insulin resistance is with dietary changes, exercise, and sufficient sleep.

In some cases, insulin resistance is part of a condition formerly known as syndrome X and now known as metabolic syndrome. Metabolic syndrome is usually characterized by insulin resistance along with obesity and elevated levels of cholesterol and triglycerides. The official diagnostic criteria for metabolic syndrome include any three of the following factors:

- Overweight, with a body mass index (BMI) greater than or equal to 25
- Abdominal obesity (waist circumference greater than 40 inches in men and 35 inches in women)
- Triglyceride levels above 150 mg/dL
- Low HDL (high-density lipoprotein) cholesterol levels (less than 40 mg/dL in men and 50 mg/dL in women)
- High blood pressure (greater than or equal to 130/85 mm Hg)
- High fasting glucose level, with fasting blood sugar more than 110 mg/dL

Some experts estimate that as many as one in four adults in the United States has metabolic syndrome.

LEPTIN AND LEPTIN RESISTANCE

Leptin is a hormone that communicates the status of your food intake, delivering instructions about the need to store or burn fat. Leptin is released by fat cells after food intake. Normally, after you eat, the fat cells release leptin, blood levels of leptin go up, and this communicates with your hypothalamus, which then sends out the message that you're full. The message is supposed to tell your body hormonally, "There is enough fat stored now to avoid starvation, so you can stop eating." The "stop eating" message is translated into a reduction in appetite and a speeding up of metabolism. Then leptin drops back down.

When someone chronically overeats in terms of volume or in terms of an excess of simple carbohydrates, circulating levels of leptin become higher. But just as in insulin resistance, over time the cells can become less and less responsive to leptin, a situation that is referred to as leptin resistance. In that situation, the leptin message is not getting through to the hypothalamus, so more leptin is produced in order to try to deliver the message.

When the body faces real starvation—or when it perceives starvation, such when calories are substantially reduced—leptin release can slow or stop. This communicates to the brain that there is insufficient fat stored to prevent possible starvation, and food intake should be increased. Appetite will rise, and the metabolism will shift toward more effective fat storage. This is the mechanism that makes you feel hungry when you go on a particularly low-calorie diet.

Kent Holtorf, MD, a leading physician studying leptin resistance, explains:

> The hormone leptin has been found to be a major regulator of body weight and metabolism. Leptin is secreted by fat cells and the levels of leptin increase with the accumulation of fat. The increased leptin secretion that occurs with increased weight

normally feeds back to the hypothalamus as a signal that there are adequate energy (fat) stores. This stimulates the body to burn fat rather than continue to store excess fat, and also stimulates thyroid-releasing hormone (TRH) to increase thyroid-stimulating hormone (TSH) and thyroid production.

Studies are finding, however, that the majority of overweight individuals who are having difficulty losing weight have varying degrees of leptin resistance, where leptin has a diminished ability to affect the hypothalamus and regulate metabolism. This leptin resistance results in the hypothalamus sensing starvation, so multiple mechanisms are activated to increase fat stores, as the body tries to reverse the perceived state of starvation.

The mechanisms that are activated include diminished TSH secretion, a suppressed T4-to-T3 conversion, an increase in reverse T3, an increase in appetite, an increase in insulin resistance, and an inhibition of lipolysis (fat breakdown). These mechanisms may be in part due to a down-regulation of leptin receptors that occurs with a prolonged increase in leptin.

The result? Once you are overweight for an extended period of time, it becomes increasingly difficult to lose weight.

Logic would dictate that giving leptin as a treatment might help with weight loss, but in a rush to create leptin-based drugs this theory was tested and failed, because, as Dr. Holtorf explained, people who are overweight tend to have very high levels of leptin. The real problem appears to be that if you are overweight, it's not a shortage of leptin that causes difficulties; rather, it's that your brain is not getting the message. In essence, the brain is leptin-resistant, meaning that your brain and metabolism think you are starving even while you are eating enough or too much food.

If the brain isn't getting the right message about leptin in the first place, the metabolic circuit becomes broken. The brain cannot tell the body, "Enough fat is stored, food intake can slow down, appetite can drop, and energy expenditure can rise." Instead, the brain tells the body, "You're at risk of starvation. Accumulate more fat, slow down the metabolism."

Are you getting the picture? The leptin feedback process is also the mechanism that explains why some people can eat very little yet not lose weight, or even gain weight. The hypothalamus never sends out the message that sufficient fat is stored, so the body becomes incredibly efficient at converting even a low-calorie diet into stored fat, and the mechanism that activates fat burning can be almost entirely shut down.

Testing for Leptin Resistance

Leptin resistance can be measured by a blood test for the leptin level. While many labs show a level under 25 ng/mL as normal, Kent Holtorf, MD, diagnoses leptin resistance in overweight patients with leptin levels above 10. According to Dr. Holtorf, the higher the number, the more significant the leptin resistance.

Sara Gottfried, MD, notes that ideally, the leptin level should be between 4 and 6. At this level, the hypothalamus is receiving the message from, and responding appropriately to, the body's leptin. The target range of 4 to 6 comes from looking at the population of lean people who don't have a problem with insulin resistance and obesity.

Dr. Gottfried also agrees that a level above 10 is evidence of leptin resistance.

If your level is above 10, your leptin receptors are fatigued. The result? Metabolism slows inappropriately because the hypothalamus is interpreting the messages inappropriately.

Dr. Gottfried believes that when leptin is high, free T3 and reverse T3 measurement become especially important for thyroid patients.

If your leptin is high, TSH less reliably reflects your tissue level of thyroid hormones. For example, in diabetics, who are almost universally leptin-resistant, T4-to-T3 conversion is cut in half without a change in TSH. While you may not be diabetic, you may still experience a significant reduction in your conversion before your TSH picks it up. This is where, yet again, measuring your free T3 and reverse T3 can help elucidate the issues.

Ron Rosedale, MD, explains why he believes leptin testing is crucial:

Leptin will not only determine how much fat you have, but also where that fat is put. When you are leptin resistant you put that fat mostly in your belly, your viscera, causing the so-called "apple shape" that is linked to much disease. Some of that fat permeates the liver, impeding the liver's ability to listen to insulin, and further hastening diabetes. Leptin plays a far more important role in your health than, for instance, cholesterol, yet how many doctors measure leptin levels in their patients, know their own level, even know that it can be easily measured, or even what it would mean?

Treatment for Leptin Resistance

There are a variety of ways that leptin resistance is approached, including lifestyle and dietary changes, nutritional supplements, and prescription medications.

From a lifestyle standpoint, some ways to combat leptin resistance include:

- Practice active stress reduction
- Get sufficient sleep
- Get regular, moderate exercise

Some general food guidelines:

- Avoid large meals in general, or overeating at a meal
- Avoid or eliminate processed and simple carbohydrates
- Avoid or eliminate foods high in sugar
- Avoid desserts, especially after larger meals
- Eat a high-protein breakfast
- Eat more calcium-rich foods

Timing is also extremely important.

- Eat slowly, and chew your food well.
- Avoid eating after dinner, including bedtime snacks.
- Finish your dinner at least three to four hours before you go to bed.
- Allow ten to twelve hours between dinner and breakfast.
- Eat two to four meals a day, maximum, and allow five to six hours between meals.
- Do not snack between meals.

A number of specific supplements may be helpful in reducing leptin levels or reversing leptin resistance, including:

- Calcium
- Melatonin
- Anti-inflammatory oils, including fish oil and gamma-linolenic acid (GLA) supplements
- Pantethine, a form of pantothenic acid (vitamin B_5)
- Acetyl-L-carnitine, a derivative of L-carnitine
- Chromium

Dr. Sara Gottfried says that if leptin is elevated, use nutrition as a first strategy:

I find that 70 to 80 percent of my patients are successful just by making the nutritional changes that are recommended for reversing leptin resistance, such as Dr. Ron Rosedale's *Rosedale Diet* program or Byron Richards' five-step plan.

Byron Richards is a nutritionist, and his five-step nutritional approach to leptin is featured in his excellent book *Mastering Leptin.*

Kent Holtorf, MD, an expert on hormonal imbalances, metabolism, and weight loss, is using the injectable medications Symlin, Byetta, and Victoza, typically prescribed for type 2 diabetes, as off-label prescription treatments for leptin resistance. These medications are administered in conjunction with a diet that limits carbohydrates, and in particular high-fructose corn syrup.

ADRENAL HORMONES AND ADRENAL RESISTANCE

The adrenal glands, two small peanut-shaped glands located above the kidneys, produce hormones that help to manage stress. Your hypothalamus, via the pituitary gland, directs the adrenal glands to secrete the stress hormones cortisol and adrenaline. Cortisol is released as part of your daily hormonal cycle, and adrenaline is typically released when the body perceives itself to be in a stressful or crisis situation—generating the flight-or-flight response that is essential for survival. Adrenaline makes you energetic and alert and quickly increases metabolism. It also helps fat cells to release energy. Cortisol helps your body become more effective at producing glucose from proteins and is designed to quickly increase the body's energy in times of stress.

Adrenal hormones help balance blood sugar, which helps your body to manage daily ebbs and flows of energy. When blood sugar drops, the adrenals release hormones that cause the blood sugar to rise, increasing energy. The adrenals also release hormones when you're under stress, thus releasing energy. It's the fight-or-flight response from the days when humans needed to run away from wild animals. Today, it kicks in for everyday stressors such as traffic jams, arguments, and work pressures. But being consistently under stress takes a toll on the adrenal glands, and eventually they run out of steam and stop producing sufficient hormones.

In rare cases, underlying disease causes the adrenal glands to produce excessive amounts of cortisol. This is a rare but serious disease known as Cushing's syndrome.

More commonly, however, when excessive simple carbohydrates have been eaten, the body generates a strong insulin response, which then causes blood glucose levels to fall. That fall can trigger an adrenaline surge, which in turn can cause nervousness, anxiety, irritability, and even palpitations. (This is the phenomenon observed in some children when they've had too much sugar.) In some people, chronic stress—either physical, emotional, or both—can cause chronically elevated levels of stress hormones to circulate. Over time, cells can become less responsive to cortisol and adrenaline, less able to produce cortisol and adrenaline when needed, or less able to produce them in proper balance—a situation that is referred to as adrenal resistance.

In his book *Mastering Leptin*, nutritional expert Byron Richards explains this process well:

In an effort to stimulate metabolism, the brain releases adrenaline. This is magnified by too much stress. Such adrenaline should stimulate fat cells to release energy which in turn should cause weight loss. However, when adrenaline is too high too often, fat cells develop adrenaline resistance. From a fat cell's point of view, it is like being yelled at too often. After a while, the fat cells go numb to the adrenaline, and adrenaline resistance develops. This causes metabolism of fat cells to stay locked in a "hibernation metabolic rate." It also causes weight gain around the middle, high blood pressure, and sleep problems.

The problem is that many of us are under a constant state of stress—physical, emotional, or both—for many reasons. Poor nutrition, insufficient sleep, hormone imbalances, chronic infections, emotional issues, exposure to toxins in food, water, or air—these sorts of chronic stress lead to what's known as "sympathetic dominance," which can include a state of almost constant and excessive production of cortisol. This excess cortisol stimulates glucose production. The excess glucose is then typically converted into fat, and ends up as stored fat. This is the premise behind some of the late-night supplement infomercials that declare, "Stress causes belly fat!" There is some truth to that claim, as research studies have shown that high levels of circulating cortisol increase the risk of obesity and increased fat storage—particularly abdominal obesity, which is one of the most dangerous types of obesity.

In some cases, the adrenal gland is unable to produce a sufficient level of adrenal hormones. When this develops due to an underlying disease process, it is an acute situation known as Addison's disease, a potentially life-threatening condition. When adrenal resistance and chronic stress are the underlying cause, however, the resulting condition is referred to as adrenal fatigue. Some other names for this condition include non-Addison's hypoadrenia, subclinical hypoadrenia, and hypoadrenalism.

Symptoms of adrenal fatigue include:

- Excessive fatigue and exhaustion
- Nonrefreshing sleep (you get sufficient hours of sleep but wake fatigued) or sleep disturbances
- Feeling overwhelmed by or unable to cope with stressors
- Feeling run-down
- Craving salty and sweet foods
- Feeling most energetic in the evening
- Experiencing low stamina, being slow to recover from exercise
- Being slow to recover from injury, illness, or stress

- Having difficulty concentrating, brain fog
- Poor digestion
- Low immune function
- Food or environmental allergies
- Premenstrual syndrome or difficulties that develop during menopause
- Consistent low blood pressure
- Extreme sensitivity to cold

Testing for Adrenal Imbalance

Adrenal disease may be suspected based on a serum cortisol level, but a diagnosis of Addison's disease is typically confirmed using the ACTH stimulation test. Cushing's syndrome is confirmed with a dexamethasone suppression test or a twenty-four-hour urinary cortisol evaluation. A CT scan, MRI, or other imaging of the adrenal glands may also be performed as part of a diagnosis of adrenal disease.

Conventional endocrinologists and conventional tests don't diagnose adrenal fatigue, because they are prepared to diagnose only extreme dysfunction in the adrenals. An integrative, holistic, or complementary practitioner is more prepared to evaluate symptoms and signs of milder or more subtle adrenal dysfunction, using the twenty-four-hour saliva cortisol test.

Treating Adrenal Imbalances

Sara Gottfried, MD, recommends that one of the first-line efforts to combat adrenal excess be to start a regular stress-reducing practice, a shift in diet, and nutritional supplementation.

You can modulate your cortisol with even eight minutes of meditation or a fifteen-minute yoga practice. Protein, especially at breakfast, also is increasingly important when the adrenals are out of balance. Starbucks and a muffin is not an acceptable breakfast. I also find that most people will feel better if I start them on supplements such as B vitamins, vitamin C, B_5 (pantothenic acid), and in some cases the adaptogenic herbs.

Dr. Gottfried says that she typically finds that there are three levels of treatment for adrenal fatigue.

I prefer to start with the first-level treatment, herbals. But don't just grab a formulation off the shelf. You need to be careful. My favorite is a double adaptogen, something to both balance and tonify, like ashwagandha or maca. I also like Cortisol Manager by Integrative Therapeutics. My second-level approach would be to go to adrenal glandular supplements. And when needed, my third-level approach is to use prescription hydrocortisone.

Adrienne Clamp, MD, has a similar approach:

In cases of adrenal excess, I use herbal adrenal adaptogens and lifestyle modifications, as well as phosphatidylserine, to calm an overactive adrenal response. In the case of hypofunction, I first attempt treatment with adaptogens and, if there is positional hypotension (low blood pressure), licorice root. If this doesn't yield good results, I use low-dose natural cortisol (hydrocortisone), which may take the pressure off of the adrenal gland and give it some time to recover its function. Cortisol, however, is not a benign drug and can have side effects. I usually reserve it for more resistant cases.

Another recommendation is to avoid stimulants, such as caffeine. They put further stress on the adrenals to work harder and produce more energy, which ends up further depleting the glands. Things to avoid besides caffeine include ephedra, guarana, kola nut, and prescription stimulants.

MELATONIN DEFICIENCY

Melatonin, a hormone produced by the brain's pineal gland, helps regulate sleeping and waking. Melatonin levels typically rise in the evening, stay high during the night, then decline in the morning as you awaken. Melatonin typically declines with age and can become almost undetectable in some older people. Reduced light during the winter months and too much light in your bedroom can also imbalance melatonin, which can interfere with your sleep. Some experts believe that low-dose melatonin supplementation (0.5 to 3 mg per night) can be safe and effective at helping replace low levels of melatonin. Typically, the recommendation is to take the melatonin an hour before you go to sleep, but no later than 11:00 p.m., so as to trigger a melatonin surge at the appropriate time.

OTHER HORMONES

In addition to thyroid, adrenals, and the metabolic hormones such as leptin and insulin, there are other hormonal factors that can affect your ability to lose weight.

- Both progesterone deficiency and progesterone excess can cause weight gain. In particular, excess weight gain in the abdomen is associated with progesterone imbalances.
- Estrogen excess, or estrogen dominance (a predominance of estrogen in the estrogen/progesterone ratio), is associated with weight gain.
- DHEA and testosterone deficiency are associated with reduction in muscle mass and slower muscle building, which can contribute to weight gain or slow weight loss.
- DHEA and testosterone excess can be associated with weight gain or difficulty losing weight.

- Pregnenolone deficiency can be associated with imbalances in all the sex hormones.
- Melatonin imbalance or deficiency can interfere with weight loss.

For women, perimenopause and menopause add additional hormonal burdens to metabolism and weight loss. During menopause, women become more effective at storing fat and less able to burn fat. After menopause, an enzyme called adipose tissue lipoprotein lipase (AT-LPL) is more active. AT-LPL breaks fat down so that fat cells can absorb it. One study actually found that fat in the buttocks of postmenopausal women was 75 percent less metabolically efficient than similarly located fat in perimenopausal women.

Testing Other Hormones

If you suspect imbalances, deficiencies, or excesses in estrogen, progesterone, DHEA, pregnenolone, testosterone, or melatonin, the answer is not to head off to the store and start self-treating with over-the-counter hormones. (Progesterone, DHEA, pregnenolone, and melatonin are available in over-the-counter forms in the United States.) Instead, you'll want to first get baseline levels of these hormones. You can have a knowledgeable practitioner oversee those tests for you. Or, if you want to take the step of having these levels tested yourself—or your doctor or insurance won't run the tests or cover their costs—you can order these tests yourself using reliable self-testing services, such as MyMedLab or ZRT Laboratory. Information on these services is in the Resources section.

Treating Hormone Imbalances

Whether you've had the tests run by your practitioner or done self-testing, you should work with a practitioner to decide on sensible approaches for balancing and supplementation, whether using over-the-counter hormones, prescription hormones, or a combination of both. It's important to remember that whether or not they require a prescription, hormones have powerful effects . . . and side effects. If you do not have imbalances or deficiencies, adding hormones willy-nilly on the basis of your own self-diagnosis can be detrimental to your health; it can also destabilize your thyroid and ultimately derail your weight-loss efforts.

Dr. David Brownstein, author of *The Miracle of Natural Hormones* and a number of books on thyroid disease, believes that balancing the entire hormonal system may be a key to weight loss for some people.

> This can include the use of the adrenal hormones (i.e., DHEA and pregnenolone), ovarian hormones (i.e., using natural progesterone and natural estrogens and natural testosterone), growth hormone, melatonin, and others. I find using small amounts of each of these hormones in combination much more effective than using one hormone individually. Sometimes, patients need a combination of treatments to help them achieve their optimum health.

TOXINS, ALLERGIES, AND SENSITIVITIES

In addition to hormone imbalances, there are other factors—including toxins, allergies, sensitivities, stress, mind-set, and lifestyle—that make it more difficult for thyroid patients to lose weight.

At the core of many issues is inflammation. The role of inflammation in metabolism and weight issues is really just beginning to be understood, but we know that inflammation is a sign that your immune system is fighting off some sort of infection or attempting to heal an injury. So, for example, when your nasal passages swell during a respiratory infection, your immune system is sending white blood cells and other substances to help fight off viruses and bacteria.

Anytime we are sensitive to a particular substance, whether it's due to an intolerance, an allergy, or a sensitivity—or when that substance is a bacterium, virus, parasite, or toxic chemical or substance—the body responds with inflammation.

Some kinds of inflammation are signs that the body is in a state of imbalance. For example, when you regularly eat foods to which you are allergic or sensitive, you can inflame the mucosal lining of your intestines. Eventually, the lining can become less and less able to prevent large molecules from passing into your bloodstream— a condition known as leaky gut syndrome. This condition is connected to the development of various forms of autoimmune disease, including thyroid disease, as well as other conditions.

Research is recognizing the role of chronic inflammation in weight gain. One study in the *Journal of the American Medical Association* found that a particular inflammatory marker known as C-reactive protein (CRP) was increased by more than 50 percent in obese women whose fat concentration centered mainly on their hips and thighs (i.e., pear-shaped distribution) and was increased by more than 400 percent in obese women whose fat was centered on the waist and abdomen (i.e., apple-shaped distribution).

Clearly, avoiding substances that are toxic, or to which we have sensitivities and allergies, becomes an important way to reduce inflammation and create a situation more conducive to weight loss.

TOXINS

There are so many different toxins in our food, water, and air— including toxins that specifically affect the thyroid, impair our metabolism, and cause inflammation—that it's impossible to list them all.

Just a few of the many substances to be aware of include the following:

- *Teflon.* Teflon is the brand name for polytetrafluoroethylene (PTFE), a synthetic substance used as a nonstick coating on pans. Another chemical, perfluorooctanoic acid (PFOA), is used in the manufacture of PTFE. People with higher levels of PFOA in their bloodstream have a higher risk of thyroid disease.
- *Stain- and water-resistant carpets and fabric coatings.* PFOA is an ingredient in stain and water-resistant coatings used on many carpets and fabrics.
- *Microwave popcorn bags.* PFOA is used in microwave popcorn bags.
- *Fluoride.* When ingested, fluoride can act in the body as an antithyroid agent, slowing thyroid function.
- *Perchlorate.* This by-product of rocket fuel and fireworks production is contaminating water supplies around the nation, particularly in the western United States. Produce grown in these areas may be irrigated with perchlorate-contaminated water, and may be sold all over the United States. Perchlorate can negatively affect thyroid function.
- *Antibacterial soaps and toiletries.* The ingredients triclosan and triclocarban may impair thyroid function.
- *Plastics.* Avoid cooking in or storing food in plastic, especially those that contain thyroid-damaging bisphenol A (BPA) and phthalates.
- *Pesticides.* Resmethrin and sumithrin, the pesticides used to kill West Nile virus–carrying mosquitoes can be toxic to the thyroid.

Clearly, some things are more avoidable than others. You can stop using nonstick pans and microwave popcorn; choose products without stain-resistant coatings; make sure your soaps and toiletries don't include triclosan or triclocarban; and avoid plastics for serving, storing, and microwaving. If you have the resources, you can invest in a reverse osmosis system to filter fluoride, perchlorate, and other antithyroid chemicals out of your tap or well water.

Another little-known toxin that is starting to gain attention is electromagnetic frequencies and what is known as "dirty" electricity. Dr. Ann Louise Gittleman talks about the latest research and the toxic effect that these exposures have on hormones, the endocrine system, and the adrenal system in her book *Zapped*.

You don't have to do without electric lights, satellite TV, your microwave, cell phone, or BlackBerry as long as you are reducing exposure, prudently avoiding overuse, and implement some cutting-edge and grounding lifestyle therapies.

I would suggest reading *Zapped* for a detailed protocol of recommendations to reduce exposure.

FOOD ALLERGIES AND SENSITIVITIES

Sensitivities or full-scale allergies to particular foods or pathogens can cause inflammation in your intestinal system, making weight loss difficult if not impossible. Food sensitivities and intolerances are quite common, but full-scale food allergies are less so. One report found that while a third of people think they have a food allergy, only one in fifty actually does. An allergy is defined as a reaction to a food or substance that could potentially trigger a life-threatening response such as anaphylactic shock, airway swelling, or difficulty breathing. A food sensitivity is more likely to cause migraine headaches, fatigue, bloating, skin rashes, or diarrhea.

The most common allergenic foods include:

- Wheat and gluten
- Dairy foods
- Corn
- Soy
- Fish (especially shellfish)
- Tree nuts
- Peanuts
- Fruits

Inflammation occurs when you have a food allergy or sensitivity. This sort of inflammation gradually wears away the ability of your intestinal surface to filter out pathogens and toxins. Eventually, like a window screen that has developed holes, bigger particles can pass through your stomach and intestinal lining directly into the bloodstream, which triggers inflammation and irritation, interfering with your body's ability to optimally absorb nutrients.

You may already know which foods are problems for you. I'm allergic to non-citrus tree fruits (such as apples, pears, cherries, peaches, and plums) and certain tree nuts such as walnuts, pecans, and cashews. I know I have an actual allergy, because my throat gets tight and sometimes my lips swell when I eat these foods. (An aside: I also have seasonal hay fever, and these particular fruit and nut allergies are more common in people who have hay fever. Interestingly, it's not the fruit per se but an enzyme on the fruit, one that is destroyed by cooking, that triggers the allergy. So I am able to eat applesauce, baked fruits, canned fruits, and nuts that have been cooked.)

If you suspect but aren't sure if you have food sensitivities or allergies, you don't need to head off for expensive allergy testing. One of the primary ways to assess them is to try an elimination or rotation diet. Stop eating a particular food for about a week, then reintroduce by eating a substantial quantity. Keep track of any symptoms you have over the next several days including aches, pains, headache, fatigue, stomach upset, skin eruptions, itching, mood swings, and other strong reactions.

If you're going to do an elimination diet test, start with some of the most common allergens for people with thyroid problems: wheat, dairy, corn, soy, and fish. Check the ingredients list of supplements and processed foods to make sure you're avoiding all sources of the allergen being tested. It can be difficult, because some ingredients, such as wheat flour, corn oil, hydrogenated soybean oil, and soy protein, are in everything from meal replacement bars to breakfast cereals.

You can also pursue more formalized testing with an integrative or functional medicine expert or an allergist. A specialized blood test known as an enzyme-linked immunosorbent assay (ELISA) is considered a state-of-the-art way to diagnose food sensitivities.

Obviously, if you discover a food to which you have a sensitivity or allergy, one of the key things you can do is eliminate it from your diet, to see if it aids you in your weight-loss efforts and helps alleviate other symptoms.

In some cases, immunotherapy—a fancy name for allergy shots—may be a help. On the holistic front, some practitioners and patients report success with a technique known as NAET, short for Nambudripad's Allergy Elimination Techniques. I have, however, tried the technique myself, receiving treatments for my apple and tree fruit allergy, and found it had no effect.

CELIAC DISEASE (GLUTEN SENSITIVITY)

Celiac disease, also known as celiac sprue, celiac sprue dermatitis, or gluten intolerance, is a chronic disease of the digestive system that prevents absorption of nutrients from food. People who have celiac disease have an inappropriate response to gluten, a protein that is found in grains such as wheat, rye, barley, and possibly oats. Eating these foods causes damage to and destruction of the mucosal lining of the intestine, which leads to an inability to properly digest and absorb nutrients and, frequently, to immune system dysfunction.

According to the National Institutes of Health, more than two million people in the United States have the disease, or about 1 in 133 people. Among people who have a first-degree relative—a parent, sibling, or child—diagnosed with celiac disease, as many as 1 in 22 may have the disease. The majority of people with celiac disease are undiagnosed. Celiac disease is also on the rise; according to a Mayo Clinic study, it is four times as common today as it was fifty years ago.

Celiac disease and gluten sensitivity can affect both men and women, but is slightly more common in women. The incidence of celiac disease in various autoimmune disorders is ten to thirty times higher compared to the general population, so autoimmune thyroid patients are much more likely to have celiac disease or gluten intolerance.

Celiac disease and gluten sensitivity can first appear in infants when they begin to eat gluten products. However, it may not be diagnosed at that time, and symptoms flare and diminish through adolescence and into adulthood, when symptoms reappear again. Most cases are diagnosed in people in their thirties and forties.

Symptoms of full celiac disease and gluten sensitivity include:

- Diarrheal, watery, odorous stools
- Abdominal bloating, cramps, excessive or explosive gas
- Weight loss or gain
- Failure to gain weight and growth retardation in infants and children
- Weakness, fatigue, including muscle weakness
- Bone pain
- Tingling and numbness in hands and feet
- Absence of menstrual periods, delayed start of menstrual periods in adolescents
- Infertility in women and men
- Impotence
- Orthostatic hypotension, where blood pressure drops upon standing or sitting up in bed; this can cause dizziness or fainting

The main noninvasive way to diagnose celiac disease is with a blood test to measure circulating antibodies to gluten—antigliadin, antiendomysium, and antireticulin. A home or office finger-prick test that does an analysis known as an IgA tissue transglutaminase (tTG) autoantibody assay can be done to help diagnose celiac disease. In some cases, endoscopic examination of the small bowel or a biopsy is necessary to make an accurate diagnosis.

Many adults with celiac disease spend years being misdiagnosed; commonly they are told they have irritable bowel syndrome, and so they are not treated with a gluten-free diet. It's particularly important to get a diagnosis of celiac disease as early as possible, because the more delayed the diagnosis, the riskier the disease can be.

People with celiac disease must stay on a gluten-free diet for the rest of their lives or risk damaging their small intestine and further losing the ability to absorb nutrients. One Italian study found that the death rate for those who failed to stay on a gluten-free diet was six times higher than for those adhering to the diet. A gluten-free diet means total avoidance of all wheat, rye, and barley and products made from them. There is some disagreement as to whether oats are also to be avoided, as some people with celiac disease are sensitive to oats as well. Be careful to avoid hidden glutens such as vegetable protein and malt, modified food starch, some soy sauces, and distilled vinegars, among other food items. A good support group can help you learn how to eat gluten-free among today's variety of food options.

Some experts estimate that a substantially larger percentage of the population also has sensitivity to or allergy to gluten and wheat that, while not characterized as full celiac disease, can cause numerous symptoms, contribute to or even trigger autoimmune disease, and prevent weight loss.

There are many reports from patients who have found that, independent of any confirmed diagnosis of celiac disease, they have been able to reduce symptoms such as fatigue and bloating, reduce their thyroid medication dosage, and lose weight by following a gluten-free diet. In fact, a few practitioners I've spoken with have wondered if the success of grain-free, low-carbohydrate diets for some thyroid patients may be due to the fact that they are naturally almost gluten-free, and it is the elimination of the gluten—rather than the carbohydrates per se—that may be responsible for weight loss.

Certainly, if someone has symptoms of celiac disease, or is a thyroid patient struggling to lose weight—especially if your thyroid condition is autoimmune in nature—celiac testing should be performed.

CANDIDA (YEAST)

Thyroid patients seem to be more susceptible to candidiasis, a chronic overgrowth of the fungus candida. Also known as chronic yeast infection, the condition was brought to the public's attention by the late Dr. William Crook in his 1983 book, *The Yeast Connection*, and is considered to be the cause of many hard-to-diagnose chronic illnesses (or at least is more common in people with these illnesses). We also know that chronic yeast infection can be a factor that prevents weight loss in some people, who discover that they are able to lose weight only after the yeast overgrowth is addressed.

If you have been on long-term antibiotic therapy, have a diet high in sugars, have used steroids, or have a suppressed immune system, you are at higher risk for developing candidiasis. There are a number of other risk factors, and the topic of chronic yeast is too big to tackle in depth here, but they are outlined at length in Dr. Crook's several definitive books on the topic.

The symptoms of candidiasis are fairly wide-ranging, and include:

- Frequent vaginal yeast, "jock itch," and athlete's foot infections
- Frequent oral yeast infections (thrush)
- Frequent infections of the nipple or breast when breast-feeding
- Chronic ear, upper respiratory, allergic, or sinus problems
- Urticaria (hives, wheals, or welts), itching, or burning sensation in the skin
- Stomach, digestive, and elimination problems
- Fluid retention, swelling, and bloat
- Skin problems
- Difficulty losing weight, or inappropriate weight gain

These are just a few of the dozens of other symptoms attributed to candida overgrowth.

Detecting candida involves one or more tests, including:

- *Candida immune complex assay test.* This is a blood test that can detect the presence of antibodies that fight off yeast infections.
- *Stool test.* An exam of stool under a microscope may reveal the presence of candida. One of the most reliable tests is the stool analysis done by Genova Labs (see Resources), which tests for candidiasis and dysbiosis.
- *Candida culture.* In the case of oral, genital, or nipple thrush, a culture can be taken and analyzed.

Treating candidiasis can be a complex process and may require monitoring by a good nutritionally oriented doctor or practitioner. Treatment is typically multifaceted and may include the following tactics:

- *Changes to diet.* Dietary changes depend on the severity of symptoms. Some of the most extreme candida diets suggest eliminating the foods that "feed" yeast, including anything with yeast itself (such as bread), plus sugar, flour, fruits, dairy, certain meats, mushrooms, and fermented products such as vinegars and alcoholic drinks. Other suggestions include eliminating only those foods that are particularly troublesome. (Again, Dr. Crook's books cover the entire yeast issue and provide specific guidelines on the diets.)
- *Supplements.* Antiyeast supplements are sometimes recommended, including garlic, biotin, caprylic acid, pau d'arco, and others.
- *Probiotics.* Probiotics are supplements that contain live bacteria—the "good" bacteria—and experts say that probiotic bacteria can help train the immune system to resist allergic reactions, including candidiasis.
- *Antifungal drugs.* Prescription antifungal drugs may be necessary in order to completely eliminate the candida infection. Some of the drugs your doctor can prescribe include fluconazole (Diflucan), terbinafine (Lamisil), nystatin, and itraconazole (Sporanox).

Interestingly, some of the physicians that I've interviewed have speculated that some of the people who respond to gluten-free and low-carbohydrate diets by losing weight may have underlying yeast issues, and by going gluten-free and eliminating processed carbohydrates, they are also following a diet that is unfriendly to yeast.

PARASITES

There are a variety of parasitic infections, ranging from microscopic parasites such as giardia, amoebas, cryptosporidium, and *Blastocystis hominis* to larger parasites such as various worms, flukes, and parasitic insects. You can pick up these parasites from a variety of sources, including improperly cooked foods, raw foods such as sushi, water, poor sanitation or hygiene, travel to tropical climates, exposure to animals or their feces, insect bites, and other means.

The symptoms of various parasitic infections vary but often include intestinal problems and can include difficulty losing weight. Diagnosis depends on the suspected parasite and may include a physical exam, stool samples, urine samples, blood tests, biopsies, ultrasound, X-ray, and tape tests (applying tape around the anal region to examine for microscopic worms).

Treatments depend on the type of infection and can include antiparasitic drugs, steroids, pain relievers, anti-inflammatories, antihistamines, and antibiotics for relief of symptoms or to treat various infections. Some herbal remedies are fig, andrographis root, garlic, wormseed, turmeric, and pumpkin seeds, among others. There are also a number of parasite cleansing systems and herbal combination remedies available.

Parasites are a complex issue, so you should not self-diagnose or self-treat. If you suspect that you may have any risk factors or symptoms of parasites—and many of us don't realize how pervasive parasitic infections are—you should start by reading one of the definitive books on the topic, such as *Guess What Came to Dinner? Parasites and Your Health* by Dr. Ann Louise Gittleman, then consulting with a practitioner who can help you diagnose and treat the infection.

COPPER-ZINC BALANCE

One overlooked but important consideration for thyroid patients is copper overload. Dr. Gittleman, in another key book, *Why Am I Always So Tired?* explores this issue.

> Copper and zinc tend to work in a seesaw relationship with each other in the body. When the levels of one of these minerals rise in the blood and tissues, the levels of its counterpart tend to fall. Ideally, copper and zinc should be in a 1:8 ratio in favor of zinc in the tissues. But stress, overexposure to copper, or a low intake of zinc can throw the critical copper-zinc balance off, upsetting normal body functioning.

Dr. Gittleman believes that a copper-zinc imbalance can slow weight loss and impede conversion of T4 to T3 even in people whose thyroid hormone levels are normal.

To determine whether you have excess copper or a copper-zinc imbalance, you should have your doctor or practitioner run a trace elements analysis. This test uses a small hair sample to assess your nutritional levels of various minerals and metals. Laboratories that perform TEA testing are included in the Resources section.

Dr. Gittleman recommends that if you are found to have high copper levels, you should avoid foods that are rich in copper, including soy products, yeast, wheat bran and wheat germ, chocolate, mushrooms, nuts, seeds (except pumpkin), shellfish, organ meats, and tea. She also recommends avoiding foods and drinks that deplete zinc, including alcohol, coffee, sugar, and excessive carbohydrates, while emphasizing zinc-rich foods such as eggs, chicken, turkey, red meats, game, and pumpkin seeds. Dr. Gittleman's *Why Am I Always So Tired?* includes additional detailed recommendations for managing copper-zinc balance.

PART 3

THE THYROID DIET

REVOLUTION

CHAPTER 6

Your Thyroid Diet:
What and How to Eat

Tell me what you eat, and I will tell you what you are.
— JEAN-ANTHELME BRILLAT-SAVARIN

When you're dealing with a metabolic issue such as thyroid disease, as well as the many other possible impediments to weight loss, finding a successful approach that will work for you is part science and part instinct. You and your body know how to lose weight; it's just a matter of trying out the likeliest approaches, observing your body's responses, and monitoring how you feel until you find an approach that works, then tweaking it so that it fits you.

We all know people who stay slender and don't vary in weight, and let's face it, we can be green with envy about them sometimes. But if you're really honest about it, except for the rare freak of nature or teenage athletes with a supercharged metabolism, you will rarely see them wolfing down everything in sight and loading up on junk food. They've most likely come up with a way of eating that works for them, and they are usually physically active in some way.

My friend Jane is like this. Jane used to wear a size 18, and as a gourmet cook, she regularly entertains and makes the most amazing meals for friends and family. But she also listened to her body and figured out what it needed. She cut almost all processed foods out of her diet and increased her protein, fiber, green vegetables, and good fats. She regularly purchases fresh organic produce, and she started her own vegetable garden, where she grows tomatoes and other produce all summer. She almost always cooks from scratch, using whole foods. She almost never eats fast food, and when she does dine out, she often chooses a big salad, with a grilled meat or fish as her entree. She rarely snacks between meals, and she rarely eats after dinner. She drinks purified water all day long—friends laugh at the giant travel cup she carries around, which she refills multiple times a day—but she is drinking at least 100 ounces of water daily. I don't know if I've ever seen Jane have a soft drink.

Jane also made a major change—she started moving. Jane's not an exercise hound or gym rat, but she walks daily. She started with shorter walks around the neighborhood. Now, she power-walks several miles every morning. She rarely misses a day. As a concession to cold weather, she got an elliptical machine for her family room, and uses that when it's too cold to walk outdoors.

In two years, Jane walked and ate her way from a size 18 to a size 6. She has low cholesterol and terrific blood pressure, and at this point she doesn't count calories, weigh herself daily, or watch what she eats.

The key for her is consistency. Almost every day she eats well, in a way that allows her to maintain her healthy weight loss. And when she has a treat here and there, she goes right back to eating regularly the next day. She's following what some people call the 90/10 (or sometimes 80/20) rule of weight management—because she maintains healthy eating habits and activity levels at least 80–90 percent of the time, she can enjoy an occasional splurge at other times.

People who didn't Jane know before look at her now and say, "Oh, you can eat anything you want and not put on weight," or "You're skinny, you have such a good metabolism—you're so lucky." Jane is not a metabolic miracle; nor is she luckier than anyone else. She simply found the precise formula that takes care of her body in the best way possible. Your job is to find the system that is going to work best for you.

So let's take a look first at the structure, and then what to eat.

THE PLANS

I have not set out one specific plan and presented it as the plan that will work for you and everyone else with a thyroid problem, because I've discovered that there simply isn't one plan that will work for everyone. Some thyroid patients are carbohydrate-sensitive and find that they can only lose weight when strictly limiting starchy foods. You could potentially be a thyroid patient who actually gains weight on a low-carb Atkins approach. Or you may be more calorie-sensitive and find that you only lose weight when you take your calorie levels lower. Or you may need a very balanced approach of proteins, starches, vegetables, fruits, fat, and so forth.

If all this sounds confusing, relax, because I've outlined a number of approaches that you can try. Your objective is to find the plan that works best with your unique metabolism.

WHICH PLAN IS RIGHT FOR YOU?

Complete the following checklists to help determine which one of the plans is the best starting point for you.

____ You have tried a low-carb diet such as Atkins, or a low-glycemic diet such as South Beach, and gained weight while following it.
____ You truly enjoy eating vegetables and fruits.
____ You feel your best after a meal that contains protein, starch, fat, and some vegetables or fruit.
____ You need variety in your diet.

If you have checked two or more of the previous statements, then you should start with the Free-Form Plan.

_____ You frequently crave things such as pasta, bread, rice, potatoes, sugary drinks, and desserts.

_____ Once you get started eating things such as pasta, bread, rice, potatoes, sugary drinks, and desserts, you find it hard to stop.

_____ After you eat things such as pasta, bread, rice, potatoes, sugary drinks, and desserts, you find yourself feeling hungry again fairly quickly.

_____ You find that after you eat a piece of cake or a bowl of pasta, you temporarily end up a pound or two heavier on the scale the next day.

If you checked two or more of the above statements, then it's likely that carbohydrates are a problem for you. You should start with the Carb-Sensitive Plan.

_____ You have tried a calorie-controlled diet such as Weight Watchers and gained weight while following it.

_____ You have tried a low-glycemic plan such as South Beach and gained weight while following it.

_____ You suspect that you probably eat too much, but you don't keep track.

_____ You find that you can gain weight on what others would consider a diet or "cutting back."

If you have check two or more of the above statements, then you should start with the Calorie-Sensitive Plan.

If you found yourself agreeing with many of the statements in all of the categories, then start out with the Free-Form Plan.

While the checklists can help you choose a plan to start with, read through all the plan guidelines. You will probably have an instinctual sense of which plan may be the best for you to try first. If we really listen, we know what our bodies really need.

As you can see, recipes are not included in this book. There are thousands of popular cookbooks out there, and hundreds of thousands of recipes available on the Internet, featuring low-carb, vegetarian, low-fat, low-glycemic, and other sorts of foods, as well as every possible category of food from every possible cuisine. Given the variety of foods thyroid dieters will eat, there's no possible way that one book can provide recipes to cover everyone's preferences and needs. Instead, I encourage you to develop a list of a few favorite go-to cookbooks or websites. The Resources section has some you can investigate as a start.

Follow the plan suggested by your checklists, or try whichever plan makes the most sense for you. Give it at least four weeks. I mean it—four weeks. I know the temptation is to try it for four days, and if you don't notice the scale going down, you'll abandon it for the next plan. But give it four weeks. See how you do. Note how you feel. Keep a food journal and track types of foods, carbohydrate intake, fat (including saturated fat), your moods, exercise level, menstrual periods, water, supplements, and daily weight so that you can see how you're doing and what might be affecting your weight.

After four weeks, if you've lost a few pounds (and remember, when you're dealing with a thyroid problem, consider it a resounding success if you have lost one pound in a week), you'll want to stick with the plan you're on. But go back and look at the notes you've kept. Did you find that you didn't have any weight loss on the days after you ate dairy, or you even bloated up and gained a bit? Think about cutting down on dairy as you move forward. Did you notice that if you met your goal for drinking water one day, the next day you saw some weight loss on the scale? This tells you that you really need to keep your water intake high. In contrast, if you felt terrible quite a bit of the time, or haven't lost anything or have even gained weight, then try one of the other plans. And give that plan four weeks.

I'm not offering a quick fix. If there were a miracle diet, you and I wouldn't need to be here. It usually takes quite a bit of time to become hypothyroid and for metabolism to get off track. It can take just as much time or more to get your thyroid back toward balance and help reenergize your metabolism so that you start losing weight. And once you're hypothyroid, you're likely to remain that way, so we're looking for a way of eating that is going to work for life.

But have faith. You will find that one of the plans featured in this book has an approach that will work for you!

THE FREE-FORM PLAN

The Free-Form Plan is straightforward and gives you quite a bit of leeway. It's a balanced, healthy starting point. If you already know you are extremely carbohydrate-sensitive, this may not be the place to start, but if you're not sure, this is a good plan to follow. Daily charts to help you keep track of your progress are available to download at the website ThyroidDietRevolution.com.

- *Protein:* each meal should include a seving of lean protein, and you should eat 4 to 6 serving of lean protein total per day
- *Low-glycemic vegetables:* eat all you want, and make sure you're getting at least 6 servings a day
- *Low-glycemic fruits:* 1–2 servings a day maximum
- *Low-glycemic starches:* 2–3 servings a day maximum
- *Good fat:* a serving with each meal and snack
- *Snacks:* 1–2 per day only if needed (and avoid eating after 8:00 p.m.)
- *Water:* 64 ounces, minimum
- *Fiber:* 25 grams, minimum
- *Supplements:* your choice, as per your practitioner's recommendation

You don't need to count calories with this diet, but focusing on lean proteins, plenty of vegetables, good fats, and limited starches and fruits naturally keeps the calories at a healthy level.

CARB-SENSITIVE PLAN

- *Protein:* some lean protein at each meal, for a total of 6 to 8 servings of protein a day
- *Low-glycemic vegetables:* eat all you want, and make sure you're getting at least 6 servings a day

- *Low-glycemic fruit:* 1 serving a day
- *Good fat:* a serving with each meal and snack
- *Snacks:* 1–2 per day, only if needed (and avoid eating after 8:00 p.m.)
- *Water:* 64 ounces, minimum
- *Fiber:* 30 grams, minimum
- *Supplements:* your choice, as per your practitioner's recommendation

While you don't want to go overboard with calories on the carb-sensitive plan, you don't have to be particularly concerned about them, either. One pilot study followed three groups: one on a low-fat calorie-controlled diet, the second on a low-carbohydrate diet at the same calorie levels, and the third on a low-carbohydrate diet at 300 more calories per day. Statistically, all the groups lost about the same amount of weight, despite the fact that the third group technically should have lost seven pounds less than the other groups.

THE CALORIE-SENSITIVE PLAN

Some people simply can't lose weight without cutting calories. With the calorie-sensitive plan, you'll need to do more tracking of foods, and unless you're a math whiz, you'll want to invest in a computer program or smartphone app that will help you keep track of your intake fairly closely. (A number of recommendations are featured in the Resources section.)

Your aim is to stay around your calorie target and to get approximately 35 percent of your calories from lean protein, 20 percent from low-glycemic vegetables, no more than 15 percent from low-glycemic fruits and starches, and 30 percent from good fats.

How Many Calories Do You Need?

Ultimately, the number of calories you need to eat daily in order to lose weight depends on several factors:

- Your targeted body weight
- Your activity level
- Your metabolic efficiency

The rough rule is that to get your calorie target, you take your targeted body weight in pounds and multiply it by a number that's based on your activity level.

- Sedentary (you get no exercise; you sit at a desk all day; you're a couch potato): 10 × target weight = calories per day
- Moderately active (you get some gentle or moderate form of exercise three to four times a week): 12 × target weight = calories per day
- Highly active (you get regular intense exercise more than four times per week): 14 × target weight = calories per day

Let's say your target weight is 140 pounds. Here are some sample calculations:

- Sedentary: 10 × 140 = 1,400 calories a day
- Moderate: 12 × 140 = 1,680 calories a day
- Active: 14 × 140 = 1,960 calories a day

Keep in mind that these are rough numbers. Computer tools and smartphone apps have more sophisticated calculators that can help you determine a much more specific calorie target. An even more valuable tool is a metabolic assessment. Bariatric physicians, health clubs, fitness coaches, and weight-loss counselors have elaborate and accurate metabolic test equipment that can calculate your resting metabolic rate (RMR). This sort of stand-alone metabolic testing typically costs between $100 and $200, but it's very useful to get a picture of what is actually going on in your body.

Keep in mind that experts recommend never going below 1,200 calories a day. If you are at 1,200 calories a day with a moderate level of activity and you are not losing weight, then you are likely suffering from an abnormally low metabolic rate or some sort of hormonal resistance—including potential thyroid resistance—that will require treatment and medical intervention.

If you are a repeat dieter or a yo-yo dieter, or if you are insulin- or leptin-resistant, your metabolic efficiency also may be substantially reduced, which means that weight-loss success ultimately will require that you medically address the underlying metabolic dysfunction.

Dr. Kent Holtorf checks the resting metabolic rate in his weight-loss patients, and he notes:

> Interestingly, many of our overweight patients, and in particular those with elevated leptin levels indicative of leptin resistance, have RMRs that are consistently below normal. These patients are often burning 500 to 600 calories less each day than someone of equal body mass.

IMPLEMENTING YOUR PLAN

What Is Your Optimal Weight?

I can't tell you at which weight you'll feel the best, and there are many different expert opinions. One of the simplest formulas is this: for women, allow 100 pounds for the first five feet and 5 pounds for each additional inch; for men, allow 110 pounds for the first five feet and 5 pounds for each additional inch. More sophisti-cated charts take into account height and frame size. I have links

to various calculators to identify your optimal weight at the website
ThyroidDietRevolution.com.

Ultimately, I know you have a number in your mind. It may
be based on a calculation. More likely, it is based on a weight at
which you felt and looked your best in the past. Now, I want you
to put that number in the back of your mind. It may be your final
goal, but you need to set realistic goals along the way. One of the
best ways to decide on a target weight is by identifying your current and target body mass index, or BMI. Take a look at the chart
below and identify your BMI. (You can also use the calculator at
ThyroidDietRevolution.com.)

BMI BY WEIGHT

Height	21	22	23	24	25	26	27	28	29	30	31	40
4'10"	100	105	110	115	119	124	129	134	138	143	148	192
5'0"	107	112	118	123	128	133	138	143	148	153	158	205
5'1"	111	116	122	127	132	137	143	148	153	158	164	212
5'3"	118	124	130	135	141	146	152	158	163	169	175	226
5'5"	126	132	138	144	150	156	162	168	174	180	186	241
5'7"	134	140	146	153	159	166	172	178	185	191	198	256
5'9"	142	149	155	162	169	176	182	189	196	203	209	271
5'11"	150	157	165	172	179	186	193	200	208	215	222	287
6'1"	159	166	174	182	189	197	204	212	219	227	235	303
6'3"	168	176	184	192	200	208	216	224	232	240	248	321

- Generally, a healthy BMI is 19–25.
- Overweight BMI is 26–30.
- Obese BMI is 31–40.
- Morbidly obese is above 40.

Identify your current BMI. If you're a 198-pound person, for
example, and you are five feet seven inches, your BMI is 31. That

would be considered overweight to slightly obese. Your target weight should be no higher (and possibly lower) than 159, which is a BMI of 25, the top end of the healthy range for that height.

If you belong to a gym, work with a fitness trainer, or see a nutritional expert, they can also perform more detailed BMI calculations that take into account important fat measurement spots.

Excess fat in the abdominal area is a risk factor for insulin resistance and other diseases. The waist measurement at which there is a definite increase in risk is 40 inches or more for men and 35 inches or more for women. So you should also focus on reducing waist size.

Setting Realistic Goals

- *Phase 1:* If you have a BMI over 30, your first goal should be to lose enough weight to get into the BMI range of 25–29. This will automatically reduce the risk of various diseases and help make your metabolism more efficient. You should also target a waist measurement reduction of 5 percent.
- *Phase 2:* If you're in the 25–29 BMI range (or if you've lost enough weight in Phase 1), then your goal should be to get down to a BMI of just below 25, plus an additional reduction in waist measurement. At this point, you are no longer overweight. You have greatly reduced your health risks and improved your metabolism; no doubt you look and feel better, and have more energy and greater fitness.
- *Phase 3:* If your ultimate goal weight is less than where you are with a BMI of a little under 25, then keep working on weight loss until you reach that objective.

In each phase, you should target a 5 percent reduction in waist measurement. The following chart may be a help:

Waist Measurement Reduction Targets			
Waist (in inches)	Phase 1 5 percent less	Phase 2 5 percent less	Phase 3 5 percent less
28	27	25	24
29	28	26	25
30	29	27	26
31	29	28	27
32	30	29	27
33	31	30	28
34	32	31	29
35	33	32	30
36	34	32	31
37	35	33	32
38	36	34	33
39	37	35	33
40	38	36	34
41	39	37	35
42	40	38	36
43	41	39	37
44	42	40	38
45	43	41	39

ABOUT THE TIMING

Did you know that just thinking about eating can actually trigger changes in your insulin levels and hormones that stimulate appetite? So your goal is to stop thinking about eating. (These days, I even switch off the television when I see the beginning of a particularly enticing food ad, so that my hormones don't get interested!) But one of the most important ways you can stop thinking about eating is to know when you're going to eat. If you eat on a fairly predictable schedule, you won't have to think about food between meals.

Most of the experts in the area of insulin and leptin resistance are now recommending that, rather than frequent mini-meals or grazing, people who are overweight focus instead on eating two or three meals a day. This allows enough time between each meal for the appropriate hormonal response to occur so that food is properly digested and nutrients absorbed, followed by an appropriate metabolic shift into fat burning before the next meal appears.

Research studies have also found a correlation between more meals per day and obesity. Studies found that women who were obese ate one meal more per day on average than those who were not obese. The overweight women tended to eat more between-meal snacks than the women who were of normal weight.

Another critical component to timing is not to eat after dinner if at all possible—ideally, nothing after 8:00 p.m. You should even try to go to bed a bit hungry—not so famished that hunger pangs will keep you awake, but your stomach should feel nearly empty. Your body is looking for fuel to burn during the night, and rather than have it burn undigested dinner or after-dinner snacks, you really want it to pull from your fat stores. Nutritional psychologist Marc David says that allowing time between eating and going to bed means that "you'll also do what you were meant to do while lying in bed—healing, detoxifying, rebuilding, and so forth—without side-tracking vital metabolic force into digestion."

If you go to bed with your stomach nearly empty and insulin levels are low, your body is much more likely to go to your fat stores and start burning. But if you have a big meal or a large snack before bed, you have insulin flooding your system and glucose circulating all night that will be stored in your fat cells.

According to experts, how or why a person gains weight is very complicated, but it clearly is not just calories in and calories out. One study found that eating a high-fat diet during the typical sleep period results in far greater weight gain than eating the same high-fat diet during normal waking hours. Another study comparing obese women and women of normal weight found that the over-weight women tended to eat more food later in the day and evening than their normal-weight counterparts.

Given how often we hear about "stoking the metabolism with frequent eating," this may sound quite radical. But we now know more about how food is processed in people (and cultures) where low metabolic efficiency is rampant, versus those with less of a problem. Look at the French, for example, who do not have nearly the obesity problem that we have in the United States. Experts studying the French diet have found that the French tend to eat three meals a day, slowly. The French rarely snack, and they take in fewer calories at a meal than most Americans. The typical slim French person is simply not having six mini-meals and additional snacks throughout the day to keep the metabolism "stoked."

In the beginning, you may still need to snack. But try cutting back to one snack a day, and eventually see if you can give up your snack entirely. And if you absolutely must have a snack between meals or in the evening before bed, make it a small one, and consider a handful of nuts or a small serving of protein.

In my own case, I had to get used to not snacking before bedtime. Before, I could easily down a dozen crackers and a piece of fruit before bed (and wake up bloated and up half a pound on the scale). But I adjusted to going to bed with an empty stomach, and I started waking up with no bloating and with the scale showing some weight loss. After switching to two to three meals a day, I also noticed that I feel more energetic than when I was eating multiple mini-meals. I also find that knowing generally when I will eat made me stop thinking about what snack I could have between this meal and the next, what time I should snack, and so on.

THE MOST IMPORTANT THING ABOUT YOUR FOOD

If there is a most important factor that you should consider when choosing your food, it would be the advice of nutritionist Marc David, author of the book *The Slow Down Diet*. David says, "No matter what food you eat, choose the highest-quality version of that food."

There are many reasons for this, and he explains them thoroughly in his terrific book and in his coaching, but here's the quick version. The highest-quality versions of foods—fresh, organic, local, hormone-free, and pesticide-free, and foods that are raised and grown under positive situations, for example—are more nutritious and in the end may have fewer negative effects on your weight than their lower-quality counterparts. There is so much to say about this, and it's more than we can get into here in *The Thyroid Diet Revolution*. But it's an important guiding principle.

WHAT TO EAT: LEAN PROTEINS

One of the key components of your diet should be lean proteins. These can include animal proteins, seafood, dairy products, eggs, and plant proteins.

Animal Protein

When choosing animal proteins, your objective is to choose lean proteins, from hormone-free, free-range, organically raised, grass-fed meat whenever possible. For beef, lamb, and bison (buffalo), grass-fed meat is particularly important, because grass-fed meats are substantially lower in saturated fat than feedlot-fattened animals. Some of the best proteins include:

- Lean cuts of beef (sirloin, top round, tenderloin)
- Bison (all cuts)
- Poultry (skinless): turkey breast (including ground), chicken breast, turkey bacon, ostrich
- Lean pork (pork loin)
- Lean cuts of lamb (loin, shank, leg)

Some of the proteins you want to avoid, or eat rarely, include:

- Beef brisket, liver, ribeye steaks, and other fatty cuts of beef
- Bacon, other fatty cuts of pork, honey-baked ham, processed cold cuts
- Lamb blade, ground lamb
- Chicken and turkey wings, legs, and thighs
- Duck and goose

One of the least familiar meats on the recommended list may be bison, also known as buffalo. If you haven't tasted bison, don't discount it! Bison tastes like rich, lean beef, with a bit of the savory aspect of lamb. Bison, however, is leaner, much lower in fat, and higher in protein than beef, making it a healthier option. Much of the bison available on the U.S. market is also organic and grass-fed. My local Trader Joe's and Whole Foods markets have precooked bison burger patties—two minutes in the microwave, and they're ready. They're absolutely delicious, and one burger with a salad fills me up for hours.

While we're on the topic of meat, let's look at pork loin. This is lower in fat, calories, and cholesterol than many other meats and poultry; in fact, any cut from the loin—such as pork chops, pork roast, and pork tenderloin—is actually leaner than skinless chicken thigh, according to U.S. Department of Agriculture data. I love cooking a pork loin roast as a special Sunday dinner. It's easy (a dash of Worcestershire, some garlic, and a few tablespoons of olive oil, and I pop it into the oven to roast, basting periodically while it's cooking). And if you make a large enough roast, you'll have terrific leftovers for lunch or dinner.

Keep in mind that in addition to natural foods stores, kosher and halal markets may be good sources for higher-quality, natural meats and seafood.

Seafood

Fish and shellfish can be complicated, because one day we hear how healthy they are, and then the next we hear about mercury, toxins, and cholesterol levels in some favorite seafoods.

Generally, healthy seafood choices that have the lowest level of contaminants include:

- American shad
- Anchovies
- Atlantic croaker
- Atlantic haddock
- Atlantic pollock
- Butterfish
- Canned salmon
- Catfish
- Chub mackerel
- Clams
- Crab
- Crawfish (crayfish)
- Flounder
- Hake
- Herring
- Mussels
- North Atlantic mackerel
- Ocean mullet
- Ocean perch

- Pacific oysters
- Pacific sole
- Plaice
- Sardines
- Scallops
- Shrimp
- Squid (calamari)
- Striped bass (farmed)
- Tilapia
- Trout
- Whitefish
- Whiting
- Wild salmon (coho, sockeye, Atlantic)

Some fish do contain higher levels of mercury, so they are best eaten in moderation—several servings a month maximum for adults—and most experts recommend that children and pregnant women avoid them entirely. They include:

- Chilean sea bass
- Spanish mackerel
- Bluefish
- Canned light tuna
- Cod
- Grouper
- Halibut
- Lobster
- Snapper
- Yellowfin tuna

Mercury and PCB contamination have resulted in some seafood being so contaminated that experts recommend you avoid it entirely. Seafood to avoid includes:

- Ahi (bigeye) tuna
- Canned white albacore tuna
- King mackerel
- Marlin
- Orange roughy
- Salmon (farmed)
- Shark
- Swordfish
- Tilefish
- American oysters (wild)
- Eastern oysters (wild)
- Striped bass (wild)

Eggs

Eggs, in particular organic omega-3 eggs, are a healthy protein source. Omega-3 eggs are from regular chickens that have been fed a diet of grains high in flaxseed. As a result, the eggs are high in alpha-linolenic acid, an omega-3 essential fatty acid that can have positive health effects. Omega-3 eggs are not genetically engineered. In studies, even eating two a day did not raise LDL cholesterol and actually was shown to raise HDL (the "good" cholesterol) and lower triglycerides. Eggs also rank high on satiety—they're filling. One study found that dieters who ate two eggs for breakfast typically ate as many as 300 fewer calories per day on average, compared to those not eating eggs.

Eggs are actually considered a near-perfect protein, because they contain a wealth of amino acids. Omega-3 eggs are somewhat more expensive than regular eggs, but the health advantage justifies the cost. They are available at many grocery and health food stores.

Dairy Foods

With dairy, one of the key issues is to make sure that you choose organic, hormone-free dairy products whenever possible.

There are various forms of dairy that you can use as healthy proteins. Remember that some dairy products (particularly nonfat versions) may include additional sugars and carbohydrates, so check the label. Some of the best dairy proteins include:

- Low-fat cottage cheese
- Plain yogurt and Greek yogurt
- Lebneh (yogurt cheese—a thickened, strained form of yogurt popular in Middle Eastern cuisine)
- Low-fat cheeses
- Feta cheese, goat cheese, Indian paneer cheese, and Neufchatel cheese (lower in fat than other types of cheese)

Laughing Cow also has a line of lower-fat cheeses that come packaged in little triangular wedges, and they're delicious.

Plant Proteins

Plant foods are a healthy source of protein. Some of the highest-protein plant foods include the following:

- Soybeans and soy products such as tempeh, tofu, miso, and natto
- Lentils
- Peanuts and peanut products
- Beans, including broad beans, kidney beans, lima beans, and chickpeas (garbanzo beans)
- Seeds, including pumpkin, squash, flax, sunflower
- Nuts, including walnuts, pine nuts, almonds, pistachio nuts, cashews, walnuts, hazelnuts, and brazil nuts

- Grains: quinoa, oats
- Protein powders based on plant proteins such as peas, rice, or hemp

While nutritionally, we know that these foods can be healthy, you'll need to determine whether your particular circumstances will allow you to lose weight while using fermented soy products (miso, tempeh, natto, certain kinds of tofu), beans, and grains. And generally, when it comes to plant proteins, it's wise to avoid unfermented soy products (including unfermented tofu), processed soy products (soybean oil, soy flour, soy lecithin, soy-based meat substitutes and burgers, soy cheese, soy ice cream, dried soybeans, soy milk, soy protein shakes or bars, soy protein powders), and peanut products.

The Debate over Animal Protein Versus Plant Protein

Some experts are now suggesting that the truly optimal diet for health is a diet that eliminates meat and fish and instead gets its protein only from plant-based sources. This has been an ongoing debate for several decades, with experts making convincing cases and studies offering convincing evidence on both sides of the argument.

As far as weight loss is concerned, what we do know is that depending on the dieter and his or her physiology, both animal- and plant-based diets can result in successful weight loss. So that aspect of the diet wars needs to be put to rest. We also know that low-carbohydrate diets—as compared to low-fat, higher-carbohydrate diets—can also be an effective way to lose weight. In some cases, controlling carbohydrates appears to be more effective than higher-carbohydrate diets in terms of the amount of weight lost and maintained over time.

But the diet wars still rage over whether a low-carbohydrate diet that relies on animal protein can be healthy, even if it's a successful weight-loss strategy. Some experts say yes, pointing to changes in cholesterol levels that suggest improved cardiovascular health. Others say no, suggesting that the evidence points to plant-based protein being healthier.

The compromise solution? A modification to low-carbohydrate diets that replaces animal protein with plant-based protein. Labeled "Eco-Atkins," it's a vegan diet that limits carbohydrates to 100–150 grams a day (high by Atkins standards, but lower than the typical 300 grams a day of the typical American diet). And those carbohydrates are primarily vegetables and fruit; processed carbohydrates such as bread, rice, potatoes, sugar, and pasta are not included. In the Eco-Atkins diet, the protein sources are primarily gluten, soy, and nuts.

One study compared Eco-Atkins to a lacto-ovo-vegetarian low-carb diet, where tofu, eggs, and cheese were the main sources of protein. It found that the Eco-Atkins group had significant improvements in risk factors for heart disease, plus a drop in bad cholesterol.

One of the more recent additions to the debate is a study reported on in the *Annals of Internal Medicine* in September 2010, which looked at the long-term risk of mortality for people following animal-based and vegetable-based low-carbohydrate diets. The focus was not on whether cholesterol was lowered or triglycerides improved, but simply on mortality. They found that "diets that emphasized animal sources of fat and protein were associated with higher all-cause, cardiovascular, and cancer mortality, whereas diets that emphasized vegetable sources of fat and protein were associated with lower all-cause and cardiovascular mortality." They concluded that the health effects of a low-carbohydrate diet may depend on the type of protein and fat, and a diet that includes mostly vegetable sources of protein and fat is preferable to a diet with mostly animal sources of protein and fat.

It would seem to be case closed, then: plant-based protein wins over animal-based protein.

But is it closed?

I would argue that what we really need to compare—apples to apples, so to speak—is a plant-based, carbohydrate-controlled diet with a diet that includes sufficient—but not excessive—amounts of protein that is organic, hormone-free, pesticide-free, and grass-fed, as well as a controlled amount of organic, low-glycemic carbohydrates. A low-carb diet where the protein sources are grass-fed organic beef, wild salmon, and organic locally grown vegetables, for example, is likely to have a very different impact on overall health, inflammation, hormones, cancer risk, and mortality than a diet where the protein sources are fatty cuts of hormone-laden beef, processed cold cuts, additive-riddled sausages, mercury-laden fish, poultry pumped full of toxins, and vegetables and fruits coated in pesticide residues and loaded with perchlorate.

There are also two key issues to consider regarding the thyroid impact of an Eco-Atkins type of diet that relies on gluten, soy, and nuts as primary proteins. First, we know that gluten is a common allergen, and sensitivity to it—or even a complete intolerance, such as seen in celiac disease—is on the rise and is at the root of many cases of thyroid and autoimmune disease. An increasing number of physicians are now advocating a gluten-free diet to help calm thyroid autoimmunity and to aid in weight loss. For those who have sensitivity or celiac disease—most of whom are undiagnosed at present—shifting to a diet that relies on gluten as a key form of protein could worsen underlying health issues.

Second, soy is a phytoestrogen, and it can in some cases block the body's ability to absorb thyroid hormone. In small quantities—for example, as a condiment—and in its fermented forms, it can probably be a safe part of the diet. But in the high quantities necessary for it to be a primary protein in a protein-sufficient diet, soy can function as an goitrogen in those who still have a gland, meaning that it can slow the thyroid down and promote formation of a goiter. Soy can also impair absorption of thyroid medication in anyone on thyroid hormone replacement medication whether or not they have a gland. Add to that two other issues: much of the soy available these days is genetically modified, and soy too is a common allergen.

So if thyroid patients switch to a diet based entirely on plant protein, will they find its health benefits cancelled out by worsening hypothyroidism or by sensitivity to gluten, soy, or nuts? I think we need a far better understanding of whether such a diet is beneficial in the long term for weight loss and overall health for people with thyroid issues. And until we have definitive information, if you are a thyroid patient who wants to eat only plant-based proteins, I recommend that you carefully monitor your response, not only in terms of weight loss but also in terms of your thyroid antibodies and thyroid function. If you are including meat in your diet, try to choose the best-quality meats—lean, grass-fed, organic, and hormone-free—whenever possible.

WHAT TO EAT: LOW-GLYCEMIC CARBOHYDRATES

The term *low-glycemic* refers to the glycemic index (GI). The GI basically is a measure of how quickly your blood sugar levels will rise after you eat a particular food. Both a food's chemical composition and its fiber content typically affect its GI rating—how quickly your body takes that carbohydrate and converts it to glucose.

To determine a food's GI rating, portions of the food are given to people who have fasted overnight. Their blood sugar is then monitored over time, and the rise in blood sugar is calculated. Foods with a lower glycemic index will create a slower rise in blood sugar, and foods with a higher glycemic index will create a faster rise in blood sugar.

Low-Glycemic Vegetables

Some of the lowest-glycemic vegetables that you can safely include in your diet are:

- Artichokes
- Beans and legumes
- Brussels sprouts
- Celery
- Eggplants
- Green peppers
- Mushrooms
- Tomatoes
- Asparagus
- Broccoli
- Cauliflower
- Cucumbers
- Green beans
- Lettuce
- Spinach
- Zucchini

The higher-glycemic vegetables that you should limit are:

- Beets
- Celery root
- Parsnips
- Rutabaga
- Turnips
- Winter squash
- Carrots
- Corn
- Red potatoes
- Sweet potatoes
- White potatoes
- Yams

A great way to get your veggies is by starting meals with a healthy vegetable soup. Researchers have found that blending vegetables and water into a soup makes you feel full and satisfied, compared to eating the soup's ingredients—i.e., the solid foods and water—separately. It sounds strange that eating vegetables and water together as a soup can make you feel more full than eating the same vegetables with a glass of water, but according to scientists, after you eat a meal, the pyloric sphincter valve at the bottom of your stomach holds food back so that digestion can begin. Water passes through the sphincter to the intestines, so water on its own doesn't help fill you up. But mix the water with other ingredients into a soup, and the whole mixture stays in your stomach, because the stomach "reads" the soup as a food. This keeps the stomach fuller for longer and helps reduce hunger. The full, stretched stomach also communicates to the hypothalamus to stop producing the hunger hormone ghrelin, so the longer the stomach remains full, the longer you feel satisfied and the less you are likely to eat.

And don't forget that capsaicin, the compound responsible for the heat in cayenne, jalapeño, and other hot peppers, can stimulate metabolism—by as much as 40 percent in the short term, according to some experts. So pile on the peppers!

Low-Glycemic Fruits

The best fruits generally for thyroid dieters are berries—including strawberries, blueberries, blackberries, raspberries, and other types. They have a lower glycemic index than other fruits, and they are rich in antioxidants. Choose organic berries whenever possible, however, as berries can carry pesticide residues, and do not have a peel or skin to protect the fruit.

Some other low-glycemic fruits include:

- Apples*
- Cantaloupes
- Grapefruits
- Peaches*
- Apricots
- Cherries*
- Nectarines
- Plums

Fruits that you should limit or avoid, because they have a higher glycemic index, are:

- Bananas
- Grapes
- Oranges
- Papayas
- Tangerines
- Clementines
- Honeydew melons
- Pineapples
- Watermelon
- Raisins, dates, other dried fruits*

* These fruits are higher in fructose, and may have a more glycemic effect on some individuals.

Low-Glycemic Starches

Your best choices are low-glycemic-index starches, including:

- Sprouted bread (try the Ezekiel line of products)
- High-fiber multigrain bread
- Bulgur
- Whole-grain wheat bread
- Whole-grain rye bread
- Pumpernickel
- Whole-grain crispbreads, such as Wasa, Ak-Mak, and Kavli
- Low-carb bread
- Quinoa
- Amaranth
- Wild rice

Note that millet, while considered a low-glycemic grain, is highly goitrogenic and is not recommended.

Slightly higher-glycemic starches that may be eaten on occasion, depending on how sensitive you are to them and whether they slow or stall weight loss for you, include:

- Plain cooked oatmeal (old-fashioned, steel-cut, or Irish; not instant)
- Spinach pasta
- Brown rice
- No-sugar-added, high-fiber cereals

Starches you should avoid:

- Bagels or breads that are not high-fiber
- Cakes
- Cold cereals (except high-fiber)
- Cookies

- Corn bread, corn tortillas
- Crackers
- Granola, granola bars
- Muffins
- Pretzels
- Refined flours
- White rice
- Rice cakes
- Pasta (from white or wheat flour)
- White sugar

When you're looking to cut out sugar, don't forget about sugar-sweetened drinks—they are pretty much like mainlining sugar straight into your veins. You know the drill: there are 10 teaspoons of sugar in one can of cola. And don't overlook the macchiatos and sweetened coffee drinks at your favorite coffee bar—these drinks can be as sugary and high-calorie as a milk shake. Even pure fruit juices can be problematic. If you must have a glass of orange or other fruit juice in the morning, consider juicing it yourself and leaving the pulp in so that you get some fiber and more nutritional value from it. Or if you are using prepared juice, consider diluting it with half water to help cut the sugar content. You'll still get some flavor from it, but with less of the sugar and calorie impact.

One option for juice lovers is to get unsweetened fruit juice, then add your own no-calorie sweetener. For example, I buy unsweetened cranberry juice concentrate (which is rather sour as is), but I add stevia and water and have a low-cal, low-carb, nutritious cranberry juice cocktail. Occasionally I like to mix a bit of stevia with unsweetened fruit juice and seltzer and make my own sugar-free "soda." Or try Emergen-C drinks, which are single-serving vitamin drinks that come in small packets. You add water, and you have a slightly fizzy, naturally sweetened, low-carbohydrate, low-calorie vitamin drink that contains 1,000 mg vitamin C, along with potassium and other nutrients.

WHAT TO EAT: FATS

Fat in your diet can be of several types:

- *Monounsaturated fatty acids (MUFAs).* Monounsaturated fats lower total cholesterol and LDL cholesterol (the bad cholesterol) while increasing HDL cholesterol (the good cholesterol). Nuts (walnuts, almonds, and pistachios), peanuts, seeds, avocados, and olive oil are high in MUFAs. MUFAs have also been found to help in weight loss.
- *Polyunsaturated fatty acids (PUFAs).* Polyunsaturated fats fall into two categories: omega-6 fats and omega-3 fats. Omega-6 PUFAs are found primarily in vegetable oils such as sunflower oil and cottonseed oil. Omega-3 PUFAs are considered the heart-healthiest and are concentrated in fatty cold-water fish (such as salmon, mackerel, and herring) and fish oil. They are also found to a lesser extent in flaxseeds, flaxseed oil, and walnuts.
- *Saturated fats.* Saturated fats are mainly found in animal products such as meat, eggs, dairy products, and seafood. Some plant foods are also high in saturated fats, including coconut oil and palm oil. There is a continuing controversy as to whether saturated fats are dangerous to health or in fact heart-healthy.
- *Trans fats.* Trans fats are chemically created fats that are used because they provide a longer shelf life for processed and packaged foods. Trans fats are found in many commercial baked goods (such as crackers, cookies, and cakes), many commercially fried foods such as french fries and doughnuts, packaged snacks such as microwave popcorn, and some types of vegetable shortening and stick margarine.

Fats are a contentious, controversial topic, and if you talk to different nutritional experts, you'll hear very different stories. The conventional wisdom is that saturated fat is bad because it raises total cholesterol and LDL (bad cholesterol) while lowering HDL (good cholesterol). Conventional nutrition thinking urges us to avoid all saturated fat and trans fat and get our dietary fat from MUFAs and PUFAs.

At the same time, some nutritionists are pointing to cultures that traditionally have diets high in saturated fat yet also have low rates of heart disease. Furthermore, there are increasing numbers of respectable studies showing that diets rich in saturated fat can result in a lower or unchanged concentration of total and LDL cholesterol and an increase in HDL cholesterol.

So the advice you get on fat will probably depend on whether you're reading something from the generally dietary-fat-phobic American Heart Association or Dr. Dean Ornish, or the dietary-fat-friendly Weston A. Price Foundation or researcher and writer Gary Taubes.

What should you do? My recommendations are as follows:

- Make the majority of fat in your diet healthy MUFAs and PUFAs.
- Don't be afraid of some saturated fat in whole foods, but eat them in moderation as part of a calorie-controlled diet.
- Avoid trans fats. Everyone agrees they have no place in a healthy diet or a diet designed for weight loss.
- Avoid corn, soy, canola, safflower, and sunflower oils, especially in cooking, due to their risk of contamination, rancidity, and inability to remain stable at high temperatures.

You can't go wrong with olive oil as a key fat in your diet. And while we're on the subject of olive oil, let's mention vinegar.

Vinegar has been a folk remedy for obesity for many years, and it appears that the old wives' tale may have some truth to it, based on some studies of vinegar's properties. Various studies have shown that vinegar may help slow down fat accumulation and weight gain. Some animal studies conducted in Japan have shown that animals fed a high-fat diet plus acetic acid, the ingredient that gives vinegar its strong smell and sour taste, developed 10 percent less body fat than animals not receiving the acetic acid. Another recent study found that diabetics who took 2 tablespoons of apple cider vinegar before bed lowered their morning glucose levels by 2 to 4 percent.

Apple cider vinegar, red wine vinegar, and balsamic vinegar have a great deal of flavor with minimal calories, so you may want to regularly mix up a fresh olive oil vinaigrette for your salads or vegetables.

WHAT TO DRINK: WATER

Even if you're eating exactly the right things and working out, if you're not getting enough water you may find it difficult, if not outright impossible, to lose weight. This is because the liver, which converts stored fat into energy, acts as a backup to the kidneys in detoxifying the body. If the kidneys are not functioning optimally because they are deprived of water, then the liver is diverted away from fat conversion and toward detoxification.

Drinking enough water:

- Helps the metabolism work efficiently
- Helps reduce appetite
- Helps skin appearance and tone
- Helps muscles work more efficiently
- Helps digestion, reduces constipation, and encourages regular elimination

Ideas about how much water you should drink depend on whom you ask, but many agree you should get eight 8-ounce glasses a day. Some experts say that you should drink an additional 8-ounce glass for every twenty-five pounds of weight you need to lose. So if you are fifty pounds overweight, you should drink two more 8-ounce glasses of water, for a total of ten 8-ounce glasses. If it's particularly hot out or if you are exercising intensely, the American College of Sports Medicine suggests drinking even more—adding 6 ounces for every fifteen minutes of activity. Philip Goglia, author of *Turn Up the Heat: Unlock the Fat-Burning Power of Your Metabolism*, recommends drinking 1 ounce of water per pound of scale weight. For most of us, this is substantially more than eight glasses. If you are a 160-pound woman, for example, that's 160 ounces a day, which is equal to twenty 8-ounce glasses a day, or the equivalent of almost three 2-liter bottles. And if you are a 200-pound man, that's twenty-five 8-ounce glasses a day.

I know that for the first few days after increasing water intake, you feel as if you're living in the restroom. But this will calm down. As your body begins to recognize that you are finally taking in enough water, it gives up the water it's been holding on to. This is also the mechanism behind the counterintuitive but true theory that if you want to stop feeling bloated and retaining water, you need to drink more water! You'll know you're getting enough when your urine is pale yellow or nearly colorless. If it's darker, increase your water intake. (Keep in mind, however, that certain vitamins darken your urine, even if you're getting enough water.)

Spread out water consumption during the day as much as possible. One rule that some experts recommend is that you not drink water while you are eating. The theory is that if you are drinking water with your meal, you may be using it to help swallow food without fully chewing your food. You may want to drink a glass of water before your meal. It's even better if you can have a big glass of water with some sort of fiber (e.g., psyllium, or Dr. Levine's Ultimate Weight Loss Formula) before you eat. (Don't forget, however, to make sure that supplemental fiber is taken several hours apart from your thyroid medication.)

Ideally, you want to make sure that your water is as clean and pure as possible. At a minimum, filter your drinking water. You can get decent, inexpensive, quality pitcher or sink-based filters, such as

Pur or Brita. If you want a more elaborate system, reverse osmosis systems purify water and remove many toxins.

Some people find electrolyte-enhanced water to be especially helpful. Electrolyte-enhanced water contains extra amounts of minerals, including magnesium, potassium, and sodium. It's a bit like Gatorade, though without calories and flavor, in terms of helping to replace minerals and rehydrate the body. You may recognize the brand SmartWater by Glaceau, which is a popular electrolyte-enhanced water. Many grocery and natural food chains also have their own house brands of electrolyte-enhanced water. Typically, these waters start with purified water, which is then vapor-distilled and enhanced with minerals.

Finally, should you drink your water cold or at room temperature? There is anecdotal evidence that the stomach absorbs cold water more quickly and that cold water may enhance fat burning. The idea is that your body has to use extra energy to heat the cold water up to body temperature—98.6 degrees—so this may help you burn more calories. However, there is also some thinking that cold water stimulates appetite and that warmer water is far easier to drink in large quantities. Since there is no real agreement, the right temperature is the one you like best and find easiest to drink. Personally, I have found that I can drink far more room-temperature water, and I am quite used to it this way. My favorite? Room temperature SmartWater.

WHAT TO EAT: FIBER

Fiber is essential to digestion and will optimize your weight-loss efforts. Sometimes called roughage, it is the part of plant foods that is not digestible. Fiber comes in two forms: (1) soluble, which dissolves in water, and (2) insoluble, which does not. Foods that are high in soluble fiber include oats, barley, beans, and citrus fruits. Soluble fiber is also found in psyllium seed and oat bran. Good sources of insoluble fiber include wheat bran and certain vegetables.

Fiber:

- Absorbs water and helps create softer, larger stools, promoting regularity
- Can help prevent or minimize digestive tract problems and their consequences, such as hemorrhoids, diverticular disease, irritable bowel syndrome, and even rectal cancer
- Can slow the digestive process, preventing dramatic swings in blood sugar
- Can help lower cholesterol

There is evidence that fiber helps with weight loss. Fiber has minimal calories but can fill you up by adding bulk. When consumed with carbohydrates, it helps modulate the insulin response and normalize blood sugar. There is a fair amount of scientific support for fiber's ability to increase the feeling of fullness after you eat. One study found that adding 14 grams of fiber per day was associated with a 10 percent decrease in calorie intake and a weight loss of five pounds over four months.

In another study of fifty-three women who were moderately overweight and followed a 1,200-calorie-a-day diet over twenty-four weeks, half were given a fiber supplement and half received a placebo. The fiber group was given 6 grams of fiber a day to start, then 4 grams. The fiber group lost a mean of 17.6 pounds versus 12.76 pounds in the placebo group.

Fiber can be incorporated into food, but you need to keep in mind the trade-offs between fiber-rich foods and the calorie or glycemic impact. Some ways to incorporate fiber into your diet include:

- Raw fruits and vegetables, which have more fiber than cooked or canned

- Dried fruits, especially dried figs (note, however, that dried fruits are high in natural sugar and can have a high glycemic index, so use them with caution)
- Whole grains (such as quinoa) or whole-grain bread
- High-fiber cereals (a ½-cup serving of All-Bran, for example, has 90 calories and 10.4 grams of fiber)
- Nuts—many are high in fiber (¼ cup almonds, for example, provides 2.4 grams of fiber)
- Beans (1 cup black beans provides a whopping 19.4 grams of fiber)

Other high-fiber foods include apples, oranges, broccoli, cauli-flower, berries, pears, Brussels sprouts, lettuce, prunes, carrots, and potatoes.

Men younger than fifty require 38 grams of fiber a day, and women should get 25 grams. Men over fifty should get at least 30 grams and women at least 21 grams. The typical American diet, however, includes 10 grams of fiber a day or less. You'll probably have to add a fiber supplement, in addition to emphasizing fiber-rich foods. Start slow because you need to give your intestinal system time to adjust. Adding too much fiber too quickly can cause discomfort.

Some fiber supplements to consider include

- *Psyllium.* One study found that women who took 20 grams of psyllium before a meal ate less fat and felt full more quickly during that meal, helping with weight reduction. Psyllium husk is found in Metamucil products (but watch for sugar or artificial sweeteners such as aspartame in these products). I prefer plain psyllium powder, but even better is psyllium in capsule form. Taken with a big glass of water before a meal, the fiber helps slow the glycemic response of your food and helps you feel full longer than usual.
- Guar gum (i.e., Benefiber), which dissolves with no grit or bulk into drinks

- FiberCon tablets, which use polycarbophil, a synthetic fiber; it has the filling and stool-softening effects of fiber but may not lower cholesterol or blood sugar like other types of fiber

Important warning: If you switch from a low-fiber diet to a high-fiber one, be very careful that you are taking your thyroid medication at least an hour before eating in the morning so that absorption of the medication is not impaired. High-fiber diets can change your dosage requirements, so six to eight weeks after starting a high-fiber diet, you may wish to have your thyroid function retested.

In addition to fiber supplements, a great high-fiber food product is Gnu Bars. These are bars that contain 12 grams of fiber each—the fiber in one bar equals three to four doses of most fiber supplements. Gnu Bars come in a variety of flavors, including Chocolate Brownie (the only one I've actually tasted). They're decent. They don't taste like brownies, but they are chewy and chocolatey, and definitely do *not* taste like they have 12 grams of fiber. You can get Gnu Bars at local health food stores or online.

My favorite fiber product is Dr. Levine's Ultimate Weight Loss Formula (which I'll call DLUWLF for short). It's the highest-fiber supplement I've found on the market—one serving provides 35 grams of fiber, which comes from five different healthy fibers, including psyllium. It has no calories and comes in a variety of flavors. I have more information on DLUWLF in chapter 7.

WHAT IS A SERVING SIZE?

I can almost guarantee you that the recommended serving size of whatever food you are eating is probably smaller that you think it is! When I first started keeping track of serving sizes, I was amazed to find that my idea of a serving of pasta was actually two to three servings. That plump chicken breast? Two servings. And one of those really nice, big, fat-free blueberry muffins from Starbucks? Four servings of starch! The fundamental truth here: you will often overestimate the serving sizes of foods, but you'll rarely underestimate them.

You can walk around with a food scale in your pocket (not particularly practical) or you can learn to fairly accurately eyeball a serving by comparing certain foods and serving sizes with common objects. Let's start with the definition of a meal-size serving.

One serving of vegetables is basically:

- ½ cup raw, chopped, or cooked
- ¾ cup vegetable juice (try to stick with the low-sodium varieties, or juice it yourself)
- 1 cup raw leafy greens (salad, spinach, etc.)

One serving of starch is basically

- 1 slice whole wheat bread
- ½ whole-wheat bagel or muffin
- ½ cup cooked whole-grain cereal, pasta, brown rice, beans, corn, potatoes, rice, or sweet potatoes
- ½ of a small white potato or sweet potato, or 1 red potato
- 2 slices unseasoned Melba toast
- ½ Ak-Mak cracker
- ½ small corn tortilla
- 2 cups popcorn

For protein, one serving is:

- 3 ounces beef, pork, or lamb
- 5 ounces fish
- 6 ounces poultry
- 1 ounce regular cheese, or 2 ounces low-fat cheese
- 2 eggs

One serving of fat is:

- 1 tablespoon oil (i.e., olive, flaxseed, coconut)
- 1 tablespoon low-fat mayonnaise, or 1 teaspoon regular mayonnaise
- 1 tablespoon oil-and-vinegar dressing
- 5 large olives or 7 smaller olives
- 1/8 medium avocado
- 1 pat or 1 teaspoon butter
- 1 ounce of nuts without the shell; 2 tablespoons of peanut butter

One serving of fruit is:

- 10 fresh cherries
- 2 small tangerines or clementines
- 1 cup berries
- 1 small peach, apple, or orange
- 1 medium plum or nectarine
- ½ medium-large grapefruit
- ½ cup canned fruit
- ½ cup cut melon or papaya
- ¾ cup juice
- ¼ cup dried fruit

One serving of dairy is:

- ½ cup low-fat milk
- 1 cup low-fat plain yogurt
- ½ cup lowfat ricotta or cottage cheese

Not quite convinced that you're underestimating how much food you're eating? How many cups of popcorn do you think there are in one medium-size container of movie popcorn? Would you be surprised to hear that it has 16 cups of popcorn, which is eight full

2-cup servings? Have you ever shared a medium popcorn with eight people? More likely, you've eaten a whole bag yourself (I have)!

How about that prime rib and baked potato dinner out? The typical restaurant gives you 13 ounces of prime rib, or more than four servings of beef. And the large baked potato on the side? It's equivalent to four actual potato servings. So your restaurant plate is enough to feed a family of four!

What about those giant cinnamon buns that assault us at malls and airports? One is the equivalent of four starch servings (not to mention all the extra sugar).

How to Eyeball Portions

Now that you're more familiar with the concept of a real portion size versus portions in our supersized food culture, let's talk about how to eyeball portions.

AMOUNT	IS THE SIZE OF...
1 cup	A closed fist
1/2 cup	An ice cream scoop
2 tablespoons	A ping-pong ball
1 teaspoon	The top of your thumb from tip to joint
Meat, 3 ounces	A deck of cards or a cassette tape
Cheese, 1 ounce	Four stacked dice
1 medium piece of fruit	A tennis ball

Finally, here are two important tips to remember about portions:

- Be careful when you're dealing with any prepackaged foods that you assume are single servings, such as bottled juices, sweetened teas, a bag of chips, and so forth. Read the food label to see what the serving size is, then check to see the total size of the product. You may be looking at calories for a serving of juice or chips only to discover that the bottle or package you have is actually two servings.

- Whenever you can, measure out one serving and put it on a plate. Don't put the entire box, bowl, bag, or platter on the table in front of you, or you will overestimate the serving amount. If a serving of cereal is ½ cup, take the time to measure it in a measuring cup, because until you are very good at eyeballing and are familiar with sizes, if you just shake the cereal into a bowl, you're likely to over-estimate.

OTHER ISSUES

Sweets and Treats

Generally, good health and weight loss mean that most "desserts" will need to go by the wayside. Ideally, as you retrain your taste buds and balance your blood sugar, those raging cravings for sugary, carbohydrate-rich treats will diminish. When you must have a treat or dessert, try a small bowl of berries, a piece of low-glycemic fruit, a yogurt parfait, or a small piece of good-quality dark chocolate. Eat your treat slowly, and savor every bite.

Snacks

Ideally, you'll want to focus your approach more toward three meals a day, and eliminate frequent snacking, But when you do need to snack, avoid processed carbohydrates and typical snack foods—chips, popcorn, and so on—and instead reach for some of the following foods, which are primarily protein and good fat:

- Low-fat cottage cheese
- Celery with cream cheese or nut butter
- Hard-boiled eggs
- Seeds
- Guacamole
- A handful of nuts
- A handful of olives and a small piece of cheese

Coffee and Tea

Coffee, to be honest, is a huge question mark. Some studies have shown that coffee may help with blood sugar and therefore potentially aid in weight loss. Recent studies comparing coffee and caffeinated water found that both drinks had positive effects on insulin sensitivity and fatty liver. One study also found that while drinking caffeinated water lowered "leptin expression in adipose tissue," coffee was not found to have the same effect. Researchers are looking into this discrepancy.

A number of recent studies have shown specifically that consumption of coffee may help reduce the risk of developing type 2 diabetes. It's now thought that coffee may function as an antioxidant and anti-inflammatory as well.

Regular coffee also contains caffeine, which is proven to raise metabolism.

At the same time, in people with diabetes, coffee can sometimes cause a short-term increase in blood sugar levels, and some dieters may find that reducing coffee intake or even eliminating coffee may actually help with weight loss.

Nutritionist Marc David says that people who drink coffee regularly should know that coffee can actually mimic the body's own stress response and cause abdominal weight gain. In his book *The Slow Down Diet*, David says:

This doesn't mean coffee is bad. It just means that when you combine lack of food (survival response—elevated cortisol), anxiety (stress response—elevated cortisol), and caffeine (mimics stress response—elevated cortisol), you have three factors that powerfully synergize to send cortisol production through the roof, suppressing digestive metabolism and depositing weight.

My advice? Coffee puts additional stress on what is usually already an overtaxed adrenal system, and I've heard so many anecdotal reports from thyroid dieters—myself included—who simply don't lose weight when we overdose on coffee daily. I think a normal-size cup or two (and no, a cup is not a 32-ounce mug, or a venti triple espresso) is probably manageable, but pay close attention to how you feel after you've had a cup of coffee. If you later feel shaky, jittery, or hungry, that's your sign to cut back on coffee or cut it out entirely.

As for tea, if you're a heavy tea drinker, you may want to watch your intake of black tea. One study has found that the high concentration of fluoride in black tea may be a thyroid risk for those who drink more than 3 or 4 cups of black tea daily. (Note to southerners: that includes iced tea as well!)

At the same time, research suggests that green tea may aid in weight loss. One study found that green tea resulted in a significant increase in energy expenditure—known as thermogenesis—plus also had a significant effect on fat oxidation. Specifically, people who drink 5 cups of green tea a day typically burn 80 more calories over a twenty-four-hour period. The component responsible for the increased fat-burning is epigallocatechin gallate (EGCG), which is also a potent anti-inflammatory compound.

Oolong and white tea have also been the subjects of studies, some of which have found that these types of tea may help prevent fat accumulation and stimulate fat burning.

If you're a tea drinker, you may want to think about switching from black tea to green, oolong, or white tea.

Sweeteners

Should you use sweeteners on your diet? Ideally, your best choice would be to avoid all sweeteners—nutritive and non-nutritive—entirely, or as much as possible. A nutritive sweetener has 4 calories per gram and provides energy like other simple carbohydrates. Nutritive sweeteners include white and brown table sugar, molasses, honey, maple syrup, agave, and corn syrup. Sugar alcohols are also nutritive. These are derived from fruits or produced commercially and include sorbitol, mannitol, xylitol, and maltitol.

Generally, you'll want to avoid sugar products—including honey and agave—as much as you can. As far as sugar alcohols, some experts suggest that these are metabolized somewhat more slowly than straight glucose-based sugars, but they can still affect your blood sugar, and may cause abdominal discomfort in some people.

As for artificial low- or no-calorie (non-nutritive) sweeteners, including those in diet sodas, we now know that they may actually sabotage your efforts to lose weight. There is still ongoing controversy over the safety of the various artificial sweeteners, including saccharine (Sweet'n Low), aspartame (NutraSweet, Equal), and sucralose (Splenda), however, because of alleged relationships with cancer, neurological problems, and other symptoms including headaches, nausea, insomnia, dizziness, diarrhea, depression, anxiety, memory loss, and even vision changes.

Purdue University's Ingestive Behavior Research Center did animal studies showing that eating yogurt sweetened with saccharin caused more calorie consumption, weight gain, and later gain of body fat than eating yogurt sweetened with plain sugar. It seems counterintuitive, but if you look at the idea behind it, it makes sense. Sweet foods provide a very specific stimulus that causes digestive reflexes to prepare for the intake of higher calories, including an increase in metabolism and raised body temperature. But when an artificial sweetener is used, the taste of sweetness is "false," meaning that it isn't followed by a higher-calorie food. When this happens, the system gets confused. Over time, this leads to a blunted response to *any* sweet-tasting calories. So even after eating a sweet-tasting, high-calorie meal that does not use artificial sweeteners, the blunted digestive reflexes don't kick in, metabolism doesn't increase, and body temperature does not change, which translates to impaired fat burning and more weight gain. Basically, artificial sweeteners train your body to overconsume refined carbohydrates.

The more you get blood sugar under control, the less you will likely crave sweet foods and drinks. Ideally, you should focus on re-training your taste buds away from sweet foods, even those that are artificially sweetened. But if you do occasionally need a sweetener, what should you use? For the occasional cup of coffee, some experts suggest that you use an actual teaspoon of a nutritive sweetener such as sugar, so that the body does not become acclimated to the idea that sweet tastes are associated with low or no-calorie foods and beverages. As for the artificial sweeteners, almost every natural health expert I know recommends that you stay away from aspartame. They are less adamant about saccharine and sucralose, and very occasional use of these products is probably not a problem for you. Some experts feel that sugar alcohols are a good choice. Personally, I get stomach upset from all of them, including xylitol, so I avoid them. Many healthy eating proponents are suggesting that for occasional use, stevia may in fact be the safest no-calorie sweetener.

Stevia has no calories and is not a carbohydrate. It comes from a plant native to Paraguay. I use a little bit in my tea or coffee. Stevia is versatile and can be used in hot and cold beverages, on fruit and cereals, and as a sugar replacement in baking and cooking. I also occasionally use stevia to naturally sweeten plain yogurt. If you take plain low-fat or fat-free yogurt and mix in fruit and some stevia, you have healthy, low-fat fruit yogurt without a chemical sweetener.

With stevia, just like when you first switch to any sweetener besides sugar, it takes a few days to adjust to the flavor. But once you're used to it, it tastes fine and satisfies your sweet cravings. You may want to carry single-serving packets of powdered stevia to work, to restaurants, and when you travel.

For the most part, experts have concluded that stevia and the derivatives of stevia are safe. The World Health Organization conducted a thorough evaluation of all the research and said that stevia shows no evidence of being a cancer risk. Other studies show that stevia may improve insulin sensitivity and lower blood pressure.

Fruit and Fructose

One of the reasons you won't find recommendations in *The Thyroid Diet Revolution* to eat many servings of fruit each day is that fruit is high in fructose, a type of sugar that is easily and quickly converted into body fat. High-fructose corn syrup—made up of half glucose and half fructose—is even more problematic, and is a key ingredient in many processed and fast foods.

Recent studies have shown that the liver is less able to prevent fructose (as compared to glucose) from being converted to fat. In one study, individuals had to drink a breakfast drink that was 100 percent glucose, then in another test a drink that was half glucose and half fructose, and in a third test a drink of 25 percent glucose and 75 percent fructose. The research showed that lipogenesis, the process by which sugars are turned into body fat, increased substantially at the point when even half the glucose was replaced with fructose. Interestingly, even if the fructose was given at breakfast, the body still stored fat more easily as late as lunchtime.

If you want to minimize fructose, there's one key thing to do: if you see high-fructose corn syrup listed as a packaged food's ingredient, cut that item out of your diet completely. You will also want to eliminate processed and packaged foods that list crystalline fructose, honey, or sorbitol as key ingredients.

Don't forget drinks—commercial drinks are loaded with high-fructose corn syrup. You'll find it in sodas, fruit juices, sports drinks, lemonade, iced tea, and almost every sweet drink on the market. Apple juice, apple cider, and pear juice are made from higher-fructose fruits, so you may want to limit them or avoid them entirely. Also watch your intake of pears, cherries, peaches, plums, grapes, dates, prunes, and apples, as these fruits are higher in fructose.

Alcohol

Alcohol is empty calories, and whether it's a part of your diet plan is going to be up to you. If you do choose to drink, the heart-healthiest option is a glass of red wine. And make it a point to avoid liqueurs, cordials, and frozen restaurant drinks—such as margaritas—which can have hundreds of calories a glass and sometimes are loaded with sugar. Alcohol may slow or even stall your weight-loss effort, so if you think you are doing everything right but you're still not losing weight, try even a week or two without any alcohol and see if it gets the scale moving again.

CHAPTER 7

Popular Diet Programs: Making Them Work for You

A balanced diet is a cookie in each hand.

—Unknown

What if the guidelines from the last chapter are not enough for you? Do you want a specific diet to follow? Would you prefer shakes and bars, shopping lists, recipes, smartphone apps, in-person centers, a week away to get things started, food delivery, or other services and support to help provide a system, structure, and specific plan that you can follow?

The challenge is that there are always hundreds of different diets and diet programs that are popular at any given time. Just follow Oprah's highly publicized efforts to lose weight, and you can get a snapshot of the diet trends of the last two decades. Oprah has done everything from liquid protein diets to high-carb/low-fat diets and vegan cleanses. (And we all know how *that* has worked out for her.) If you go online, walk into a bookstore, turn on the television, or open a magazine, you can't get away from someone—a doctor, actress, chef, even Dr. Phil—telling you how to lose weight, what books to buy, what special diet products to eat, what workouts to do, and so on. It's an ever-changing cast of characters and an ever-changing list of options. Should you eat like Gwyneth, Jen, or Angelina? Take weight loss and fitness advice from Jackie, Jillian, or "The Situation"? Detox, fast, master-cleanse, or go macrobiotic? Be a carblover, a carb-cycler, or carb-controlled? Go four-day g-free, or just be "you" on a diet? Be a "skinny bitch" or smash some fat? How about whole foods, raw foods, vegan, vegetarian, or caveman diets?

Is your head spinning? Mine is! Maybe we should just move to France—after all, French women don't get fat!

Seriously, who has time to figure it out?

The truth is, I have looked at hundreds of popular diets, heard from thousands of thyroid patients who have tried to lose weight, and talked to dozens of the nation's best thyroid, hormone, and nutrition experts, and based on that research, I have identified several approaches that I think you want to consider.

My criteria? The programs I highly recommend:

- Are fundamentally healthy and balanced
- Offer a way of eating that can be maintained relatively easily and without more exotic ingredients, as in you won't be living on raw bok choy juice or ostrich burgers
- Do not require purchase of their own proprietary foods or supplements
- Do not involve your joining a multilevel marketing pyramid company
- Are not promoted by shady middle-of-the-night infomercials
- Are suited for and adaptable to thyroid patients

I've evaluated them in terms of what we know about effectiveness, general good health, and, perhaps most important, how they fit for us as thyroid patients, especially given that many of us are struggling with the challenge of an inefficient metabolism, compounded by insulin and leptin resistance.

What I have found is that a variety of programs that may be good fits for thyroid patients who want to lose weight and enjoy good health. These recommendations include:

- Dr. Ann Louise Gittleman's Fat Flush Diet
- Dr. Ron Rosedale's Rosedale Diet
- Kat James' Truth About Beauty approach
- Mark Sisson's Primal Blueprint Diet
- Dr. Mark Hyman's UltraMetabolism Diet
- Dr. Arthur Agatston's South Beach Diet

In this chapter, I'll tell you a bit more about these diets and why I'm recommending them. But my recommendations do not mean to exclude other approaches or systems. In fact, I've also included a number of other popular approaches and systems that I feel have merit for thyroid patients and may be the right fit for you. And just because a diet or way of eating is not mentioned here or I don't highly recommend it does not mean that it may not work for you individually.

Remember: for thyroid patients, one size does not fit all. That applies as much to choosing the optimal diet plan as it does to thyroid medications.

RECOMMENDED PROGRAMS

Fat Flush Diet: Ann Louise Gittleman, PhD, CNS

Ann Louise Gittleman, PhD, CNS, is a naturopath and nutritionist who has tremendous insight into weight-loss challenges, particularly those facing women and thyroid patients. Dr. Gittleman herself has thyroid imbalances, and she has been a leader in understanding the relationships that connect hormones, allergies, parasites, metabolism, and weight loss.

The centerpiece of Dr. Gittleman's weight-loss advice is found in her book *The Fat Flush Plan,* which focuses on supporting, cleansing, and detoxifying the liver while eating essential healthy fats, balanced proteins, and quality carbohydrates. *The Fat Flush Plan* specifically looks at what Dr. Gittleman refers to as the "five hidden factors that sabotage weight loss and vitality: liver health, food sensitivities and resulting waterlogged tissues, fear of eating fat, excess insulin/excess inflammation, and stress."

Fat Flush has a two week jump-start period, followed by Phase 2, the active fat flush, along with an eating plan for ongoing weight management.

For those who struggle to lose weight and also have significant gastrointestinal issues such as irritable bowel symptoms, her book *The Gut Flush Plan* is a good starting point to help calm and rebalance the intestinal system.

Her website, AnnLouise.com, has information about her books, a health blog, weight loss and health resources, and information about recommended products. She also has an active community that connects and shares information at her website's forums, and many of her fans are women with thyroid conditions.

Dr. Gittleman herself is very thyroid-savvy and is on the record as not recommending unfermented soy products or excessive raw goitrogens.

You can follow the Fat Flush Diet using foods readily available at your grocery, and no special products or supplements are required for the diet.

Dr. Ann Gittleman is the formulator of the protein powder that I personally find the best on the market for thyroid patients. It's called Body Protein, and it's a plant-based protein powder for use in smoothies. It's soy-free, dairy-free, gluten-free, lactose-free, low-glycemic, carbohydrate-controlled, and suitable for vegans and vegetarians. She has assembled a terrific combination of weight-loss supplements that I personally like and use that she calls the Fat Flush Kit. The kit includes her Dieters' Multivitamin and Mineral, a multivitamin that provides key nutrients helpful when dieting and for general health. (There is an iron-free version for thyroid patients who want to take the vitamin at the same time as their thyroid medication.) The kit also includes GLA-90—which contains the essential fatty acid gamma-linolenic acid—and her Weight Loss Formula contains chromium and acetyl-L-carnitine. The GLA and Weight Loss Formula are taken with meals, to help stabilize blood sugar and enhance metabolic efficiency.

Books: Selected books by Ann Louise Gittleman include: *The Fat Flush Plan, The Gut Flush Plan, Fat Flush for Life, Get the Sugar Out, The Fast Track Detox Diet, Zapped,* and *Guess What Came to Dinner: Parasites and Your Health.*

Websites: www.annlouise.com, www.unikeyhealth.com

The Rosedale Diet: Ron Rosedale, MD

Ron Rosedale, MD, is a physician with expertise in nutritional and metabolic medicine who says his goal is to eliminate or reduce the need for insulin in diabetics and reduce heart disease in patients, without drugs or surgery. Weight loss is not, therefore, Dr. Rosedale's primary objective. At the same time, as one of the more hormone-savvy doctors working in the field of nutrition, he has created a diet that is carbohydrate-controlled, yet also extremely healthy, in that it encourages sufficient but not excessive healthy protein, nutritious vegetables, and good fat.

Dr. Rosedale also focuses very specifically on reversing insulin and leptin resistance, and has some very specific approaches that are designed to help balance these hormones and activate the body's own ability to burn fat more effectively. Dr. Rosedale sums up the reason for his diet quite clearly:

> The idea of the medical profession to go on a high complex carbohydrate, low saturated-fat diet is an absolute oxymoron, because those high complex carbohydrate diets are nothing but a high glucose diet, or a high sugar diet, and your body is just going to store it as saturated fat.

The basic rules of the Rosedale Diet are straightforward: avoid sugar and non-fiber-containing starch—including potatoes, bread, rice, pasta, cereal, corn, and for the first several weeks whole grains. He generally suggests a diet heavy on vegetables (excluding starchy or sugary vegetables such as beets, yams, carrots, or tomatoes). He also advocates sufficient lower-fat protein, such as fish or poultry, but in a controlled, portion limited way. This is not in any way an "all the steak and bacon you can eat" diet.

Dr. Rosedale recommends limiting protein based on a person's size. His basic guideline is to estimate your optimal lean muscle weight in kilograms, and eat about 1 gram of protein per kilogram of desired weight per day, divided up in three servings per day. According to Dr. Rosedale, most people will require around 40 to 60 grams of protein a day.

Here's an example. If your target weight is 140 pounds, with 20 percent body fat, that means that your target lean muscle weight is 112 pounds (20 percent of 140 is 28, and 140 − 28 is 112), and 112 pounds is 50.8 kilograms. So you would be aiming for three servings of around 17 grams of protein each.

He recommends limiting fruit to a small serving of berries daily, limiting red meat, and snacking on nuts and olives. Also to be avoided: artificial sweeteners. Eating slowly, not eating for at least three hours before bedtime, and gentle exercise (including a walk after dinner) are also part of his approach.

Dr. Rosedale explains the science behind his recommendations very well, and his rules, while somewhat stringent by some standards, make for a healthy, carbohydrate-controlled diet.

Dr. Rosedale does not have a diet empire or a support system at his website. However, at his site you will find enough information to start the diet right away. I recommend his book for greater detail, explanation, and background. (Also, health advocate Kat James' Total Transformation workshops and teleseminars generally follow many of Dr. Rosedale's principles, and Dr. Rosedale has publicly supported Kat's approach, which is discussed later in this section.)

Book: *The Rosedale Diet*

Website: www.drrosedale.com

The Truth About Beauty and Total Transformation: Kat James

I've included Kat James, her book *The Truth About Beauty*, and her in-person and teleseminar-based Total Transformation program because she has an incredibly sensible, basic, and grounded view of food, eating, diet, and fitness. Kat is not a physician or health care practitioner—she actually started out in the world of beauty as a makeup artist in New York City. Kat battled an eating disorder and weight gain until she had her own "total transformation," completely changing the way she thought about her body, the way she ate, the way she exercised and moved, and her overall mind-set. The result? Kat dropped ten sizes and now maintains a slim size 4 figure without rigorous diet and exercise. And Kat is hypothyroid herself.

Kat's secret? A balanced, mindful eating program based on whole foods and incorporating many of the principles of Dr. Ron Rosedale's *Rosedale Diet*, along with some recommended supplements and life-style changes.

Frankly, I think every woman should own a copy of *The Truth About Beauty*, simply because Kat explains, in a sensible, no-nonsense way, how beauty really is from the inside out—and that applies not only to body shape and weight loss but also to skin, hair, nails, and aging.

I would have to describe Kat's dietary approach as much more Zen—it's not a structured "eat this and here's how to make it" book. There are no phases, and Kat does not have a line of protein bars or supplements for sale. I don't think there's even a single recipe in it.

The book is inspiring, featuring stories of transformations and how they happen. Kat gets right down into the nitty-gritty of the fact that most people who need to lose weight—even those who have thyroid conditions—also have an unhealthy relationship with food, and addressing that dysfunctional relationship needs to be the first step of any successful effort to lose weight.

You can follow Kat's approach simply by reading her book, which also includes an information-packed resources section featuring some of her favorite and recommended products and tools.

Kat also offers the opportunity to jump-start a transformative weight-loss effort by participating in one of her five-day Total Transformation programs in person, or one of her Total Transformation teleseminars. The in-person program includes food, drinks, and personal coaching. Both programs include educational information and one-on-one time with Kat herself.

In addition to her book and programs, Kat also hosts a weekly syndicated radio program, *The Kat James Show*, focusing on health issues.

Book: *The Truth About Beauty*

Website: www.informedbeauty.com

Total Transformation Program: www.totaltransformation.com

Radio Show: www.totaltransformation.com/kat_james_radio .html

Primal Blueprint (Paleo) Diet: Mark Sisson

A Paleolithic diet is a carbohydrate-controlled approach, focused on eating like a "caveman," so to speak. The idea is to return to the way that our earliest ancestors ate, focusing on meat, fish, vegetables, fruits, roots, and nuts and excluding grains, legumes, dairy products, salt, refined sugar, processed oils, and processed foods in general.

Loren Cordain started the trend with his book *The Paleo Diet*, but the book I think is the best on the topic is Mark Sisson's *Primal Blueprint* and his popular website, Mark's Daily Apple.

Sisson explains his basic premise: "The *Primal Blueprint* is a set of simple instructions (the blueprint) that allows you to control how your genes express themselves in order to build the strongest, leanest, healthiest body possible, taking clues from evolutionary biology (that's the primal part)."

Sisson's book combines science and common sense. Sisson is a former world-class endurance athlete, marathoner, Ironman, and now a health and fitness consultant, so he knows his stuff. In *Primal Blueprint*, he challenges what he calls "Conventional Wisdom"—always using the capital *C* and *W*—by outlining the science behind his recommendations that we follow some basic rules. These rules include eating animals and plants, moving a lot at a slow pace, lifting heavy things, running fast once in a while, getting a lot of sleep, playing, getting daily sunlight, avoiding trauma, avoiding poisonous things, and using your mind.

Sisson goes into much greater detail and provides guidelines on how to apply these rules to daily life. But the end result is a healthy, carbohydrate-controlled diet that does not involve measuring, calorie counting, or portion control.

One of Sisson's key tenets is that low-fat, grain-based diets are actually the root cause of many illnesses, diseases, and weight problems, and that excessive exercise may suppress the immune system and sabotage weight loss.

Book: *The Primal Blueprint*

Websites: www.primalblueprint.com, www.marksdailyapple.com

UltraMetabolism Diet: Mark Hyman, MD

Integrative physician Mark Hyman's healthy, sensible weight-loss program prepares the body for automatic weight loss. His book *UltraMetabolism* takes you through an eight-week program that promises to reboot your metabolism by focusing on improving the fundamental health problems that cause obesity and disease. For

Dr. Hyman, that means optimizing your brain chemistry, especially by eating healthy fats such as omega-3s and avoiding processed carbohydrates. Dr. Hyman also believes in eliminating gluten and supporting the thyroid. His book *The UltraSimple Diet* describes an accelerated seven-day plan to revitalize your health and is a simplified version of *UltraMetabolism*.

Keep in mind that Dr. Hyman's program does suggest incorporating soy protein, which can sabotage the thyroid in some people or impair a thyroid patient's success at weight loss, so you may want to substitute other options.

But generally, UltraMetabolism can be a healthy way to follow an eight-week program that takes a good look at a cross-section of health issues in order to optimize your health.

Books: Dr. Hyman has a number of books, but the two key books are *UltraMetabolism: The Simple Plan for Automatic Weight Loss* and *The UltraSimple Diet: Kick-Start Your Metabolism and Safely Lose Up to 10 Pounds in 7 Days*.

Websites: www.ultrametabolism.com, www.drhyman.com

South Beach Diet: Arthur Agatston, MD

South Beach Diet is an empire, with many millions of books sold, a series of cookbooks, a Web-based paid membership program, and a line of South Beach convenience foods and products.

If you shift away from the processed convenience foods and use the South Beach guidelines to follow a more whole-foods-based diet, South Beach can be a healthy, low-glycemic program that is not confusing to follow.

When starting South Beach, the first phase of the diet, which usually runs for two weeks, is designed to detox somewhat, help eliminate carbohydrate cravings, and kick-start the weight-loss process. During the first phase, a goal is also to help stabilize blood sugar and insulin levels, making it a good fit for thyroid patients who are insulin-resistant, prediabetic, or diabetic. In Phase 2, healthy low-glycemic carbohydrates are added to the Phase 1 food list. Phase 3 is maintenance and allows for a wider range of foods. It can be continued as a general way of eating for a lifetime.

The South Beach website is packed with features, including meal planners, a shopping list generator, a recipe finder, discussion groups, support forums where dieters interact with each other, guides for dining out and fast-food restaurants, a weight tracker, and much more.

Books: There are numerous South Beach books, including recipe books, restaurant dining guides, and more, but the key book is *South Beach Diet Supercharged: Faster Weight Loss and Better Health for Life.*

Website: www.southbeachdiet.com

CARBOHYDRATE-CONTROLLED AND LOW-CARB DIETS

Atkins Diet

The Atkins Diet conquered the planet more than thirty years ago with a new concept in dieting: replace carbohydrates with protein and fat. There is much controversy as to whether or not low-carb, high-protein, high-fat diets are healthy. This famous diet program has a free website, which explains the four-phase plan with interactive tools, food ideas, recipes, success stories, an active online community, a food journal, a shopping list, a recipe box, a BMI calculator, and Atkins food products.

Atkins emphasizes protein and fat in the diet, with carefully controlled carbohydrates. Atkins does not count total carbs, but rather a concept called "net carbs," where you subtract the fiber grams from the total carb grams, to come up with the net level. The Atkins

Diet uses this net carb calculation on the premise that fiber-rich carbohydrates do not affect blood sugar the same way as simple carbohydrates do.

In the early stages of the diet, most carbohydrates come from high-fiber, nonstarchy vegetables, while low-glycemic fruits, starchier vegetables, and legumes are introduced later.

Atkins has suffered from the reputation that it's an all-you-can-eat steak-and-bacon diet. Jimmy Moore, a professional health blogger and author—and founder of the Livin' La Vida Low-Carb website, book, and podcasts—has advocated for low-carbohydrate diets like Atkins for a number of years. Says Moore:

> The Atkins Diet never said anything about just eating meat and bacon—they *always* promoted vegetables, and never encouraged people to gorge on meat and bacon. This idea of unlimited steak and cheese and fatty food became the media's shorthand to mock Dr. Atkins. That's why, when people say to me, "I went on the Atkins Diet," but they ate only meat, eggs, and cheese, I say, "That's the media version of the Atkins Diet."

The *New Atkins for a New You* book and approach are attempting to shift that perception, and now include a daily requirement of a substantial amount of high-fiber vegetables, what the program calls "foundation vegetables." But keep in mind that Atkins is still primarily a low-carbohydrate diet that focuses on animal protein and does not attempt to limit saturated fat.

Note that the Atkins Diet may not be suited for vegan or vegetarian thyroid patients, as soy protein is often recommended in large quantities to those who wish to modify the Atkins Diet to exclude meat and fish. Also note that the shakes, bars, and other food products sold under the Atkins name are frequently highly processed, and often use soy as their primary protein.

Book: There are many books that outline the Atkins Diet, but the most recent is Dr. Eric Westman's *New Atkins for a New You: The Ultimate Diet for Shedding Weight and Feeling Great.*

Website: www.atkins.com

Livin' La Vida Low-Carb Diet

Jimmy Moore is a one-man low-carb empire. After successfully losing more than a hundred pounds himself with a modified version of the Atkins Diet, Moore turned his own health triumph into a mission as a professional health blogger and author. He now has a successful book, website, blog, podcast, and video series that focus on all aspects of following a low-carbohydrate lifestyle—or, as Moore calls it, Livin' La Vida Low-Carb.

Moore's books outline the approaches he has used over the years to successfully lose weight and maintain the weight loss, and his community is a hub of support and information for low-carb dieters, including an active group of thyroid patients.

According to Moore, "You can do everything to fix your thyroid, but if the diet isn't under control, you won't get the weight-loss results you want." At the same time, Moore recognizes the role of thyroid treatment in successful weight loss. "As much as I love and support low-carb, it's not the be-all and end-all—some people definitely also need thyroid treatment."

There is no official diet to follow—followers of Livin' La Vida Low-Carb follow general low-carb principles, and Moore and his readers exchange ideas, support, and information about the low-carb lifestyle. "Controlling insulin levels is the primary theme song of Livin' La Vida Low-Carb," says Moore.

In addition to his website, books, and a video series on YouTube, Moore hosts a popular podcast, where he interviews some of the nation's leading voices on nutrition, healthy eating, and the low-carb lifestyle. Moore also hosts an annual Low-Carb Cruise, which features a number of doctors, authors, and experts on the low-carb lifestyle as speakers.

Books: *21 Life Lessons from Livin' La Vida Low-Carb: How the Healthy Low-Carb Lifestyle Changed Everything I Thought I Knew;* and *Livin' La Vida Low-Carb: My Journey from Flabby Fat to Sensationally Skinny in One Year*

Website: www.livinlavidalowcarb.com

Moore's list of low-carb-friendly doctors: www.lowcarbdoctors. blogspot.com

SUPPORT SYSTEMS

Weight Watchers

Weight Watchers is both a diet and a support system.

The organization has been around for years, and started out primarily as a support group, where people got together for meetings, shared their successes, talked about strategies, and got advice regarding diet.

Basically, with the Weight Watchers approach, you're keeping track of what you're eating, and categorizing it in various food groups. Weight Watchers has always been a largely calories-in, calories-out sort of approach, and it is not a pioneer in understanding insulin resistance, leptin issues, or the physiology of weight loss. (You'll find Weight Watchers recommending popcorn, pasta, and other higher-glycemic-index starches, for example.) I've also heard many stories from thyroid patients who, like me, tried Weight Watchers at some point, followed it to the letter, and gained weight. I even had a Weight Watchers leader suggest to me that I must not be following the program when in fact I was, including exercise. This was before my thyroid diagnosis. Even after my thyroid diagnosis, losing weight on Weight Watchers required that I avoid recommended snacks and eat at the absolute lowest possible number of points to lose even a small amount of weight each week.

The challenge is that Weight Watchers is not inherently a low-glycemic or carbohydrate-controlled diet, which is why some thyroid patients may not find themselves losing much weight on the program. If you want to control carbohydrates, you'll have to tweak the diet recommendations to cut back on or eliminate bread, pasta, rice, and other simple carbohydrates that are regularly featured as part of Weight Watchers' menus and recipes.

That said, Weight Watchers can be a great resource for someone who has not tried to lose weight before and who needs to start off with the idea of portion control, balance in the diet, and incorporating gentle exercise; in particular, it's good for someone who knows he or she will respond best to a support-oriented community. Weight Watchers—whether in meetings or online—offers easy-to-follow instructions, many ideas on what to eat, and recipes for preparation.

In addition to the option of attending in-person meetings, Weight Watchers online offers a host of tools, including a journal, a weight tracker, meal plans, point calculators, recipe search, an active online community, and more.

Keep in mind that some of the Weight Watchers prepared foods sold online and in grocery stores are highly processed, and some do contain soy.

Kay had her thyroid removed twenty years ago and has slowly and steadily gained weight since then:

> Doctors told me that it would be impossible to lose weight. Just after topping 200, I decided that it was time to do something. I joined Weight Watchers online (no meetings, no weigh-ins). Now, after six months, I have lost twenty-four pounds. I'm not there yet, but I am losing. Slowly, but I'm losing. Being on Weight Watchers has made me very aware of the hidden calories in my diet. I have already noticed an increase in my energy level (okay, a slight increase!) and an improvement in how my knees feel. More exciting

for me, I have gone down one full size in my clothes. I have tried other diets before but none have worked.

Books: *Weight Watchers Eat! Move! Play!*; *Weight Watchers New Complete Cookbook Momentum Edition*; *Weight Watchers New Complete Cookbook*; *Weight Watchers Annual Recipes for Success 2010*; *Weight Watchers in 20 Minutes*; and *Weight Watchers All-Time Favorites*

Website: www.weightwatchers.com

Telephone: 800-651-6000

Take Off Pounds Sensibly (TOPS)

Established in 1948, Take Off Pounds Sensibly (TOPS) is a nonprofit weight loss and wellness organization with 170,000 members, age seven and up. TOPS has ten thousand chapters in the United States and Canada.

There is a very low annual fee (usually less than $30) for TOPS membership, which gives you full access to all areas of the TOPS website, including My Day One (a ready-set-go guide); a one-year subscription to TOPS News; plus membership in a local chapter of your choice for weekly weigh-ins and support.

The TOPS program rests on support for choosing and keeping track of a healthy diet, based on portion control and the Exchange System, which divides foods into six food groups. The ratio of carbohydrate, protein, and fat determines the placement of a food into a specific food group. Within the TOPS program, the exchange portion of a food is determined by each food's weight in grams. Foods within a group are considered "equivalent." Any specific food may be substituted for or exchanged for another food from the same group.

TOPS offers a broader program, not necessarily minute-by-minute instruction. The success of this diet is in teaching portion control and providing a support community for encouragement, guidance, and accountability. If you are someone who finds strength in a shared journey, you may benefit from this approach.

Book: *The TOPS Way to Weight Loss*

Website: www.tops.org

Telephone: 414-482-4620

Overeaters Anonymous

Overeaters Anonymous (OA) is a program of recovery from compulsive eating using the familiar "twelve steps" approach to addiction. OA addresses dysfunctional behaviors such as binge eating, obsession with body image, starvation, obsessive tryouts of many diet programs, use of laxatives or diuretics, and bulimia. With meetings around the world, OA provides a fellowship of experience, strength, and hope.

OA is not a weight-loss organization and does not promote a particular diet. Rather, OA focuses on physical, emotional, and spiritual well-being, and offers support for curbing behaviors that result in overeating. It is not a religious organization. OA charges no dues or fees and is self-supporting through member contributions. The only requirements to attend a meeting are mutual respect and a desire to stop compulsive eating. There are currently 6,500 meeting places in seventy-five countries.

If emotional eating, eating disorders, obsessive eating, or obsessive dieting is an obstacle to weight loss, support from OA may be a helpful adjunct to a healthy diet and exercise program.

Books: *Letting Go of Compulsive Eating: Twelve Step Recovery from Compulsive Eating—Daily Meditations; Recovering Compulsive Overeater—Daily Meditation; Overeaters Anonymous; Overeater's Journal: Exercises for the Heart, Mind and Soul; Abstinence: Members of Overeaters Anonymous Share Their Experience, Strength, and Hope; Recovery from Compulsive Eating: A Complete Guide to*

the Twelve Step Program; Compulsive Overeater: The Basic Text for Compulsive Overeaters; and *Twelve Step Workbook*
   Website: www.oa.org
   Telephone: 505-891-2664

OTHER DIETS

Weight Loss Centers

Physicians Weight Loss Centers and Diet Center are both franchise companies that have a number of local centers, along with online programs. Both programs feature a number of different diets, plus extensive lines of nutritional protein supplements, bars, shakes, snacks, and supplements.

Online, their sites have BMI and body fat calculators, support communities, and other resources.

Physicians Weight Loss Centers claim that 1.5 million clients have completed their program, and Diet Center's website says its program has helped 15 million people.

If you like one-on-one support, the local centers may be a help to you, though each local center is only as good as its employees, and some of the counselors or consultants may have only several weeks of training, making them glorified salespeople, not experts in weight loss.

For in-center services, these programs can also be costly, running from $400 to $1,000 for a three-month period, not including signup and program fees. At in-person centers, you are also likely to experience "upsell," where counselors attempt to sell you supplements that are usually fairly high-priced compared to similar supplements available elsewhere.

Thyroid patients need to be aware that many of the foods and supplements offered by these companies contain soy protein. This is a serious consideration, as many of these products are intended to be meal replacements.

Websites: www.pwlc.com, www.dietcenter.com

Residential Centers or Spas

If you have money and time to spare and you're looking to kick-start a diet program, you may want to look into a residential or spa-based diet program. There are many residential weight-loss programs; some run for five days or a week, others are multiweek programs. Some are more spa-based and luxurious, while others are more medically oriented, with a more intensive focus on fitness.

Some of the premier medical or fitness-oriented programs include:

- Duke Diet and Fitness Center, Durham, North Carolina
- Hilton Head Health, Hilton Head Island, South Carolina
- The Pritikin Longevity Center, Aventura, Florida
- Cooper Wellness Program, Dallas, Texas
- New Life Hiking Spa, Killington, Vermont
- Red Mountain Spa, St. George, Utah

Some of the premier spa-oriented programs include:

- The Oaks at Ojai, California
- Cal-a-Vie, Vista, California
- The Greenhouse, Arlington, Texas
- Canyon Ranch, Tucson, Arizona
- Canyon Ranch, Lenox, Massachusetts

Needless to say, these programs can be expensive, ranging from several hundred dollars a day to thousands of dollars a day, depending on where you go. Two weeks at the prestigious Duke Diet and

Fitness Center in Durham, North Carolina, can run $4,000, and a week at the luxurious Cal-a-Vie Spa near San Diego, California, is more than $8,000. The New Life Hiking Spa in Vermont and Red Mountain Spa in Utah, however, have all-inclusive programs of accommodations, meals, and fitness hiking for weight loss that run from $200 to $300 a day.

For a residential program to kick-start a healthy eating program, I also recommend Kat James' Total Transformation Program, which takes place in Lake Lure, North Carolina. The five-day program includes a one-on-one educational session, group educational sessions, all meals, drinks, and snacks, a makeover and photo shoot, excursions and hiking, and accommodations, and costs around $3,000. Kat's nutritional guidelines are in part based on the Rosedale Diet's carbohydrate-controlled approach.

A detailed list of residential weight-loss centers and weight-loss spas is featured at this book's website at ThyroidDietRevolution.com.

Prepared Food: Jenny Craig and Nutrisystem

In the United States, two popular, heavily advertised diet programs compete for the prepared food diet market: Jenny Craig and Nutrisystem. The programs are similar, offering prepared meals and snacks along with support for changes in diet and activity level.

Both programs offer at-home or center-based programs and involve working with a consultant to help guide and motivate. There are customized programs specifically for seniors and type 2 diabetics. Jenny Craig also has special programs for men and teens. Nutrisystem has a vegetarian program. Online, program members have access to an active support forum, articles, tips, recipes, a menu planner, a progress planner, a journal, and an activity planner.

Generally, the idea is that by following the program menus, participants practice habits such as portion control and learn strategies to manage emotional eating, so that eventually they are ready to take over preparing their own menus and maintaining weight loss.

The strength of these programs is also their weakness—if you do not want to have to really think about what to prepare or how to prepare it, prepared foods take that out of your hands. But reports suggest that many of the meals are not especially tasty. And while they may be healthier than what you are currently eating, keep in mind that the prepared meals rely on a fair amount of processed foods, and some of the prepared foods may have soy protein, so read labels carefully before purchasing.

According to Jenny Craig's website, "Jenny Craig clients, on average, spend just a $1 a day more on Jenny's Cuisine than the typical American spends on food." That's their way of saying that their program can be a bit pricey.

For both Jenny Craig and Nutrisystem, expect to pay somewhere in the range of $300 to $400 or more per month for program food, not including signup and program fees, supplements, additional snacks, and other food items such as fresh vegetables.

Books: There are a number of books published by the Jenny Craig and Nutrisystem organizations, including cookbooks and overviews of the program.

Websites: www.jennycraig.com, www.nutrisystem.com

Meal Replacement Programs

Optifast, Medifast, and Lindora are diet programs that combine diets of their specialized foods—for Optifast it's shakes, soups, and bars, while Medifast and Lindora have a wider variety of foods—along with counseling on lifestyle changes and exercise. The LA Weight Loss program, which used to have in-person centers, is now LA to Your Door, a Web-based meal replacement plan featuring shakes and bars, snacks, juices, and supplements.

Optifast claims their patients typically lose fifty-two pounds over a twenty-two-week program period. (They also say, however, that for many dieters, weight loss is only temporary.) Medifast cites clinical studies that indicate that most people lose an average of up to two to five pounds a week on their program. Lindora, which has a forty-year history, has clinics in Southern California, along with an online program.

Optifast and Lindora use soy in some of its products, and Medifast foods have fructose and soy as well.

Pricing for Optifast is vague, but it's estimated that a twenty-two-week program costs from $1,000 to $2,000, which includes medical supervision, weekly therapy sessions, and lab work. The cost of food products is extra and can run $100 a week or more.

Medifast tends to run about $300 or more per month, with no enrollment or membership fees.

Lindora's clinic costs can run $1,000 for a ten-week program, and its online programs may run in the $500 range.

For LA to Your Door, soy protein is central to almost every one of their food products, and the products tend to be pricey. It's actually quite easy to find protein shakes, protein bars, and supplements for weight loss that are not only free of soy products but far less expensive.

Websites: www.optifast.com, www.medifast1.com, www.lindora.com, www.latoyourdoor.com

Biggest Loser Diet: Jillian Michaels

Let's face it—we've all seen her on television. And if you've seen her, then like most people, you have an opinion—either you love her or you definitely don't. Jillian Michaels, known as the "tough trainer" on NBC's *The Biggest Loser*, is a controversial figure. While she manages to whip people into shape on various television shows she appears on, she does so with an aggressive style that doesn't work for everyone.

Michaels' diet plan is generally sound and emphasizes organically grown and unprocessed foods. In addition to her book *Master Your Metabolism*, her membership website has a variety of online tools: an interactive weight tracker, fitness advice videos, a calorie calculator, weight-loss buddies, hundreds of recipes and menus, printable exercises, and a community with interactive message boards. Some thyroid patients are understandably drawn to Michaels because of her high-profile television shows and larger-than-life personality, but also because Michaels herself is hypothyroid and writes about the importance of supporting the thyroid in her book. This means that Michaels also does recommend avoiding soy, and understands how to navigate the issue of goitrogenic vegetables.

At the same time, there are some reasons to be wary. There have been issues and lawsuits about Michael's line of supplements and their side effects, suggesting that being a personal trainer does not necessarily translate into safe and knowledgeable formulation of nutritional supplements. Michaels once told a women's magazine that while she would like to be a mother, she would adopt rather than give birth, because "I can't handle doing that to my body." Michaels is also a proponent of hours of intensive exercise a day. On *The Biggest Loser*, she takes pride in making her participants pass out or vomit from exercise.

My opinion? Maybe I'm playing amateur psychologist here, but Michaels has talked about how she was overweight as a teen and how traumatized it made her feel. She may not be overweight now, but I don't believe Michaels herself has an especially healthy or balanced attitude about weight or her body, hence her aggressive attitude about weight loss and excessive exercise.

The truth is, exercise is not supposed to make you nauseous. Chronic intense exercise is interpreted by the body as stress, and it raises cortisol levels, exacerbates the body's stress reaction, and can actually sabotage weight loss.

If an intense, boot-camp-style, in-your-face, shame-driven approach to weight loss and your body appeals to you, then Jillian Michaels might be a good fit. But do keep in mind that her fitness recommendations may actually be counterproductive to weight loss for people with hormonal imbalances.

Book: *Master Your Metabolism: The 3 Diet Secrets to Naturally Balancing Your Hormones for a Hot and Healthy Body*
Websites: www.jillianmichaels.com

The Zone Diet

The Zone Diet was the big diet on the scene before South Beach came along and simplified the idea of balancing fat, protein, and carbs. The Zone Diet still has its adherents, however, who believe in the diet's principle that an optimal diet has a precise balance of fat, protein, and carbohydrates that allow you to be "in the zone."

The Zone was one of the first diets to go against the conventional wisdom that unlimited amounts of low-fat carbohydrates were healthy and effective for weight loss, instead focusing on high-fiber carbs and balancing any carbohydrates with protein and good fat to lower the glycemic effect. The challenge with the Zone is that it can be very complicated to calculate the ratios, and some have accused the diet of being so complicated that it's "worse than an itemized tax return."

For those who are interested in the Zone approach, along with the book, the program has a full-featured website and various Zone food products, including shakes, bars, and other meal replacements. Note, however, that prepackaged foods—such as the bagels, granola, rolls, bread, pasta, and grain-based snacks found in the Zone Fast Track two-week program of food delivery—may be too carb-intensive for some thyroid patients. The delivery program offers complete prepared meals and snacks, following the Zone principles, delivered to your home, for around $40 or more a day.

Books: *The Zone Diet, The Anti-Inflammation Zone, Mastering the Zone,* and more
Website: www.zonediet.com, www.inthezonedelivery.com

Eat Right 4 Your Type (Blood Type) Diet

In *Eat Right 4 Your Type*, naturopath Peter D'Adamo makes a case that diet should be matched to individual blood types: A, B, O, and AB. D'Adamo's basic idea is that different blood types react differently with components of foods, and that these differences are based on evolution of the blood types over time. D'Adamo offers recommended foods, vitamins, and supplements for different blood types, for both weight loss and health.

This idea is controversial, to say the least, and most dieticians, physicians, and scientists say that D'Adamo's theory is unsupported by scientific evidence. Yet I have heard from some patients who have found this approach useful when all else failed.

Book: Peter J. D'Adamo, MD, *Eat Right 4 Your Type: The Individualized Diet Solution to Staying Healthy, Living Longer and Achieving Your Ideal Weight*, and others

Website: www.dadamo.com

Cookie Diets: The Cookie Diet, Smart for Life

Diets that rely on hunger-controlling meal replacement cookies and shakes to keep calories low while claiming to suppress hunger have been around for a long time—in the case of Sanford Siegal's Cookie Diet, more than thirty years. The food purchases average $100 a week.

Siegal's Cookie Diet has been mentioned in connection with thyroid issues because Siegal, a Florida-based weight-loss doctor, wrote a book called *Is Your Thyroid Making You Fat?* In this book, Dr. Siegal has people follow a very low-calorie diet in an attempt to see if they have a sluggish metabolism and signs of an undiagnosed thyroid problem. Dr. Siegal believes, rightly, that undiagnosed thyroid disease is making it difficult for some people to lose weight. His solution is his Cookie Diet, which involves eating his special cookies throughout the day and then having a healthy dinner of a lean protein and vegetables. (Smart for Life has a similar approach, and apparently the doctor who runs that program used to work with Dr. Siegal.)

I've tasted the various cookies for both programs, and I have to tell you, I can't imagine lasting more than a few weeks on them. For someone who really needs convenience, maybe a few weeks on a cookie diet might work to help jump-start a diet, but this kind of approach is not going to teach you how to eat, how to properly use food to manage your metabolism, and how to balance your blood sugar.

They are really no different from any of the other meal replacement weight-loss programs, except the cookies are, in my opinion, one of the worst-tasting meal replacements available.

Websites: www.cookiediet.com, www.smartforlife.com

SOME HELPFUL TOOLS

Fat Flush Body Protein

My favorite protein powder is Fat Flush Body Protein, formulated by Dr. Ann Louise Gittleman, founder of the popular Fat Flush Diet. Body Protein is a high-protein, low-carbohydrate plant-based protein powder used for smoothies. It features a blend of yellow pea and brown rice proteins that provide a complete protein source of essential amino acids.

According to Dr. Gittleman:

> Clinical studies have shown that plant-based proteins can curb your appetite, support weight loss, boost metabolism, and support the thyroid as well. One study reported that low-carb dieters substantially more weight by getting most of their protein from plants, compared to meat.

Dr. Gittleman designed Body Protein to be hypoallergenic and free of any genetically modified ingredients.

Many individuals who have dairy intolerance, or a sensitivity to casein, lactose, or dairy by-products, can't tolerate even a very pure whey protein powder. That was my impetus to create Body Protein, which is soy-free, dairy-free, gluten-free, and has no eggs, sugar, wheat, salt, corn, or artificial sweeteners, colors, or flavors.

The powder comes in a mild vanilla flavor and is sweetened with stevia and inulin, a prebiotic that nourishes good bacteria in the gastrointestinal tract. It provides a low-glycemic, steady flow of energy, and is designed to provide a feeling of fullness for hours.

I've tried many different protein powders, and Fat Flush Body Protein is unquestionably my favorite. I have a mild lactose intolerance, so I can feel bloated using even a good-quality whey protein. I still have a thyroid gland and take thyroid hormone replacement medication, so I am not comfortable using a soy-based protein powder. And honestly, a smoothie made with Body Protein makes me feel full much longer than any other smoothie or shake I've tried. I regularly use it to make a breakfast smoothie. It takes less than a minute to prepare in my blender, and I feel full for at least three to four hours.

Fat Flush Body Protein is available from Uni Key Health.

Website: www.unikeyhealth.com

Telephone: 800-888-4353

Dr. Levine's Ultimate Weight Loss Formula

One of my favorite fiber products is Dr. Levine's Ultimate Weight Loss Formula, or DLUWLF for short. The formula was developed by Scott Levine, MD—who is board-certified in internal medicine and in antiaging and regenerative medicine—as a weight-loss aid for his patients. DLUWLF is a patented powder that, when mixed in water, creates a zero-calorie high-fiber beverage that features five different fibers, including pectin, locust bean, guar, psyllium, and oat. One full serving a day activates nerve fibers in the stomach to help you feel full and provides a high dose of heart-healthy, cholesterol-lowering fiber. DLUWLF also includes the B vitamins folic acid and pyridoxine, as well as antioxidants. A side benefit of this supplement is that it blunts the insulin spike that occurs when food first enters the stomach.

Dr. Levine is knowledgeable about thyroid disease, and his high-fiber supplement has no iron, soy protein, or ingredients that interact with thyroid medication. DLUWLF does not contain any stimulants, nor does it contain sugar, saccharine, or NutraSweet (aspartame). Some versions are sweetened with Splenda (sucralose), and some have no sweetener.

Note that while the product does not contain gluten, a small percentage of people who are gluten-sensitive react to oats, and DLUWLF does contain oat proteins. Also, patients taking anti-seizure prescriptions, blood thinners, and protein-bound medicines need to check with their physicians regarding interactions between high-fiber supplements and their medications.

For weight loss, Dr. Levine has found it most effective to use the DLUWLF formula before one meal a day—lunch or dinner. He recommends preparing one drink an hour before the meal, and then the second drink thirty minutes later (thirty minutes before eating the meal). DLUWLF can also be used as a calorie-free snack. Two drinks—which is considered one full serving—provide 35 grams of fiber, which is the recommended optimal fiber intake for weight loss and heart health.

DLUWLF tastes fine. (I've tried both the chocolate and raspberry flavors, and they're good, especially when compared to trying to choke down a couple of spoonfuls of psyllium husks floating around in a glass of water!)

According to Levine, many people who use his product lose one and a half to three pounds per week without doing anything else differently—a result achieved because of reduction of food intake, combined with reduced insulin resistance and blood sugar levels, due to the increased fiber in the diet. Because Levine's formula includes both soluble and insoluble fibers, it has other benefits, including reduction of cholesterol.

Says Dr. Levine: "The right kinds of fiber can be particularly helpful for insulin metabolism, especially in people who have even a few extra pounds around the middle. That abdominal weight gain—which drives increasing insulin levels, and is the start of the whole metabolic syndrome—can be helped by high-fiber consumption."

Important warning: If you start a high-fiber diet or a high-fiber supplement such as DLUWLF, be very careful that you are taking your thyroid medicine no less than three to four hours before using the fiber supplement, so that your medication absorption is not affected. Also, because high-fiber diets in general can change your dosage requirements, six to eight weeks after starting a high-fiber diet or high-fiber supplement, you should have your thyroid levels tested to make sure you don't need a dosage change to account for the dietary fiber.

Website: www.thindoctor.com

Telephone: 800-641-2907

Meal Delivery Services

Sometimes the idea of buying and preparing healthy food may seem daunting, but at the same time you can't stomach the idea of living on weight-loss cookies, protein bars, and other meal replacements while you lose weight. That's when a meal delivery service may be a good option. While delivery services can seem expensive at first look, you'll want to total up your costs to purchase fresh food and the time involved in shopping, cooking, and cleanup. The daily cost of a meal delivery service—which ranges from $20 to $40 a day for three meals, a snack or dessert, condiments and sides—actually may be a good value for some dieters.

If you are in a major metropolitan area, some of the services offer delivery or pickup of freshly prepared meals, and may even have sample tastings so you can try some of the foods and dishes. The major services also offer shipment of frozen meals by overnight delivery.

Some of the services have low-carb, low-glycemic, and even vegetarian or vegan options, and in some cases you can exclude dairy or seafood. You'll get to choose from among more than one hundred meals at eDiets, while Diet to Go typically has a five-week rotation of meals, with a fixed menu for each week.

Dieters report that if you're in one of the areas that offer fresh delivery, the food from these services can be excellent; even if you have to have the meals delivered frozen, these services generally have food that tastes better than supermarket frozen meals such as Jenny Craig and Weight Watchers.

A list of popular meal delivery services is featured online at the book's website, ThyroidDietRevolution.com, and the following are websites and phone numbers for several of the key delivery programs.

- Diet-to-Go, www.diettogo.com, 800-743-SLIM
- eDiets, www.ediets.com, 800-650-9052
- BistroMD, www.bistromd.com, 866-401-DIET
- Freshology, www.freshology.com, 877-89FRESH

CHAPTER 8

Vitamins, Supplements, and Herbs

Nature heals under the auspices of the medical profession.

— HAVEN EMERSON

There is no shortage of miracle supplements promising to help you lose weight without any effort whatsoever. We are constantly subjected to an incessant battery of hype—the never-ending late-night infomercials, bus stop advertisements and billboards, magazine and newspaper ads, e-mail spam, and multilevel marketers—all trying to sell us the latest miracle diet supplement. You know, it's the one that will finally melt your extra pounds while you sleep, allow you to eat anything you want and still lose weight—and all without exercising!

Do they work? Do we really need to ask? The truth is—and you don't need me to tell you this—there is no miraculous diet pill for anyone, much less for thyroid patients in particular. So forget about the amazing Thyro-Weight-Be-Gone or GlandUSlim or SkinnyRoid or whatever ridiculous new capsule comes along to try to take advantage of thyroid patients.

Because they're a rip-off.

I get hundreds of e-mails each week from frustrated thyroid patients who are trying to lose weight, and I guarantee you, if any of these pills worked, I would be hearing from the legions of people who are thrilled with their miracle pills. So far, in more than fifteen years of thyroid advocacy work, I haven't heard from anyone who has had success on a "miracle pill" yet. And yes, I've occasionally fallen prey myself to the overblown marketing claims and tried a bottle or two of too-good-to-be-true miracle pills, and they haven't solved the problem. No matter what, I'm always back to eating well, moving, sleeping, and managing my stress.

That said, there are some supplements and herbs that may help you in your weight-loss efforts. Keep in mind that none of these supplements replaces the need to eat well and move. And remember that when it comes to supplements to aid in weight loss, one size does not fit all. Some supplements will do nothing at all for you; some might actually have the opposite effect. (There are *always* a few people who have a completely opposite reaction to pills and supplements.) Keep in mind that some supplements have undergone various studies and trials, and others have been in use for centuries as part of traditional Chinese medicine or Ayurvedic remedies. Some are included mainly on the basis of practitioner experience and patient evidence-based medicine (known derogatorily by some conventional authorities as "anecdotal evidence").

To ensure that there are no problems with interactions between prescription medications and supplements, always remember to check with your doctor or practitioner before starting new supplements or changing your supplement dose.

FIRST, A CAUTION

When it comes to diet supplements, I need to offer a caution. Be especially careful about diet supplements sold online. While a diet supplement sold in your local drugstore may not be effective or a good fit for you, it's more likely that it has gone through some sort of quality control process. But the products that are marketed and sold primarily online—including sometimes by online natural health stores that you trust—may pose a risk. In fact, you may not hear this in the media, but the Food and Drug Administration regularly recalls different brands of unregulated, over-the-counter diet supplements—usually imported supplements sold online—because they contain what are known as "undeclared drug ingredients." This means that these so-called natural or herbal weight-loss supplements are manufactured abroad, sold in the United States, and then recalled by the FDA because they are found to contain high levels of actual prescription drugs. Usually this happens after someone has reported adverse side effects or problems after taking the supplement. In the past few years, numerous "herbal" products have been recalled because they contained one or more of the following drugs:

- *Fenfluramine:* the dangerous "fen" in the fen-phen weight prescription combination that was pulled off the American market in 1997 for causing serious heart valve damage
- *Propranolol:* a prescription beta-blocker that can pose a risk to people with bronchial asthma and certain heart conditions
- *Sibutramine:* the generic name for the prescription weight-loss drug Meridia, which is a controlled substance and may cause an increased risk of heart attack and stroke
- *Ephedrine:* a synthetic version of ephedra, a stimulant drug that can pose a heart risk

Pop a few of these "natural" herbal diet supplements, and you could end up at risk of heart damage, heart attack, stroke, or other serious and irreversible health problems.

You'll want to be especially careful with diet supplements manufactured in China, because many of the supplements containing undeclared drug ingredients that have been sold on the Internet have been from Chinese manufacturers.

Be on the lookout also for some Chinese formulations that include ephedra, also known as ma huang. Ephedra is a central nervous system stimulant and was banned as a supplement ingredient in the United States in 2004. A synthetic form of ephedra, pseudoephedrine, is legal in the United States, but only as an ingredient in decongestants.

LEVEL 1: THE BASICS

There are a few supplements that you may want to consider as basic components of a weight-loss program.

Multivitamin

Anyone who is on a weight-loss program may want to consider starting with a good multivitamin. It can help round out the nutritional balance while you're cutting back on foods, and there is some evidence that a multivitamin can help with weight loss. One study found that obese women who took a standard multivitamin, even while continuing to eat their normal diets, lost an average of about three and a half pounds over six months, compared to no weight loss for those who took a placebo. Another study found that dieters who took a multivitamin supplement during a fifteen-week calorie-restricted diet didn't lose more weight than the nondieters, but felt less hungry.

One theory on why vitamins might help is fairly simple—if you are deficient in particular vitamins or minerals, your appetite will increase in your body's effort to get you to eat to restore nutrient balance. Helping avoid deficiencies may help prevent that mechanism from kicking in.

There are many multivitamins on the market, and which one you choose will likely depend on your own preferences and budget.

Keep in mind that you should not take a multivitamin with iron or calcium within three to four hours of thyroid medication.

Two multivitamins that I specifically recommend are Dr. Jacob Teitelbaum's Daily Energy Revitalization Formula, which is made by Enzymatic Therapies. It's a powdered vitamin that you mix with water—or add to a smoothie—that replaces some twenty-five to thirty-five separate tablets a day. It's specifically formulated for people who also deal with fatigue, and with 2,000 IU of vitamin D_3 in each serving, it has substantially higher levels of that important nutrient than most multivitamins. This product is widely available at health food stores, natural groceries, and online.

Another multivitamin I like quite a bit is Dr. Ann Louise Gittleman's Dieters' Multivitamin and Mineral, which includes basic vitamins and minerals at appropriate levels. It's available online or by telephone order from Uni Key Health. An iron-free formula is available for those who want to take their vitamins closer to their thyroid medication.

Probiotics

Another supplement that I take daily and feel is important is a probiotic. Probiotics are the good bacteria that normally are present in your digestive tract, helping maintain balance by preventing growth of harmful bacteria. We know that probiotics can help support a healthy immune system, digestion, and regularity, but now obesity research is showing that probiotics may help increase a feeling of satiety (fullness) by encouraging the release of satiety-inducing hormones in the intestinal tract.

One study found that probiotics may help reduce or prevent belly fat. Another study found that probiotics helped patients who had gastric bypass surgery lose weight more quickly than gastric bypass patients who did not use probiotics. We're also seeing studies that suggest that probiotics can reduce inflammation, another key issue in the weight-loss battle.

Hormone expert Dr. Sara Gottfried also regularly recommends probiotics because recent evidence shows that probiotics limit the absorption of bisphenol A (BPA).

Some brands I like include Natural Factors, Enzymatic Therapies Probiotic Pearls, and Flora-Key from Uni Key. You will want to make sure that your supplement includes, at minimum, the probiotic bacteria lactobacillus and bifidobacterium.

Probiotics are generally considered very safe, but those with a history of mitral valve prolapse or heart valve irregularities should check with a practitioner, because there have been a few cases of heart infection linked to probiotic intake in people with preexisting heart conditions.

Omega-6 Fatty Acids: Gamma-Linolenic Acid (GLA) and Conjugated Linolenic Acid (CLA)

Omega-6 fatty acids are considered essential for survival but must be obtained through food, as the body can't produce them. Normally, these omega-6 fatty acids are converted in the body from linolenic acid, but there is evidence that nutritional deficiencies and hypothyroidism, among other factors, may impair that conversion process, leaving people deficient in gamma-linolenic acid (GLA) and conjugated linolenic acid (CLA).

GLA is an omega-6 fatty acid that is found primarily in plant-based oils such as evening primrose oil, borage oil, and black currant seed oil. Recent studies are showing that GLA in supplement form, unlike some of the omega-6 polyunsaturated oils, may help reduce inflammation in the body, support weight loss by activating the body's brown fat, and help in maintaining weight loss.

Studies of CLA have shown that it may help with reduction of body fat while increasing lean muscle mass. There is evidence that CLA may be acting to indirectly spur the metabolism to store less fat. It's also thought that CLA may help combat leptin resistance and inflammation.

Studies have shown that 3 to 4 grams (3,000 to 4,000 mg) per day of CLA may help with muscle mass and fat storage, and 6 grams a day may help with insulin levels.

All CLA is not created equal, and it's not recommended that you get a cut-rate brand. You're better off using the patented form of CLA known as Tonalin, which is found in a number of brands. Tonalin is the formulation that has been scientifically tested.

A handful of people have reported to me that CLA had the opposite effect on them and was actually making them feel more bloated and possibly causing weight gain. If this happens to you, obviously you should discontinue it.

Vitamin D

Deficiency in vitamin D is common, and it's estimated that 75 percent of Americans are deficient. The deficiency may even be higher among those with autoimmune thyroid disease and the overweight.

In addition to its benefits for bone development, immune health, and other health issues, vitamin D is increasingly being viewed as an essential in the weight-loss arsenal. It's a very important step, and one not to overlook. But before supplementing beyond the amount of vitamin D in a multivitamin, you definitely want to get your baseline level of vitamin D tested (specifically, your level of 25-hydroxycholecalciferol) and talk to your doctor about an appropriate and safe level of supplementation.

One study found that the baseline vitamin D levels in a group of obese people were directly correlated to their weight-loss success—specifically, for every increase of 1 ng/mL in their 25-hydroxycholecalciferol level, the study participants lost about a half pound more on a calorie restricted diet. Higher baseline vitamin D levels also predicted greater loss of belly fat.

Antiaging and hormone expert Rob Carlson, MD, feels that vitamin D is a crucial component of weight loss:

Clearly, vitamin D is critical in regulating our weight, and knowing the dramatic impact on thyroid function and optimizing metabolism, the correlation between rising rates of obesity and vitamin D deficiency isn't a surprise. In the absence of sufficient vitamin D the body increases the number and size of newly formed fat cells that will promote and accelerate abdominal obesity. Providing sufficient levels of vitamin D signals fat cells to shrink. This makes weight loss much easier when calories are restricted. Researchers have also found that low levels of vitamin D interfere with the function of leptin, which tells the brain when the stomach is full, and that excess body fat absorbs vitamin D, stopping it from entering the bloodstream. Vitamin D deficiency also decreases insulin sensitivity.

The target range for many physicians is a level of 30–60 ng/mL, but some hormone experts such as Dr. Kent Holtorf and Dr. Sara Gottfried believe that a level of around 80 is more effective as a weight-loss aid.

LEVEL 2: POTENTIALLY HELPFUL

Vitamin C

Vitamin C may be able to help with weight loss in those who are significantly overweight. One research effort found that in a study group of people between sixty and seventy-four years old, vitamin C infusions resulted in an increase in resting metabolism of almost 100 calories per day. That is, people burned 100 more calories on the days after vitamin C infusion without doing anything else different.

Some experts recommend that for weight loss, you take vitamin C to bowel tolerance. Basically, you start with 500 mg a day and keep adding 500 mg a day until you get to a point where you have diarrhea. Then cut back to the highest level that will not cause stomach problems. That daily dose can, for many people, be as much as 5,000 mg (5 grams).

Selenium and Zinc

Supplementation with selenium and zinc may be tried with lower-calorie diets to prevent decline of the thyroid hormone T3. You shouldn't take more than 400 mcg of selenium a day from all sources. A daily dose of 15 mg of zinc is helpful.

Cinnamon

Cinnamon is a food supplement that may help lower both glucose and insulin in the bloodstream, as well as cholesterol levels. One study in which subjects took cinnamon capsules that delivered less than 2 teaspoons a day of the spice found that the patients had better glucose metabolism and insulin balance, and levels of LDL ("bad") cholesterol dropped from 10 to 26 percent, without reducing the levels of HDL ("good") cholesterol.

Some people prefer to use cinnamon as a supplement, and this is certainly a safe and effective way to incorporate cinnamon into your diet. Be sure you pick a quality supplement.

Others would rather get their ½ to 2 teaspoons of cinnamon a day using the spice in their foods. Keep in mind that the cinnamon you find in the grocery store probably is not true cinnamon and therefore doesn't have the same health properties. The grocery store "cinnamon" is cassia—*Cinnamomum cassia*, or Saigon cinnamon—and is less expensive than the real thing, *Cinnamomum verum* (true cinnamon), sometimes called Sri Lanka cinnamon or Ceylon cinnamon.

In the supplement area, New Chapter makes a *Cinnamomum verum* supplement called Cinnamon Force. Health food stores and natural groceries are also likely to carry true cinnamon in stick and powdered form.

If you don't want to take supplements, here are some ways to use cinnamon sticks or powder:

- Steep your favorite herbal tea with a cinnamon stick
- Add ½ teaspoon cinnamon to unsweetened applesauce
- Add cinnamon to breakfast cereal or oatmeal
- Sprinkle on toast
- Add cinnamon to butter or cream cheese
- Sprinkle on coffee, cocoa, or cappuccino
- Add cinnamon to baked fruit and fruit juice, such as peaches and apples

Fucoxanthin

One potentially promising supplement is fucoxanthin, which is derived from an edible brown seaweed (*Undaria pinnatifida*, or wakame). A Japanese study showed that fucoxanthin can promote fat burning within fat cells in animals, and apparently the type of fat most affected is white adipose tissue—the kind of fat that concentrates around organs, as abdominal fat does.

Fucoxanthin appears to fight fat through two different mechanisms: by helping stimulate fat oxidation and conversion of energy to heat, and by stimulating the liver to produce an omega-3 fatty acid that helps reduce LDL (bad) cholesterol. No adverse side effects from fucoxanthin have been reported in animal studies or in human use.

If you do decide to use fucoxanthin, be careful about the formulation, because some include extra iodine, which may be detrimental to some thyroid patients.

I have periodically used Garden of Life's Living Seas FucoThin, which is a proprietary formula of fucoxanthin that also includes pomegranate seed oil. I found that when cycled with other supplements, it does seem to help increase fat burning, especially for belly fat.

Ribose

In his book *Beat Sugar Addiction Now*, Jacob Teitelbaum, MD, strongly recommends use of ribose to help with energy. Says Dr. Teitelbaum:

> When you are exhausted, your body craves sugar as it tries to get an energy boost. A special type of sugar called ribose is an excellent nutrient for energy production. In addition to its role in making DNA and RNA, ribose is the key building block for generating energy. In fact, the main energy molecules in your body (ATP, FADH, etc.) are made of ribose plus B vitamins or phosphate. Ribose does not raise blood sugar or feed yeast overgrowth, yet it looks and tastes like sugar. Consequently, sugar addicts can use it as a sugar substitute. It actually has a negative value on the glycemic index. Ribose even tends to lower blood sugar in diabetics and may contribute to weight loss as well. Ribose will give you a powerful energy boost. . . . Start with a 5,000 mg scoop of ribose three times a day for three to six weeks, then decrease to one scoop twice a day. If you get hyper from being too energized, lower the dose. . . . Any brand of ribose is okay, as long as it is in powder form and you take the proper dose. Quality control problems have occurred outside of the United States, so buy a brand that uses Bioenergy ribose.

LEVEL 3: SUPPLEMENTS TO CONSIDER

Calcium

Scientists don't yet know exactly which vitamins and minerals have the biggest influence over appetite and weight control. Calcium seems to help: a number of clinical trials have shown that consuming 1,200 mg of calcium a day can boost weight loss in dieters by up to 60 percent, possibly by binding to fat in the gastrointestinal tract, which reduces how much fat the body absorbs. The weight-loss benefits of calcium supplements, however, appear to work best for people who aren't already getting enough of the mineral.

Calcium appears to have a connection to weight loss, although studies tend to show that this connection is to calcium-rich dairy foods. However, it's still important to ensure that you get sufficient calcium, and 1,000 to 2,000 mg a day can be particularly helpful. Some experts recommend using calcium citrate, calcium malate, and calcium carbonate forms.

Irvingia

Irvingia gabonensis—often referred to as simply irvingia—is a food-based supplement that may be promising as a weight-loss aid for some people.

Irvingia is part of a family of African and Southeast Asian trees that produce both mango-like fruit—known as African mango or bush mango—and protein-rich nuts.

A double-blind, randomized, placebo-controlled clinical trial showed that supplements made with irvingia resulted in significant improvements in body weight, body fat, and waist circumference. Improvements were also seen in blood fats, including total cholesterol, blood glucose, C-reactive protein (a measure of inflammation), and leptin levels, when compared to the placebo group. According to the researchers, the study suggests that an extract of *Irvingia gabonensis* "safely and significantly reduces body weight in overweight and/or obese subjects, and has a favorable impact upon a variety of other metabolic parameters."

A number of other studies have shown that people taking irvingia as part of a weight-loss effort lost significantly more weight and had significant reductions in total cholesterol, LDL ("bad") cholesterol, and triglycerides and an increase in HDL ("good") cholesterol.

Caralluma

Caralluma fimbriata is a succulent plant from the cactus family. In India, caralluma has been eaten as a natural appetite suppressant for centuries. In supplement form, caralluma is thought not only to reduce appetite but also to block the activity of several enzymes, which then blocks fat formation and forces fat reserves to be burned. There is no evidence of toxicity with caralluma in traditional Ayurvedic use of the plant in India.

A patented, tested extract of *Caralluma fimbriata* called Slimaluma delivers a concentrated extract of caralluma. Country Life's GenaSlim line of supplements combines Slimaluma with EGCG from green tea, and Now Foods has a line of various supplements and protein powders containing Slimaluma.

Hoodia

Hoodia gordonii is a succulent that grows in the high deserts of the Kalahari region of South Africa. Hoodia contains a molecule that has similar effects on nerve cells as glucose and tricks the brain into the sensation of fullness. Results of human clinical trials in Britain suggest that hoodia may reduce the appetite.

Experts theorize that nerve cells in the hypothalamus that sense glucose are activated by hoodia, and may cause:

- A reduced interest in food
- A delay in the time after eating before hunger sets in again
- A full feeling

Prescription drugs containing hoodia or its synthetic P57 derivative are years away from being on the market. But natural hoodia supplements are currently available. You need to be particularly careful that you take a hoodia that contains the actual plant.

I have talked with some patients who have found hoodia helpful with appetite. Hoodia does not appear to have side effects.

Acetyl-L-Carnitine

Acetyl-L-carnitine is thought to have the following functions:

- Helps the hypothalamus stimulate production of growth hormone during sleep
- Helps reduce leptin resistance
- Speeds the burning of fat by delivering more fat into the mitochondria

Carnitine links with fat and moves it into the mitochondria—the cell's furnace, or power plant—for burning, converting fats and carbohydrates into energy. Low carnitine is thought to slow delivery and allow extra fat to accumulate. One study found that people on a diet and exercise program who also took 1,000 mg of acetyl-L-carnitine daily for three months lost significantly more weight than those who took a placebo. Some experts recommend taking 3,000 to 5,000 mg just once daily, around an hour before exercise, to help burn fat during a workout.

In his book *Beat Sugar Addiction Now*, Jacob Teitelbaum recommends acetyl-L-carnitine:

When you don't have enough carnitine, it also forces your body to turn calories into fat and makes it almost impossible to lose fat. Simply taking carnitine does not adequately help, however, because it does not get into cells optimally. Instead, take 1,000 mg of acetyl-L-carnitine (which does get into the cells more effectively) daily for four months, to boost energy and allow weight loss.

Alpha-Lipoic Acid

Alpha-lipoic acid is a powerful antioxidant that plays a role in helping trigger production of adenosine triphosphate (ATP) to produce cellular energy. There is also some evidence that it may help reduce insulin resistance and help control blood sugar.

Coenzyme Q_{10}

Coenzyme Q_{10} (co Q_{10}) is a soluble antioxidant that helps the cells' mitochondria—the powerhouse—to generate nearly all of the energy that the cells need to function. It's thought that sufficient levels of co Q_{10} are needed for optimum energy and functional metabolism. A minimum daily dose is considered to be 200 mg a day.

Chromium

The mineral chromium has had interesting but inconsistent results. Some studies have shown that it has no effect on weight loss but can help maintain muscle during weight loss. There is growing evidence that chromium can help with blood sugar control in people with type 2 diabetes or insulin resistance by improving the body's responsiveness to insulin.

Jacob Teitelbaum, MD, recommends chromium:

Chromium, a mineral found in tiny amounts in the human body, is especially critical for people with reactive hypoglycemia (low blood sugar during stress). Research published in the *Journal of the American College of Nutrition* in 1997 showed that taking chromium can decrease the symptoms of low blood sugar. Think of it as "taking the edge off" by optimizing insulin function. A side benefit? It may even help you lose weight. A good multivitamin will provide the necessary 200 mcg a day.

Ron Rosedale, MD, also recommends chromium. He suggests 1,000 mcg of chromium for diabetic patients and 500 mcg for nondiabetics.

DHEA

There are some clinical trials showing that dehydroepiandrosterone (DHEA) supplementation can lower fat mass without reducing total body weight. DHEA supplementation should typically not be done without testing your DHEA levels beforehand, however, as too much DHEA can cause a variety of symptoms, especially in women, including facial hair and acne.

Glucosol

Glucosol is derived from the crape myrtle tree, native to southern Asia. The main ingredient, corosolic acid, has been shown in a variety of studies to support natural glucose metabolism and to activate cell glucose transport mechanisms that balance blood glucose levels. Corosolic acid also continues to work for a time after the treatment is stopped. An oil-based corosolic acid formulation in a soft gelatin capsule, such as Glucosol, seems to be the most efficient way to lower blood glucose levels. One 24 mg Glucosol capsule before meals has been shown to lower blood glucose levels, and in one study Glucosol at daily dosages of 48 mg for two weeks produced a significant reduction (as much as 30 percent) in blood glucose levels. Definitely worth trying, but talk to your doctor first if you're diabetic or hypoglycemic.

Glutamine

Glutamine (also called L-glutamine) is an amino acid that is usually abundant in the body and is stored in muscle. There is a theory that sometimes the body's need for glutamine is greater than the ability to make it, particularly when you are exercising and building muscle; when there is insufficient glutamine, the body will down muscle tissue. Glutamine is thought to help protect muscles and reduce cravings for carbohydrates such as sweets, starches, and alcohol.

Taurine

Taurine is one of the less well-known amino acids and has a number of different functions in the body. It aids the liver in forming bile acids, helps with detoxification of toxins and toxic chemicals from the body, and is even thought to help reduce chemical sensitivity. It is also a good diuretic. A safe and effective daily dose of taurine is considered to be 500 to 1,000 mg daily.

Milk Thistle

Milk thistle is a fat-burning herb that helps support the liver and detoxification. It is a common ingredient in detoxification and weight-loss formulas. Not much research has been done on this herb to establish the validity of claims, but anecdotally and clinically it is popular with many practitioners.

Pantethine

Pantethine is a form of vitamin B_5—pantothenic acid. It's been shown to help reduce triglyceride levels and to reduce abdominal and visceral fat and obesity. The optimum dose to help with metabolizing fat appears to be 600 to 900 mg daily.

Pyruvate

Pyruvate is a compound in the body that is also found in particular fruits and vegetables. It's thought that pyruvate may increase resting metabolism slightly, can help with overall endurance, and can slightly accelerate fat loss. One trial found that pyruvate at 22 to 44 grams per day could enhance weight loss and help reduce body fat for overweight adults eating a low-fat diet. Several trials using lower doses—from 6 to 10 grams per day—along with exercise showed similar results with weight loss and body fat. Much of the research was done based on 20 to 30 grams per day, but it's thought that 5 grams per day is enough to produce results.

Spirulina

Spirulina, a type of algae, is a source of protein and a variety of other nutrients. In one double-blind trial, overweight people who took 2.8 grams of spirulina three times per day for four weeks experienced a very small and insignificant weight loss. Another study from Greece found that spirulina can increase the body's ability to burn fat by 11 percent. Spirulina is primarily a food supplement.

Fat Blockers, Starch Blockers—Mirafit, Chitosan, *Phaseolus vulgaris*, and Others

There are a variety of supplements that claim to block fat or block starch. Chitosan, made from the shells of shellfish, is reported to bind to fat, preventing you from absorbing the fat, which simply passes through your body. It's a popular ingredient in many of the so-called fat-blocker supplements. There is not much in the way of evidence that chitosan actually works for fat absorption. A proprietary corn fiber that is sold under the name Mirafit is also purposed to absorb fat. The French white bean, *Phaseolus vulgaris*, is the source of a key ingredient in carbohydrate blocker supplements. The studies and research are all over the place on these sort of supplements, but some patients have reported that these can be helpful.

LEVEL 4: THE JURY IS STILL OUT

5-HTP

5-hydroxytryptophan (5-HTP) is a precursor to the neurotransmitter serotonin. There is some evidence that 5-HTP may be able to reduce appetite and promote weight loss. One trial showed increased weight loss among overweight women who took 600 to 900 mg of 5-HTP daily. Another study found that type 2 diabetics significantly reduced their carbohydrate and fat intake after several weeks of taking 750 mg per day of 5-HTP. Other studies have found that 5-HTP taken at a daily dose of 8 mg per kilogram of body weight could reduce overall caloric intake even without subjects making any particular effort to cut food intake. It was thought that the 5-HTP was increasing the sense of fullness. In addition to weight loss, 5-HTP is also thought to help with late afternoon and evening cravings.

7-Keto

The supplement 7-keto (3-acetyl-7-oxo-dehydroepiandrosterone) is related to DHEA. One study found that when taken alongside a somewhat calorie-restricted diet with exercise, 7-keto resulted in greater weight loss and body fat reductions than a placebo. It's thought that 7-keto may be able to help make T4-to-T3 conversion more effective, resulting in higher T3 levels.

Garcinia cambogia (Hydroxycitric Acid)

Garcinia cambogia is a tree whose tropical fruit contains high amounts of the compound hydroxycitric acid (HCA). It's thought that HCA may be able to help inhibit the conversion of sugar into fat, curb appetite, and reduce sweet cravings. There are also claims that HCA can reduce the amount of excess carbohydrates that get converted to body fat. Research shows, however, that the supplement has little effect. While HCA is a common ingredient in many weight-loss supplements, the evidence is primarily anecdotal, but the supplement is considered safe, with no side effects.

Guarana

The herb guarana contains caffeine, along with theobromine and theophylline, which are all thought to potentially curb appetite and increase weight loss. Guarana has 30 percent more caffeine than coffee, so you should be particularly careful about supplementing with it, because it can be overstimulating, especially when combined with other sources of caffeine (found in some weight-loss combination formula supplements).

Gymnema sylvestre

Gymnema sylvestre is an Ayurvedic herbal remedy that is thought to particularly help with reducing sweet cravings and minimizing sugar absorption in the intestines. There really is minimal research to support use of *Gymnema sylvestre*.

Aroma-Based Supplements (Tastants): Sensa, Aroma Patch, SlimScents

There is a fair amount of slick marketing, and only a tiny bit of research, behind these aroma-based supplements. The most well-known and heavily marketed of these supplements is Sensa, which features little crystals that are shaken onto food the way you'd shake on salt. SlimScents is sprayed in your nose before meals. The Aroma Patch is worn on your hand, wrist, or chest.

Sensa, the most heavily marketed of the products, calls its crystals "tastants" and claims that they stimulate the sense of taste. Theoretically, by enhancing the senses of smell and taste, satisfaction is increased and food intake is reduced.

In one study, conducted by the manufacturer of Sensa, more than two thousand people used the Sensa crystals, and one hundred control volunteers did not. The treatment group lost an average of around thirty pounds, compared to two pounds for the control group. Controls had an average BMI decrease of 0.3.

Even the manufacturer of Sensa says they don't know if any weight lost on their product can be maintained, however, and say that tastants won't work for people who eat when they're full. They also have said that some of the same theories can be put into practice by smelling food carefully before you eat it, chewing throughout, and using seasonings on lower-calorie foods.

There doesn't appear to be much support for these products from the medical world. Dr. Pamela Peeke, a weight-loss expert and clinical professor of medicine at the University of Maryland, told ABC's *20/20*, "There's no magic bullet and there's no magic sprinkle. This isn't a diet. This is just another Pet Rock." Most of these products cost $50 to $60 a month, so they're on the costly side for a supplement.

Instead of investing in tastants or patches, you may want to follow the advice of weight-loss expert Marc David and eat slowly and mindfully. In his book *The Slow Down Diet*, David has said that failing to adequately look at, smell and taste one's food can blunt the digestive response. Says David: "The brain must experience taste, pleasure, aroma, and satisfaction so it can accurately assess a meal and catalyze our most efficient digestive force." According to David, failing to activate this response makes the metabolism function at 60 to 70 percent efficiency.

CHOOSING SUPPLEMENTS

You may want to consider the Level 1 basics as a starting point, and then consider some of the Level 2 and Level 3 supplements.

Always check with your health care practitioner to make sure that any supplements you wish to take are not going to interfere with other medications that you are already taking.

And keep in mind not to start multiple supplements at the same time; that makes it nearly impossible to keep track of what is working and what is not.

Some people like things to be simplified, and to that end, if you are looking for a good starting point for a vitamin, a weight-loss formula, and essential fatty acids, I highly recommend Dr. Ann Louise Gittleman's Fat Flush Kit. The kit includes three bottles of supplements: Dieters' Multivitamin and Mineral, GLA-90 (a GLA supplement), and Weight Loss Formula (with B vitamins, chromium, acetyl-L-carnitine, amino acids, milk thistle, and other gentle anti-inflammatory ingredients).

CHAPTER 9

Movement, Activity, and Exercise

> Albert Einstein discovered that a tiny amount of mass is equal to a huge amount of energy, which explains why, as Einstein himself so eloquently put it in a famous 1939 speech to the Physics Department at Princeton, "You have to exercise for a week to work off the thigh fat from a single Snickers."
>
> —DAVE BARRY

Notice that in the title of this chapter, I've put the words *movement* and *activity* first, while the last word is *exercise*. I don't want you to start thinking that you need an exercise plan or a gym membership, or that you should focus on an intensive, fitness-based approach to weight loss; rather, movement and activity should become a regular part of your life.

When you are trying to lose weight, particularly if you have an inefficient metabolism due to thyroid disease, movement has to be an essential part of the overall approach to weight loss and maintenance. I know that some of you are going to groan and swear to me that you have a friend, coworker, or relative who lost weight just dieting. I believe it. Ultimately, for most people, it's easier to cut calories than add physical activity.

But the question is, was that person also battling a thyroid problem? It may not seem fair, but you can't just cut out some calories and watch the pounds melt off. You'll have to work harder and may still have less success than someone else who is doing exactly what you are doing. But if you include physical activity in your program, you will see better results.

Calorie restriction or a change in the composition of the diet allows for some weight loss, but that weight loss can slow, stop, or even rebound if the metabolism also slows down in response. To keep your metabolism efficient or to make it even more efficient, you absolutely need movement. There's several reasons for that.

First, when done properly and for a sufficient time, exercise can burn some fat. During the first fifteen to twenty minutes of sustained moderate physical activity or exercise, glycogen (that's the sugar in your muscles) is burned for energy. As you continue moving, the body turns to glucose and free fatty acids from the bloodstream for energy. After thirty to forty minutes, the body starts burning fatty acids from stored fat.

Second, exercise appears to have a very direct effect on the hypothalamus and the whole chemistry of metabolism. Exercise makes tissues and cells less leptin-resistant and insulin-resistant. According to Jean-Pierre Despres, professor of medicine and physical education and director of the Lipid Research Center at Laval University Hospital in Quebec: "Exercise is probably the best medication on the market to treat insulin resistance syndrome. . . . Our studies show that low-intensity, prolonged exercise—such as a daily brisk walk of forty-five minutes to an hour—will substantially reduce insulin levels."

One study found that after ten minutes of treadmill jogging or stationary-bicycle riding, metabolites in the bloodstream go up by about 50 percent in people who are not fit, while those who are fit have a 100 percent increase, and elite athletes, like marathoners, can see an even greater increase. What this study showed is that exercise can have immediate effects on the body's fat-burning ability, as well as cumulative effects for those who become more fit over time. Another study found that exercising may help restore better sensitivity in the hypothalamus, resulting in a better balance of leptin and insulin, improved feelings of fullness, and reduction of food intake.

Third, weight-bearing exercises improve your muscle mass, which raises metabolism. The more muscle you have, the more calories you burn. And there is a substantial metabolic difference between a pound of muscle and a pound of fat. Some experts say that muscle burns at least three times more calories than fat. One study found that after resistance training, fat continues to burn after the workout for at least forty minutes.

In one study, after just twelve weeks, people who increased their muscle mass by as little as three pounds could eat 15 percent more calories a day without gaining weight. You can't take muscle for granted, either. Without weight-bearing activity to build muscle, you can lose as much as five pounds of muscle each decade.

Another study of women found that weight training was more effective than aerobics at controlling abdominal fat. Keep in mind that *weight-bearing* does not mean that you have to "lift weights" in the traditional sense. Push-ups, lunges, squats, resistance bands, or workouts such as T-Tapp and mat Pilates, and even walking are weight-bearing.

And finally, exercise improves lymphatic function. I want to talk a bit more about lymph, because few people understand it, and it's perhaps the least understood and most overlooked benefit of exercise, especially for thyroid patients. The purpose of the lymphatic system is to absorb excess fluid, fat, toxins, and waste products, filter them out, and return the filtered liquid—known as lymph—to the bloodstream. The lymph travels via the lymph vessels, which are located throughout the body. Blood vessels have the heart to pump blood through the vessels, but the lymphatic system relies solely on movement, massage, and deep breathing to pump lymph through the system.

According to naturopathic doctor, nutritionist, and weight-loss expert Ann Louise Gittleman, PhD, CNS, proper lymphatic function is critical, because if the liver can be viewed as the body's filter, lymph channels are the body's drainage system. Says Dr. Gittleman:

> The lymphatic system needs a better press agent! Because, despite its crucial importance, many women aren't aware of it. Healthy lymph is pumped, and what pumps the lymph is exercise. This is one way that we know nature intended us to be active, because the lymphatic system only works when we are moving. It's not involuntary, like our heart pumping blood. But Mother Nature didn't count on eighty-hour workweeks and sedentary jobs at desks.

When we don't move, the lymphatic system can't work. It can get clogged, backed up, and sluggish—and even more so if we're hypothyroid. This can causes us to bloat, swell, and retain water; make the immune system less effective; and worsen fatigue.

Beyond the benefits for weight and metabolism, regular movement has so many incredible health benefits. Exercise is good for your heart and cholesterol levels. Getting your heart pumping makes it stronger and healthier. It also helps reduce your risk of cardiovascular disease and stroke, improves cholesterol levels and ratios, and helps you live longer. Other health benefits of activity and exercise:

- Greater strength
- Improved mood
- Reduction in depression
- Reduced anxiety
- Better sex drive
- Better sleep

- More energy, less fatigue
- Helping redistribute weight
- Fewer body aches
- Better bone density
- Better, faster recuperation after surgery
- Fewer falls and better balance in seniors

We also now know that women who get physical activity during pregnancy tend to have easier deliveries and a faster postpartum recovery. And ladies over forty, take note: regular physical activity also has a direct effect on the number, intensity, and duration of hot flashes and night sweats.

So for those who are overweight, getting moving is important not just to help with calorie burning but also to help balance insulin and leptin levels and get the body's metabolism back to more efficient operation.

HOW MUCH ACTIVITY DO YOU NEED?

There are so many differing opinions on how much activity is necessary for weight loss. I've seen all sorts of conflicting information. A 2010 study found that women who were successful in maintaining a normal weight averaged approximately sixty minutes a day of moderate-intensity activity. The surgeon general says thirty minutes a day. And if you watch television's *The Biggest Loser*, well, you'll see people exercise hour after hour every day.

So, what's the situation? Do you need to live in the gym, or is there another way?

I believe there is another way. The most commonsense weight-loss experts I've interviewed and reviewed—experts who have worked with real people who have lost weight while living real lives and not starring in reality television shows—have found that a combination of moderate activity and a healthy change in diet seem to be key.

Primal Blueprint author and weight-loss expert Mark Sisson says, "Everyone should shoot for a bare minimum of two hours of low-intensity aerobic movement per week. . . . I'd consider three to five hours per week an optimal range for most people with busy lives."

I think Sisson has it right, and his target is reasonable. But keep in mind that three to five hours of low-intensity aerobic movement does not mean three to five hours in the gym. Aerobic movement can mean long walks with your dog, some time on the treadmill watching your favorite television program, a dance class, playing with your children, cleaning, raking leaves—whatever gets you moving and gets your heart rate somewhat elevated.

You should also aim for forty to sixty minutes of strength training a week. You can use a weight room at the local gym or exercise with hand weights, dumbbells, or resistance bands at home. You can use the T-Tapp techniques discussed later in this chapter, or even move heavy rocks and bricks in your backyard. *Primal Blueprint*'s Mark Sisson puts it simply: "Lift heavy things. This stimulates lean muscle development, improves organ reserve, accelerates fat loss, and increases energy."

Remember, it's important that you acknowledge mindfully that activity is activity. Just because you're not in a gym or wearing running shoes, that doesn't make the activity count any less toward your weekly goal. In fact, it helps if you focus on the fact that all activity counts. A fascinating research study looked at a group of women who worked as housekeepers at hotels. One segment of the group was told that their regular work was enough exercise to meet the requirements for a healthy, active lifestyle. The other women were not told anything. Four weeks later, the researchers found that the women in the informed group had lost an average of two pounds, lowered their blood pressure by almost 10 percent, and were significantly healthier as measured by body fat percentage, body mass index, and waist-to-hip ratio. These changes were significantly higher than those reported in the control group and were especially remarkable given the time period, only four weeks. Simply changing their mind-set about their daily activity had significant health effects for these women.

HOW MUCH EXERCISE IS TOO MUCH?

I'm going to say something you probably never expected in a book about losing weight: don't exercise too much!

Many people think that exercising for weight loss is summed up by *The Biggest Loser*'s trainer Jillian Michaels in her often-repeated motto: "Unless you puke, faint or die, keep going!" There's always someone out there saying these sorts of things. A few decades ago, we had Jane Fonda yelling "No pain, no gain" and "Feel the burn" throughout her exercise videos.

The truth is, puking, fainting, dying, pain, and burning are signs that you are doing something *wrong*.

Weight loss and fitness expert Mark Sisson, in his book *Primal Blueprint*, calls it "Chronic Cardio"—the sort of workout that, as he puts it, "overtaxes the stress response (commonly referred to as the fight-or-flight response) in your body." Sisson defines these as workouts that put you in sustained periods of elevated heart rate (between 75 percent and 95 percent of your maximum).

Because intensive exercise can also cause a release of stress hormones, Sisson cautions that, rather than help, it actually contributes to an increased risk of insulin resistance. Says Sisson:

> This hormonal imbalance caused by overexercising contributes to fatigue, burnout, immune suppression, loss of bone density, and undesirable changes in fat metabolism. Furthermore, the stress of Chronic Cardio increases systemic inflammation

(a strong contributing factor to heart disease, cancer, and nearly all other health problems) and increases oxidative damage (via free radical production) by a factor of 10 to 20 times normal. . . . Our bodies are simply not adapted to benefit from chronic aerobic exercise at intense or even mildly uncomfortable heart rates nor to slog through exhausting circuits of resistance machines several days a week. The mild to severe difficulty of these Chronic Cardio or strength workouts overtaxes the stress response (commonly referred to as the fight-or-flight response) in your body. Here, your pituitary gland tells your adrenal glands to release cortisol into your bloodstream.

Nutritional psychologist Marc David, author of *The Slow Down Diet* and cofounder of the Weight Loss Pleasure Camp, believes that intense exercise may actually prevent weight loss in some people:

Intense exercise can closely mimic the stress response. Yes, aerobic exercise is great for us and has a long list of wonderful metabolic benefits. . . . But in the wrong context exercise can wear us down, elevating cortisol and insulin levels, generating inflammatory chemicals, and locking us into a survival metabolism in which we vigorously store fat and arrest the building of muscle. Low to moderate intensity exercise for only thirty minutes three or four times per week is the best prescription for health, weight maintenance and fitness.

Weight-loss expert and Weight Loss Pleasure Camp cofounder Jena la Flamme agrees:

Any weight-loss strategy, no matter how sensible it appears to the mind, that is stressful to implement, for example, portion control, dieting, punishing exercise regimes, are counterproductive by nature. Simply put, stressful weight-loss strategies trigger the body's self-protection instinct, inhibiting the very thing you set out to accomplish: lasting weight loss.

Rick Ferris, a naturopath and pharmacist who provides holistic weight-loss counseling, says that some of the patients he sees are overexercising.

I have some people who come in, and it's clear that they are horribly stressed, I tell them to stop the exercise immediately, and to do nothing for at least thirty days, to allow time for the adrenals to start healing.

How will you know if you are overexercising?

- You feel fatigued to the point of needing a nap after an exercise session.
- You have excessive pain during or after exercise.
- You feel flulike symptoms after exercise.
- You are sluggish in the hours or day after exercise.
- You feel mentally exhausted in the hours or day after exercise.
- You are quick to develop aches, pains, and injuries during and after exercise, and slower to recover.

Aim for moderate activity on a regular basis, but recognize that exhausting yourself with exercise not only isn't likely to help your effort but may actively prevent you from losing weight, by interfering with your hormones and metabolism.

Ellyn, a thyroid patient, described her own issues with exercise:

When I gained weight in my mid-forties, I started exercising more, doing marathons, weight training, and Pilates—I was doing about eight to ten hours of exercise a week! I ended up discovering that all that exercising was creating stress and adrenal fatigue, and was unhealthy, so I cut back to about four to five hours a week of walking and yoga. With that and a gluten-free diet, I have kept the weight off!

THYROID PATIENT CHALLENGES TO ACTIVITY

Overexercising is not a problem for most of us, however; even the majority of people without thyroid problems aren't getting the amount of physical activity they need. But thyroid patients face a number of additional challenges that can make it especially difficult to exercise regularly.

Focus on Health, Not Weight Loss

Your motivation for exercise should be health, not weight loss. Health and beauty expert Kat James, author of the book *The Truth About Beauty*, talks about motivation:

> Don't focus on exercise as the cure for your problem, and don't feel bad if it doesn't result in weight loss. . . . Once you've switched to low-impact eating and addressed your biochemical imbalances nutritionally, you will be surprised at your desire to get moving again, and you will take joy in activity. Exercise that is properly fueled with a focus on health (not calorie burning) will have a far more positive impact than weight-loss-focused exercise.

I agree with Kat. If you focus on the general health benefits of healthy movement and activity and not on the amount of calories you think you are burning, you can't help seeing a positive result. If you exercise solely because you think it will help you lose weight, you are less likely to enjoy the day-to-day positive feedback from your body rewarding you for movement, activity, and exercise.

Fitness expert and trainer Silvia Treves suggests that a few sessions with a personal trainer in the beginning can help. She explains, "That way, you can learn the exact way to perform the exercises and movements, and learn how to protect your spine, neck, and back from injury. Clients tell me that they are likelier to continue working out if they don't always feel incredibly sore for days after exercising."

You can also follow the ten-minute rule: when you don't feel like exercising, set your wristwatch alarm or a timer for ten minutes at the start of your exercise session. If you want to quit after ten minutes, then stop. But it's likely that once you start, you'll be feeling pretty good and will continue past the ten minutes.

Be sure that you plan ahead and schedule time for physical activity. When others want to schedule something else for that time, tell them you have an important meeting. What else is more important than meeting with yourself?

Muscle or Joint Pain

Pain in the muscles and joints is a common thyroid symptom and can persist even after treatment is optimized. There are several things you can do to help with this sort of pain so that you can exercise more effectively.

You can take a high-quality fish oil supplement (2 to 3 grams a day). I particularly like Enzymatic Therapy's Eskimo Oil because it has no fish "burp"—that is, that terrible fishy aftertaste you get with some fish oil supplements.

Nonsteroidal anti-inflammatory drugs (NSAIDs), including over-the-counter options such as aspirin, ibuprofen (Motrin, Advil), and naproxen sodium (Aleve), as well as the prescription drugs celecoxib (Celebrex) can be helpful with muscle and joint pain and autoimmune-related inflammation. But note that both prescription and nonprescription anti-inflammatory drugs can have various side effects, so discuss this with your doctor.

Also, keep in mind that even for fibromyalgia patients who are struggling with chronic body pain, gentle exercise, stretching, and movement is now known to be a key treatment, and results in substantial improvement in pain for many people. So if you are doing gentle, sensible physical activity, muscle and joint pain should decrease over time.

Fatigue

Being tired is one of the most common complaints of many thyroid patients. You may find that even after treatment you feel too tired to keep up with your daily activities, much less exercise. Once your thyroid treatment is optimized, there are several things you can do to help increase energy.

Get enough sleep. It seems an obvious solution, but most people aren't getting enough sleep. The National Sleep Foundation has found that only 30 percent of adults are getting eight or more hours of sleep per night on weeknights. I personally have to get eight hours or my immune system slowly starts to degrade.

Another thing that can affect energy is a low dehydroepiandrosterone (DHEA) level. Before supplementing with DHEA, you should have your level assessed by your physician. If it is low, supplementation (usually no more than 1–5 mg a day for women and up to 25 mg a day for men, every other day, taken in the morning) can help greatly. In my case, at one point I experienced extreme fatigue in the afternoon, and my doctor found that I had particularly low DHEA levels. Within a week after she put me on a regimen of 5 mg of DHEA, I had enough energy to exercise again.

If you are suffering from flagging energy, you need to make sure that you are getting enough B vitamins. Vitamin B_{12} is essential for energy. Consider taking a B complex plus B_{12} separately in a sublingual form (one that dissolves under the tongue) for maximum absorption.

You will want to ensure that you are getting enough vitamin D, as new research shows a link between vitamin D deficiency and fatigue.

Also consider using one of the supplements that can help with energy. These include:

- The Royal brand of maca
- Panax ginseng and Siberian ginseng
- Rhodiola
- Schizandra (a Chinese herb that is used for fatigue)
- D-Ribose

Resist the temptation of a giant-size latte, multiple cups of coffee, or herbal energy supplements that contain stimulants such as caffeine or guarana. These are all like stepping on the gas pedal of your adrenal system while keeping on the parking brake. You rev things up but don't go anywhere.

Body work and energy work, such as yoga, tai chi, qigong (pronounced "chee-gung"), and reiki, can all help in adding and balancing energy. In qigong, tai chi, and yoga, gentle movements are used to move energy along the energy pathways of the body. In reiki, a practitioner helps open up energy channels. (Personally, I've found yoga and reiki to be most beneficial to my energy.)

Hyla Cass, holistic physician and bestselling coauthor of *Natural Highs*, offers these suggestions for natural energy boosters. You can start with Siberian ginseng (400 mg), licorice (500 mg), and pantothenic acid (100 mg). (The latter two are more for adrenal support than actual energy.) Or take 500 mg of the amino acids tyrosine or D,L-phenylalanine (DLPA). Depending on your response, you can add in any or all of the following to create your own personal energy formula, preferably one at a time to gauge your response. This can differ from day to day, too, depending on how you are feeling. If you do end up taking them all, reduce the dose of each accordingly, about one-third to one-half:

- Take about 100 mg of Asian (Panax) or American ginseng
- 300 mg of ashwagandha
- 3,000 mg of reishi mushroom
- 100 mg of rhodiola
- 100–250 mg of DLPA
- 100–250 mg of tyrosine

You Think You're Too Overweight or Out of Shape

If you feel you are very overweight, you may not think that you can do much of anything in the way of physical activity. It may seem daunting. Your body may feel stiff and inflexible, and you don't want to end up in pain after just one session. Paige Waehner, a personal trainer, About.com exercise guide, and author of numerous books on exercise, has these suggestions for how to get started:

First, choose something accessible. Walking is usually a popular choice because you can do it anywhere, there's no learning curve, and you don't need fancy equipment or gym memberships. Allow your body time to get used to what you're doing and make regular activity a part of each day, whether it's just walking more than usual or taking the stairs when you normally don't. The more active you are, the more comfortable you'll be and the more energy you'll have to go further and longer.

Even if all you can do to get started is walk around the block once, do a few sit-ups, or lift a two-pound hand weight a few times, that's enough. Slowly add more distance, more repetitions, or more weight. Don't try to run a mile or bench-press 100 pounds your first time out, or you'll end up sore, miserable, and swearing that you'll never exercise again. Waehner says:

One of biggest problems I see with new exercisers is that they start out too hard. Most people want to start where they want to be rather than where they are, and that almost always leads to quitting. The best way to avoid that is to do what you're comfortable with and add on to that each week.

Health and beauty expert Kat James also suggests that you stay out of gyms that are not comfortable for you. "Some gym cultures may be negative for someone who is challenged with food or body image issues, so I suggest you find an activity in an environment that will really lift your spirit, like walking with a friend, yoga, or dancing at home to music or a video."

Not Enough Time

So many of us live busy lives and feel that there's barely enough time for work, family life, and sleep, much less exercise. But if you truly want to lose weight and get in shape, you have to set aside about an hour a day, even if it's broken up into segments, and make exercise as much a priority as everything else in your life. There are no quick fixes and no miracle exercise machines that will allow you to lose weight in minutes a day. Time is your best friend!

One of the best things you can do is to get moving in the morning. Studies have frequently shown that morning exercisers are as much as three times more likely to consistently exercise than those who exercise at night. You get up, you get moving, and it's done for the day. Your morning—before work, school, and other responsibilities—is possibly the most controllable time of your day. As the day progresses, there are delays, distractions, errands, schedules, and countless interruptions that may chip away at your time, and we all know that exercise is the first thing to give when we have a schedule conflict. (Morning exercise also revs up your metabolism for your day and helps burn some extra calories.)

WALKING: THE SUPER EXERCISE

If you have to pick one exercise to get started, it should be walking. One study in the *Journal of the American Medical Association* found that women who want to lose a lot of weight should walk briskly for an hour a day while cutting calories. Researchers followed 184 sedentary women who weighed an average of 200 pounds. The women, ages twenty-one to forty-five, were told to consume 1,200 to 1,500 calories a day and exercise five days a week for a year, either continuously or in ten-minute bursts. The form of exercise used was brisk walking. After a year, here's what happened:

- The women who were walking from fifty to sixty minutes a day (either continually or in ten-minute increments) and eating 1,500 calories a day lost and kept off from 12 percent to 14 percent of their starting weight, or about twenty-five to thirty pounds. They were burning 2,000 calories or more a week with exercise.
- Those who were exercising thirty to forty minutes a day and eating around 1,500 calories lost and kept off around 9 percent of their starting weight, or about sixteen to twenty pounds. They were burning about 1,000 to 1,500 calories a week with exercise.

Remember, this is moderate-paced walking—it's not a leisurely stroll through the shopping mall, but it's also not jogging until you're out of breath. If you were on a treadmill, the speed would probably be in the range of 3 to 4 mph.

Speaking of treadmills, this is my favorite way of walking. I put on a television show, stick a movie in the VCR, or pop on my headphones and pass the time while I get my aerobic exercise. And I'm not alone—treadmills are one of the most popular exercise machines at health clubs and at home.

But with treadmill walking, it's easy to get lazy, so you need to vary the routine. One of the most effective things you can do to burn fat is raise the treadmill's incline. If you raise the incline, you can burn as much as 50 percent more calories. One simple way is to alternate five minutes of level walking with five minutes of incline, and so on. Start with a small incline (e.g., 1 percent) at the same speed, then gradually raise it. Or if your treadmill has a setting for going up and down hills, program that setting.

Walking is inexpensive, it requires no special equipment besides a decent pair of walking shoes, and even beginners can start. We've all heard the success stories of people who start out walking around the block and then gradually increase the distance until they're walking miles each day or even running a marathon.

If you're just getting into walking for fitness, you might want to follow a simple walking schedule, with five walking sessions each week, as follows:

- Week 1: start out with fifteen-minute walks that include five minutes of slow walking, five minutes of moderate-pace walking, and five minutes of slow walking.
- Week 2: add two minutes of moderate walking in the middle, for a total of seventeen minutes of walking.
- Week 3: add two minutes of moderate walking in the middle, for a total of nineteen minutes of walking.

By adding only two minutes a week, you'll be taking forty-minute walks after only twelve weeks!

As you get stronger, you can start adding periods of incline to this workout (or if you're outside, head for some hills) or switch to one of the interval approaches to make it more challenging. Intervals are short periods—even as little as 30 seconds to a minute—where you walk as fast as you can, or even run if you are able, and then go back to your regular pace.

Intervals can help give your metabolic efficiency a boost and can be used in any activity you're doing, such as stair-stepping, biking,

or swimming. One study found that women who did interval workouts on stationary bikes for two weeks burned 36 percent more fat
when they completed a continuous ride afterward, because intervals
work more muscle fibers, and the repair of muscle burns calories. As
you get stronger, you can add more intervals, make them longer, or
make them more intense.

Speaking of heading outside, Ohio State University researchers
actually found that women who walked outside reported liking their
workout better than those who did indoor treadmill walking. Another study found that outside exercise made people feel more energetic, both physically and mentally.

Music may help you keep a good pace. With an iPod, MP3 player,
or portable CD player, you can listen to your own customized play-
lists of energizing music. You may even want to try an audio walking
program. Fitness expert Joanie Greggains has a terrific one-hour
walking program called Pacewalk, which is available on a CD or by
download from the Internet. With Joanie's CD, after a warm-up segment, the music sets the pace, and you follow the beat for ten minutes, twenty minutes, or up to sixty minutes or longer, based on your
fitness level. A number of other audio walking programs, featuring
different styles of music, are also available by CD or download.

MY FAVORITE PROGRAM: T-TAPP

Besides walking, if I had to recommend one specific way to incorporate movement into your life as a thyroid patient, it would be the
T-Tapp program.

T-Tapp is a very unique system of exercises and movements created by Teresa Tapp, an exercise physiologist, expert in the science
of muscle activation, and author of a bestselling book, *Fit and Fabulous in 15 Minutes.*

When people hear about T-Tapp they sometimes think it involves tap dancing. But T-Tapp involves no dancing or Fred Astaire–style fancy footwork, and requires no grace or coordination, I promise! Rather, T-Tapp is a carefully designed series of unique movements that improve spinal alignment, flexibility, and strength; build muscle; improve lymphatic function; raise metabolism; reduce inflammation; and control glucose and lower insulin levels. T-Tapp also has a built-in focus on rehabilitation and is suitable for anyone at any fitness level.

In simple terms, T-Tapp helps your body maximize muscle movement so it can receive more benefits in less time. That's why only one set of eight repetitions is all that's ever recommended as part of a T-Tapp sequence.

In my own case, the first week I T-Tapped, I did an easy-to-follow forty-minute routine three times. I lost twelve inches in that first week alone, with three inches of it in my waist—it wasn't hard to convince me to keep T-Tapping! Over time, regular T-Tapping has helped me firm up and build muscle, stay more flexible, and wake up without aches and pains. When I go up and down the stairs, my legs feel lighter and stronger.

I used to do mat Pilates but never had the same results in terms of inch loss. Teresa Tapp explained it:

> While T-Tapp has some elements similar to Pilates and even yoga, I specifically designed the sequence of exercises in T-Tapp to provide a conditioning workout with comprehensive and compound muscle activation, meaning that it activates muscles at various points. But with T-Tapp, your muscles don't bulk up. My approach helps you develop longer, leaner, denser muscles, and these muscles act like girdles—I call it "spandex power"—to cinch in, uplift, tighten, tone, and support.

An additional benefit of T-Tapp is that it is designed to specifically optimize lymphatic function. According to Tapp, T-Tapp is not only isotonic (like most exercise) and neurokinetic (communicating mind-to-muscle, like Pilates and yoga)—but, says Tapp:

> With T-Tapp I add leverage isometrics. These are acupressure points to intensify the mind-to-muscle nerve transmission, which optimizes isometric activation. Using small added components— even something as simple as changing the position of your thumb, or keeping your knee to little toe—activates muscles better than if you are just thinking about it. Leverage isometrics help improve body alignment and metabolic function, so more muscles develop balanced density, not just mass.

A program of particular interest for thyroid patients who need to lose weight is the award-winning T-Tapp More 4-in-1 Rehabilitation Workout, available on a DVD, which is, as Tapp describes it, is "for people with more to lose, or more physical limitations, injuries and health issues." If you're not physically active, T-Tapp More is a way to ease into exercising without causing injury or exhaustion.

The T-Tapp book *Fit and Fabulous in 15 Minutes* and a variety of DVDs are available, offering a selection of different T-Tapp workouts—including workouts you can do lying on the floor, seated in a chair, using a broom for balance, and even walking. Special equipment is not needed for any T-Tapp program.

If you don't have an exercise program that you regularly follow, I would encourage you to find out more about T-Tapp and adopt it as your exercise program. And even if you participate in regular exercise, adding T-Tapp into your program can help improve your overall fitness and the results you get from your workouts.

MINI-MAX MOVES FROM T-TAPP

For readers of the *Thyroid Diet Revolution*, Teresa Tapp has shared some T-Tapp Mini-Max Moves, which help with faster inch loss, fitness, and function from the inside out. Try to perform each exercise to the best of your ability so you can achieve optimal results. Says Teresa:

> Remember, it's not what you do but how you do it! Understanding how to position your body and activate more muscles during movement is the secret to success in building a body that looks and feels better. T-Tapp is empowering because it enables you to improve your health and fit in fitness anytime and anyplace—you can do these Mini-Max moves at work, in class, while shopping, even while standing in line!

The T-Tapp Stance

Before you do any T-Tapp movements, you want to master what's known as the T-Tapp Stance. The T-Tapp Stance puts your body into alignment and activates internal muscles. Start by standing with your feet hip width apart and toes forward.

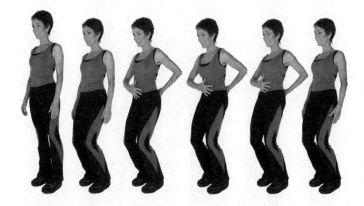

First, bend it, tuck it, and lift it! Now bend your knees. With feet forward and ankles aligned with hip joints, bend your knees. You may notice that your muscles tighten just above the knees. Straighten the knees, and feel how the thighs relax. Keep your knees bent at all times. Then tuck your butt under. This is more than just tightening your gluteal muscles. Curl your lower back—think of a dog tucking its tail between its legs. You should notice your lower back and stomach muscles activating and your belly button pressing back to your spine. Without losing your tuck, lift your ribs and bring your shoulders back in alignment with your hips. Keeping ribs up increases core muscle activation and assists cardiac function.

Next, push your knees out toward your little toe. Feel how the arches in your feel lift? The knee-little-toe (KLT) position, which is central to many T-Tapp movements, maximizes muscle activation in your lower body and provides rehabilitative benefits. Just push your knees out to the best of your ability. Then, once you have built enough strength and flexibility, also press the ball joint in your foot down and lift your big toe. This will increase the intensity and stabilize your ankles.

Now you're ready to do T-Tapp Mini-Max Moves.

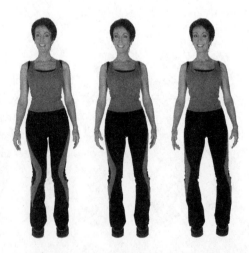

Relieve Lower Back Pain, with a Metabolic Boost

Bend it, tuck it, lift it! The very first thing you learn in T-Tapp and one of the most effective moves for pain relief, and to provide a metabolic boost, is the T-Tapp Stance, explained above. The T-Tapp Stance delivers immediate low back relief. Just standing in this position for a minute or two burns glucose and helps put your body in fat-burning mode because all your muscles are aligned and activated. "Stop to stand" the T-Tapp way for a moment or two throughout your day, and notice the changes begin!

Lift the Big Toe

If you want to have a tighter tummy, Teresa Tapp says we need to lift the big toe.

> Most of us pronate our feet and rest our weight onto the ball joint of our big toe. This is a bad habit! When we pronate, we inactivate all of the muscles along the hip, knee, thigh, and even the stomach. Whatever you're doing right now, sit or stand up straight and lift your big toe in your shoe—feel your abs activate? Do this every so often throughout your day to build better mind-to-muscle memory and a good habit. Want to take it further and increase intensity? Just add body alignment and leverage isometrics! First, sit straight on the edge of your chair with toes forward, ankles under your knees and aligned with hips and shoulders back also in alignment with hips. Now press your feet into the floor. Feel the muscles in your thighs, hips and butt activate? Now lift your big toes. Feel the difference? Adding leverage isometric activation with focus on body alignment increases intensity and effectiveness.

Knock Out Knee Fat

Do you want to get rid of knee fat? Teresa says:

> Don't walk like a duck! Walking with your feet angled out cre-
> ates muscle imbalance in your knees, ankles, and feet. Many of
> us walk with one foot more in a duck position than the other. I
> can usually tell which foot is the duck foot, simply by noting how
> much fat storage is on the inside or above the knee. Just by keep-
> ing your weight off the ball joint of your big toe along with cen-
> tering your weight to your outside three toes while you walk will
> deliver visible inch loss in your legs within ten days—especially
> knees and saddlebags.

Tame Neck Tension

The solution to neck tension, says Teresa, is "hunch and breathe."

> Seriously, any time you feel tension in your shoulders and
> neck (tight trapezius muscles), inhale deeply and lift your
> shoulders as high as you can toward your ears and hold. Then
> lift your ribs as high as you can while you exhale and reach
> down. Make sure your exhale all the way until you feel your
> ribs pull in. Repeat, but this time stretch your fingers wide
> with palms forward to increase neurokinetic and lymphatic
> flow. Repeat again, but this time, during the exhale, as you're
> reaching down, fold your fingers and point your thumbs back
> to the best of your ability. An extra bonus: deep breathing not
> only helps increase oxygen and energy, it also helps your body
> decrease inflammation.

Banish Back Fat

If you have back fat, Teresa says:

Lift your ribs and your point thumbs back! Poor posture can impair neurokinetic transmission, create muscle imbalance, and alter metabolic function. Take a look at any anatomy or physiology textbook, and you'll see that the human body is positioned with arms at the sides and palms facing forward. This is considered correct anatomical position. But when you look into a mirror at your own stance, are your palms facing backward? Although typical, this type of stance can be problematic because it causes your shoulder joints to roll forward, which ultimately creates muscle imbalance along your upper spine. Over time this can create muscle atrophy and cause your upper spine to curve forward, decrease bone health, and increase fat storage at the base of your neck.

Ready to feel the power of posture? Assume the T-Tapp Stance (bend it, tuck it, lift it) with knees out. Do four shoulder rolls back with your thumbs pointing toward your body and tune it to what you feel in your upper back and neck. Now do four shoulder rolls back, the T-Tapp way, with thumbs pointing back to the best of your ability, and feel the difference. Four shoulder rolls with thumbs back, four times a day, helps back fat melt away, and many T-Tappers notice visible results in fat reduction at the base of the neck and upper back within a week.

Whittle the Waist

If you want a slimmer waist, Teresa suggests using "mitten chops" to lift your ribs and stretch your spine.

Take a look at yourself in the mirror and lift your ribs to the best of your ability. (Don't pull your shoulders back, or you can cause muscle imbalance.) You should automatically feel your shoulders shift back and your lats activate. Additionally, you should see your torso lengthen and your waistline cinch in a bit. Tune in to how your muscles feel with this posture. Repeat, but this time press your hands in a "mitten" position with fingers together and thumbs away against your body at the top of your thighs or in front of your hips. Did your ribs move higher? Could you feel more muscles tighten? Leverage isometric activation is a primary principle of T-Tapp and is strategically used throughout all T-Tapp workouts to help optimize results.

Curl Your Core

Try to curl your core throughout the day using press, push or pull leverage isometric activation.

"Mitten chop" curls are performed while sitting with ankles under knees and knees apart in alignment with hips. Inhale and press your hands (mitten chop) into your thighs to lift your ribs and maintain this position while you exhale. Repeat, but this time during exhale, really push your hands and focus on "curling your core" (tuck tailbone and curl lower back) without dropping your ribs or shifting your shoulders. You should feel your lats intensely activate, as well as your lower back and abs. Repeat, relax, and repeat two more times, for a total of four mitten chop curls.

Next, do hunch pulls. While sitting in alignment, relax your spine and hunch. Place your "mittens" with fingers folded in front of your knee, with thumbs pointing up, and with the backs of your hands facing out. Then while inhaling, increase your hunch up and curl more by pulling and squeezing your fingertips around your kneecap (four counts). While exhaling, pull your ribs up and your shoulders back until you feel a slight arch in your back (four counts). Without relaxing this position, lift your toes, heels, and shoulders during inhale; and then during exhale, pull your ribs forward and your shoulders back, and arch your spine even more to the best of your ability (four counts) Then release and relax.

To do the core wall press, the assume T-Tapp Stance, with the back of your heels touching a wall. Then bend your knees a little deeper so you can curl your core and press your lower back against the wall (it's okay to let your shoulders come forward). Then with palms up and thumbs away in mitten position, place your elbows under your shoulders and against the wall. Inhale big, and during the exhale, tuck harder and press your elbows into the wall to help you lift your ribs and get your shoulders in contact with the wall without arching your back (this is not easy to do). Try to maintain this position throughout another big inhale and exhale (push harder during exhale), then relax and repeat as desired.

Put Organs in Place

Originally, Teresa created a sequence called Organs in Place to help improve prolapsed uterus and incontinence issues, but many T-Tappers find this to also be an effective abdominal toner.

Lie on the floor with your knees bent, toes forward, and heels aligned with hips. Press your feet into the floor until your feel your tailbone lift and your lower back curl under. Now press your fingertips deep into your abdomen by your left hip and roll your palms toward your navel. Did you feel your internal organs shift? Maintain this pressure while you activate and relax your abs four times (tighten and release). Repeat on the right side. Now place your fingertips into your lower pelvic area (below the bladder). While inhaling, press deep and roll your organs up toward your rib cage. While maintaining this pressure, exhale and then tighten and release your muscles four times. Continue maintaining pressure while you tuck, tuck, tuck, using your butt muscles to slightly lift your pelvis for a total of eight repetitions. Then slowly lower your body.

Inhale, exhale, then bring your knees toward your chest with heels in alignment with your hip joints. Now pull your knees in deep and hold (don't lift your head). Inhale and exhale as deep as you can, release, and repeat. Continue to warm up your spine with four little rock-and-rolls (knees apart and heels aligned with hips) so your spine maintains balanced muscle activation. Then pull your knees in, hold on to your knees, and open them out wide (shoulder width or to the best of your ability). While keeping your lower back pressed against the floor (no air space), lower your knees until your arms are straight.

Inhale and exhale twice, then proceed to point and flex your feet four times, then circle them out and circle them in four times each. Pull your knees in toward your shoulders until you feel your tailbone lift off the floor, and repeat another big inhale and exhale. Continue to bring your knees up and back in to the center of your body, but don't touch your knees together—keep knees and heels aligned with hip joints. Lower your tailbone and knees away until your arms are straight. Repeat spinal rocks four times and return back out to straddle position.

Organs in Place is one of the movements on the free DVD included with Tapp's *Fit and Fabulous in 15 Minutes* book, and you can also see photos of the sequence online at the T-Tapp site.

Hoe Downs

Teresa originally created Hoe Downs as an exercise that could be performed after taking medication (or after having a carbohydrate-rich treat, or a glass of wine) to help reduce blood glucose and promote fat burning and detoxification. This simple sequence will also help your body build strength, flexibility, and cardiac conditioning. Hoe Downs not only help improve physical health and drop blood glucose, they also help your mind focus because they challenge communication between left brain and right brain.

For a hoedown, you assume the T-Tapp Stance but shift your

weight to your left leg. Keep your left knee bent in KLT position, your butt tucked under, and your ribs up while you extend your hands out to the sides of your body with palms up and thumbs back. Now push your elbows forward and pull your hands back to the best of your ability. You should feel your shoulders pull back, your ribs lift higher, and every muscle tighten in your upper back. Inhale big until you feel your ribs expand, and exhale deep until your feel your ribs pull together without relaxing your shoulders forward. Now that every muscle in your body is isometrically activated, you're ready to start.

Lift your right knee up in alignment with your right shoulder (count 1) and then tap your toes to the floor (count 2). Repeat for a total of four lifts and four taps (8 counts). Try not to move your upper body when lifting your knee. Keep your butt tucked and your left knee bent in KLT at all times. Also point toe with each lift to increase activation of abdominal muscles.

Make sure you are aiming your knee toward your shoulder while lifting and keep your ankle in alignment with your knee. Allowing your foot to shift out of alignment while lifting your knee (front and side) creates inactivation of abdominal muscles and lessens effectiveness.

Without stopping, lift your right knee up and out to the right side as you bring your right hand across your body to the left (count 1) and tap your toes to the floor (count 2). Repeat for a total of four lifts and four taps (8 counts).

Repeat front and side lift-touch sequence as follows: two sets of four lifts and four taps (8 counts front, 8 counts on right side, twice), two sets of two lifts and two taps (counts 1 through 4 front, counts 5 through 8 right side, twice) and two sets of four single lifts and four taps (counts 1 and 2 front, counts 3 and 4, right side, four times)—all without stopping.

While inhaling and exhaling, do one shoulder roll back and reset to the starting position, then repeat the same sequence on the left side (two sets of four, two sets of two, and one set of four single lifts and four taps).

A number of try-before-you-buy videos featuring T-Tapp exercises are available free online. You can visit the T-Tapp site at T-Tapp. com, or visit this book's website at ThyroidDietRevolution.com for more information and links.

ADDITIONAL THOUGHTS

Move after Dinner

A tip from Dr. Ron Rosedale, author of *The Rosedale Diet*: after dinner, do some mild resistance exercise or take a fifteen-to-twenty-minute walk, ideally uphill. Since dinner is often our biggest meal of the day, planning some sort of physical activity after dinner may take advantage of the increase in metabolism after eating, and help kick-start the evening's fat burning.

Exercise It Off

Another tip from Dr. Rosedale: if you do eat something high in sugar or processed carbohydrates, exercise it off. If you don't burn off those starchy calories right away, they will raise your blood sugar, raise your leptin and insulin levels, prevent fat burning, and turn to fat, all of which get you right back to a deranged metabolism.

Teresa Tapp's Hoe Downs are actually an example of the perfect type of exercise you can do right after eating, to help get the metabolism back on track!

Incorporate Activity into Daily Life

Remember that one of the easiest ways to add to your activity level is as a normal part of your daily life. Try walking sometimes instead of driving. Walk to a local store or to a friend's house. I have a friend who loves to get espresso every weekend, but she has made a deal with herself that she needs to walk a mile to her local Starbucks to get it and then walk the mile back. She walks more than a hundred miles a year just for espresso!

One of my little tricks is that I do some exercise every time I make a cup of tea. I work at home and make a cup of herbal tea several times a day, so the five minutes it takes for the kettle to boil is exercise time for me. I do some stretching, a few sets of T-Tapp Hoe Downs, or some squats, and pretty quickly the water is boiling for teatime. Those little breaks add up to about fifteen minutes every workday, which adds up to an additional seventy-five minutes of exercising every week! Some people suggest that you do the same thing during commercials while you're watching television. Jump up and do a few T-Tapp Mini-Max Moves, or some sit-ups, leg lifts, and stretches. Keep some hand weights nearby and do biceps curls. There is an average of eight minutes of commercials for every thirty minutes of television, so if you watch two hours of television, you could end up doing a half hour of exercise. And there's almost no activity that you can't do for two minutes at a time!

Step Away from the TV

Speaking of television, get away from it! The amount of time you spend in front of the television is directly related to weight gain and mindless eating. If you're a TV fan and there are programs you just can't miss, get yourself a treadmill, stair climber, or elliptical machine and put it in front of the television. Or download episodes of your favorite shows onto a video iPod and take them to the gym. Make a strict deal with yourself that you can watch your favorite programs only if you're working out while they're on. This is a great way to get your TV and your workout, too!

Don't Obsess over the Scale

Don't be scale-obsessed. Fat takes up a lot more space than muscle, which is far denser. Typically, in middle age, most of us trade as much as one pound of muscle for up to two pounds of fat every year—the reason for the much-lamented "middle-aged spread" in both men and women. And if you do weigh yourself regularly, also be sure to take body measurements periodically as well, because as fat is lost and muscle is gained, even without a change on the scale, you may see results in terms of inches lost. You can lose ten pounds of fat, gain ten pounds of muscle, and still be far fitter, leaner, and slimmer.

Check Out Your Shoes

Some people swear by the different brands of walking or exercise shoes that claim to help tone your legs. I haven't seen much in the way of evidence that these shoes deliver in terms of any toning, but I can attest to their effectiveness at relieving foot and back pain, and in encouraging proper posture when walking. What I recommend is "physiological footwear"—shoes that are designed to help mimic the normal positions of bare feet walking on sand or grass. They often have a curved sole. You may recognize MBT, the manufacturer of many physiological footwear styles. I have a pair of Chung Shi running shoes, another brand that has a curved bottom like MBT's shoes. I love them for walking, as they almost guarantee that my alignment goes into the proper T-Tapp Stance for walking, and they keep me in better balance while I walk. If my legs, back, and feet hurt less, then I'm more likely to walk longer and more frequently. I also have a pair of FitFlops, which are flip-flops with a shape customized for support of the foot. They are extremely comfortable, and I've found that I can walk all day in them and have no resulting foot or back pain, unlike with plain flat flip-flops, which have no support for arches.

Be careful about weighted shoes, though. Some special "muscle-building" shoes have as much as one to five pounds of extra weight per shoe and are supposed to help burn more fat and build more muscle. The evidence is skimpy as to their effectiveness, and they can actually unbalance your body, throw your posture out of balance, and increase the risk of injury.

Use "Period Power"

For menstruating women, exercising later in your menstrual phase may help you burn more fat and feel less tired during your workout. Exercise may feel easier and your performance may actually improve during the later part of the menstrual cycle (the time between ovulation and the start of your menstrual period). During this time, the levels of estrogen and progesterone are highest. These hormones promote the body's use of fat as an energy supply during exercise, which helps you burn off more fat. Since the use of fat is more efficient, less waste products that cause exercise fatigue are produced.

CHAPTER 10

Medical Treatments: Prescription Drugs and Surgery

Science . . . never solves a problem without creating ten more.
— GEORGE BERNARD SHAW

By now, you probably realize that there really is no magic pill, medication, or surgery that will allow you to eat unhealthy, fatty, sugary, or starchy foods to your heart's content while you still lose weight or maintain healthy weight loss. There are, however, some medications and surgeries that may, if dietary and lifestyle changes fail, help with weight loss. But these drugs and surgeries carry varying degrees of risk and side effects, so it's important to be aware of the pros and cons. Ultimately, even with surgery or a weight-loss drug, you will still need to eat well, change your lifestyle, control your diet, and in some cases completely transform the way you eat if you want to lose weight with these interventions and keep it off.

THE HCG PROTOCOL

Human chorionic gonadotropin, or HCG, is a hormone that is normally produced in large quantities in a pregnant woman's body. In fact, a home pregnancy test is testing for the presence of HCG in the urine to confirm pregnancy. In a pregnant woman, one of the functions of HCG is to mobilize the burning of fat to ensure that energy is provided to the developing fetus and protect the pregnancy, even if the mother is facing a situation of starvation or is only able to get limited calories. As a medication, HCG is used at fairly high doses as a fertility treatment for women.

For weight loss, HCG is used in minute concentrations along with a very low-calorie diet as a way to shift the hypothalamus and trigger fat-burning. The combination of HCG and a very low-calorie diet is sometimes referred to as the HCG protocol or the HCG diet, or in some cases as the Simeons diet, after British physician Dr. A.T.W. Simeons, the doctor who first proposed it as a weight-loss method in 1954. It's occasionally referred to as the Pounds and Inches Diet after Dr. Simeons' book, which was titled *Pounds and Inches: A New Approach to Obesity.*

The theory is that the HCG is triggering the burn-off of stored fat and allows for weight loss without the normal side effects of a low-calorie diet, such as hunger, irritability, headaches, weakness, reduced muscle mass, or reduced metabolism. HCG is thought to work in a number of different ways:

• HCG causes the hypothalamus to trigger fat to move out of storage and become available for use as immediate energy. The combination of the released stored energy plus the energy from the low-calorie diet add up to several thousand calories a day of energy available for daily function. But, since much of the calories are coming from stored fat, weight is lost, and in particular body fat.

- HCG prevents the metabolism from dropping, despite being on a very low-calorie diet. The normal response to a very low-calorie diet is for the metabolism to become less efficient, which can cause fatigue and stall weight loss. The theory is that the HCG circumvents this mechanism with the hypothalamus and keeps metabolism at a stable level.
- Because HCG focuses weight loss preferentially on fat areas, muscle mass is theoretically less likely to be lost.
- After weight loss on HCG, hypothalamic balance is restored, and leptin and insulin resistance may also be reduced, making it easier to continue losing weight, or maintain weight loss.
- For patients who have been yo-yo dieters or on very low-calorie diets, hypothalamic dysfunction that has slowed metabolism or reduced their caloric needs may be reversed, and the metabolism returns to a more normal function.

Hormone expert and holistic gynecologist Sara Gottfried, MD, explains the theory behind HCG:

We are programmed to be in balance, and we're born that way, looking for homeostasis, but we have all these archaic systems, such as insulin and leptin systems, that can work against us when managing our weight. I've been interested in how we can reset the hypothalamus, remodel it so that it is appropriately interpreting signals from the thyroid and from leptin, For me, that is the greatest excitement for HCG. We don't totally understand how this works mechanistically, but we believe it remodels the hypothalamus, makes it more responsive to the thyroid, and shifts the body toward burning rather than storing fat.

Cardiac surgeon and hormone expert Dr. Rob Carlson has been prescribing HCG for more than six years and has seen hundreds of patients successfully lose up to fifty pounds during a course of HCG. Says Dr. Carlson:

Reduced-calorie diets often leave patients feeling exhausted and hungry. Coupled with a slow improvement in reshaping of their body, they quickly grow tired of the dieting process and fall back into old habits. In overweight people, HCG seems to work by making available permanently stored supplies of fat, as well as making it possible to adhere to the low-calorie diet. I've found that HCG allows patients to lose weight, preferentially from primary fat stores—double chins, protruding stomachs, and fat around the thighs are often the first to go—but also to control their appetite and reduce the "blah" feeling you get when dieting.

I also had an opportunity to speak with Dutch physician Dirk Van Lith, MD. Dr. Van Lith is a leading European proponent of HCG and author of a book on the topic. According to Dr. Van Lith, we have three kinds of fat:

Type 1 is a sort of packing material for the organs (kidneys, heart, etc.). Type 2 is a reserve of fuel, which the body can freely draw upon and distribute as needed around the body. Type 3 is the fat locked away around hips, thighs, and abdomen, which is entirely abnormal and causes obesity. Most weight-loss programs target type 1 and 2 fat, and type 3 fat is lost only as a last resort. The HCG protocol targets type 3 fat.

The Controversy

The use of HCG as part of a specific weight-loss protocol is a controversial approach.

One of the problems facing the HCG protocol is a major image problem. The HCG protocol gained visibility and public attention after pitchman Kevin Trudeau mentioned it in his book *The Weight Loss Cure "They" Don't Want You to Know About*. Trudeau is a notorious huckster, using late-night infomercials to sell various books promising natural cures, magical solutions for debt, and schemes to make money.

Not only does Trudeau have no health training, credentials, or background, but some of the health information he peddles in his books and websites is truly bizarre. For example, Trudeau asserts that AIDS is a made-up hoax and that sunscreen causes cancer. In connection with his promotional activities Trudeau is also a convicted felon, having served two years in prison for a larceny conviction related to the fraudulent use of credit cards. He has also been successfully sued a number of times by the Federal Trade Commission for fraud.

So pretty much anything Kevin Trudeau discusses is, understandably, tainted. The problem is that sometimes, in the midst of all his hucksterism, Kevin Trudeau actually does—perhaps by pure accident—manage to mix in some legitimate information, including recommendations regarding organic foods, calcium supplementation, and other commonsense ideas.

Because of Trudeau's support for HCG, some practitioners categorically dismiss HCG for weight loss, writing it off as "snake oil" or placebo. At the same time, there are practitioners who have been using HCG successfully with their patients for years, long before Trudeau came on the scene. And now, increasing numbers of legitimate practitioners, including physicians, hormone experts, and some bariatric (weight loss) physicians, are rediscovering HCG, and using it successfully themselves or with patients. Even the American Society of Bariatric Physicians includes panels and sessions on the HCG debate in its annual meetings, and recognizes that there are different positions among its members regarding the use and effectiveness of HCG.

Dr. Van Lith feels comfortable with the safety of HCG. "In twenty years," he says, "I have not seen one single side effect. Heart patients, diabetics, metabolic syndrome, thyroid patients—they all lose weight, and many have unsuccessfully tried everything else before."

Criticisms of the HCG Protocol

The main criticism of the HCG protocol is, frankly, that it's ineffective.

Critics of the HCG protocol point to research studies that have found that HCG is no more effective than placebo, and say that the effects of the diet are due to being on a very low-calorie diet of 500 to 600 calories a day, not the HCG.

There are some vague criticisms about whether HCG is safe, but typically, the concerns cite side effects that are associated with use of HCG for fertility. High-dose HCG for fertility treatments can result in ovarian hyperstimulation and rupture of ovarian cysts, among other side effects. The doses used for fertility treatment, however, are typically 5,000–10,000 IU, much higher than the 125 IU a day used in the HCG protocol.

Some critics suggest that the HCG protocol is a ketogenic diet, and what's happening is that the limited carbohydrates in the diet are sending the body into a state called ketosis, where appetite typically is suppressed. Stored fat is burned during ketosis, but there are concerns that over time, ketosis can increase the risk of kidney stones and gallstones.

Some critics say that the HCG protocol works only because it's a very low-calorie diet that is supervised and overseen by a practitioner, and that oversight by medical professionals is what is ensuring greater success.

Some practitioners have also suggested to me that one of the key reasons people lose weight on the HCG diet is not the HCG, but the fact that many people on the diet eat no starches whatsoever and are effectively on a gluten-free diet, sometimes for the first time in their lives. They attribute weight loss to the combination of eliminating gluten from the diet along with the low number of calories, not necessarily the HCG.

It's also important to note that while HCG is prescribed for and has FDA approval as a fertility treatment, its use as a weight-loss treatment is considered an "off-label" use, and the FDA requires physicians to advise patients that HCG has not been demonstrated to be an effective treatment for weight loss.

Does HCG Work?

So the question is, despite the criticism, does HCG work?

If you ask some people who have followed the HCG protocol, they will say yes. I've heard from dozens of thyroid patients who have done a forty-day course of HCG and lost fifteen, twenty, even as much as forty pounds.

I'll start with my own case. I did a forty-day course of prescription injectable HCG, along with the very low-calorie diet, and lost seventeen pounds. The weight I lost was almost all from the belly and waist area. I was not hungry on the diet, and I felt energetic. I had no difficulty staying on the diet. The injections were not painful at all. I saw steady weight loss throughout the cycle. And what was surprising to me was that even after the maintenance period and returning to a regular eating pattern, rather than the usual creep back up the scale, the weight I'd lost stayed off. In fact, the HCG seemed to reset my metabolic set point, the weight at which my body tended to want to maintain itself.

While treated for hypothyroidism, Michael went from 155 pounds and a 26-inch waist to 255 pounds and a 46-inch waist:

> I took the HCG shots for forty-five days and followed the diet and I lost about thirty-five pounds. I continued the diet but with an increased caloric intake to about 1,500 calories a day. I found that the low-carbohydrate, low-fat diet worked for me. I am now at 197 pounds and a 36-inch waist. It may not work for all, but it worked for me.

Mari, a thyroid patient, went from 115 pounds to 290 over several years and several pregnancies.

I had apnea, reflux, untreatable constipation, fourteen-day periods, prediabetes, unexplainable joint pain, muscle aches, and sinus problems. At forty-four years old, I was still looking for some viable way to lose weight. A friend of mine used HCG to lose 160 pounds, so I did three months of sublingual HCG. I lost thirty pounds, but the stress of the very low-calorie diet caused my reverse T3 to elevate. My hair fell out, and I gained six pounds of water weight. Fortunately, I changed to Cytomel, since natural thyroid meds were so rare. This was a good thing! I lost the water, my hair grew back, and I continued on to lose another twelve pounds, following Atkins. From that experience and from Atkins, I learned to count carbs and keep a fairly ketogenic diet, which keeps my weight stable and keeps me from retaining a lot of water.

With hypothyroidism and inadequate treatment from doctors, the five-foot-nine McMillan went from 140 pounds in his thirties to 298 pounds in his forties:

I started to ask doctors what was wrong with me. They told me I was depressed and gave me Prozac. They told me I had brain fog because I did not get enough sleep. I went through six doctors in seven years. Finally, once I had my thyroid somewhat in check, I went to see my naturopath about how I might lose more weight. My naturopath suggested I would be a good candidate for HCG. She explained what it was, and I read as much as I could about it. I purchased the drops and went on my way with my modified blood type diet and HCG. I followed the protocol to the letter and I am proud to say that I lost twenty pounds in forty days and I have not felt this good in ten years. I was on maintenance for three weeks, and I lost another five pounds.

I spoke with a number of physicians who are increasingly using HCG with patients who are unable to lose weight with traditional diet and exercise approaches.

So if we have some patient evidence-based medicine that shows that HCG works, and practitioners who prescribe HCG because they see it work with their patients, why don't we have research to back it up?

The truth is, one journal study showed greater weight loss with less hunger on HCG versus placebo. But a number of other studies have shown that HCG plus a low-calorie diet does not result in greater weight loss compared to the same diet without HCG.

HCG proponents explain this in part by pointing out that the studies have not looked at fat composition or body shape, and say that the key is that HCG-treated patients lose more body fat from the right places—versus muscle and fat from the wrong places—when compared to those not taking HCG.

Is that enough of an excuse? I don't know. I'll admit that while the theories behind why the HCG protocol works make sense, there is little proven research to back it up. Part of that may be due to the fact that HCG is not patentable. Large-scale studies are rarely undertaken to evaluate drugs that can't be profitably mass-produced by a drug manufacturer.

The HCG Protocol

Generally, the HCG protocol is very simple. The concept is that you follow a twenty- or forty-day cycle of using HCG, along with a very low-calorie diet composed of very specific foods, allowing you to lose a substantial amount of fat, primarily from areas of the body that have excess fat deposits.

While simple, proponents caution that HCG protocol needs to be followed very carefully. You can't take HCG and eat anything you want, or go above the calorie limits. The diet is specifically designed, at around 500–600 calories, to work with the HCG to achieve the results. According to practitioners working with the HCG protocol, the average weight loss on a forty-day course of HCG is anywhere from fifteen to thirty-five pounds.

Most practitioners who oversee the HCG protocol with patients follow a multiphase approach:

- On days 1 and 2, HCG is taken, but food is not restricted, and in fact, high-fat and higher-calorie foods are encouraged. If HCG is injected, one dose is taken in the morning; when sublingual or intranasal HCG is used, typically morning and evening doses are used.
- On day 3, the actual low-calorie diet begins, and it is followed until day 39.
- On days 40, 41, and 42, no HCG is taken, but the low-calorie diet is followed.

The foods eaten on the HCG protocol are very limited. Lunch on the HCG protocol includes the following:

- *Protein:* One 100 gram (3½ ounces, weighed raw) serving of protein, grilled or boiled without extra fat. Proteins can include veal, beef, chicken breast, fresh whitefish, lobster, crab, or shrimp. Remove all visible fat before cooking.
- *Vegetables:* One serving of spinach, chard, chicory, beet greens, green salad, tomatoes, celery, fennel, onions, red radishes, cucumbers, asparagus, or cabbage.
- *Starch:* One thin breadstick (Italian grissini) or one melba toast.
- *Fruit:* One apple, one orange, half a grapefruit, or a handful of strawberries.

Dinner is the same four choices as lunch. The fruit or breadsticks can be eaten in the morning as breakfast, or as snacks. But do not eat more than a serving of protein, vegetable, breadstick, and fruit in one meal. Also required daily is at least 2 liters of water per day.

In addition, the following are allowed:

- The juice of one lemon daily
- Seasonings: salt, pepper, vinegar, mustard powder, garlic, sweet basil, parsley, thyme, marjoram
- Tea or coffee in any quantity without sugar
- 1 tablespoon milk in every twenty-four-hour period
- Saccharin or stevia for sweetening as needed

Prohibited on the HCG protocol are salmon, eel, tuna, herring, and dried or pickled fish. No oil, butter, or dressing is permitted.

Some practitioners recommend following Dr. Simeon's original protocol, which prohibits use of all medicines and cosmetics. Other practitioners seem less concerned about medicines and cosmetics, and patients continue to take any prescribed medications and use the normal toiletries and cosmetics while on the HCG protocol.

HCG is not used while menstruating, but the diet is continued, and HCG is resumed when the menstrual period stops.

There's no recommendation to stop exercising on HCG, and most HCG protocols recommend some form of physical activity to help reset the body's weight set point.

For his patients, Dr. Van Lith recommends a slightly modified protocol. He has patients follow the high-calorie approach with HCG on days 1 and 2.

New in my routine is that, after the normal high-calorie diet on days 1 and 2, I have them stop eating on day 3, and instead take a big spoon of castor oil only. On Day 4, I recommend they take Epsom salts, to clean the body and triggers some detoxification. I then have then start on day 5 with the very low-calorie diet. I've found that this detoxification process is more effective for many patients.

Dr. Van Lith adds an unripe green pear and a thin slice of watermelon to the fruit offerings. He says that if hungry, you can eat celery, cucumber, leek, or radish at any time and in any quantity during the day. He also said that you can add celery, cucumber, leek, or radish to the main vegetable at any meal if desired. Dr. Van Lith adds Wasa crackers as an option in lieu of breadsticks and melba toast. Finally, Dr. Van Lith has his HCG patients take a serving of psyllium husk every morning, to promote regularity.

Dr. Van Lith does caution, however, that thyroid patients must remember to wait at least an hour after taking their thyroid medication to take the psyllium, and he urges having thyroid levels rechecked periodically when using a fiber supplement, to ensure the medication is being absorbed.

Maintenance and Repeat Cycles

Three days after the last dose of HCG, the low-calorie diet is stopped. At this point, for three weeks calories are not controlled, but dieters are urged to avoid processed carbohydrates, starches, and sugar in any form.

After three weeks, you can add in small amounts of carbohydrates, but you weigh yourself daily and adjust your diet accordingly. If you have an increase of more than two pounds from your final weight, you do what's known as a "steak day." This means skipping breakfast and lunch and eating a big steak and a big apple or tomato for dinner.

Typically, those who want to do multiple cycles of HCG need to wait six to eight weeks between cycles, to allow for HCG to get out of the system and restore sensitivity to the drug.

According to Dr. Van Lith, about 75 percent of his patients have little to no difficulty maintaining their weight after following the HCG protocol. But Dr. Van Lith has some specific recommendations regarding weight maintenance after the HCG protocol.

I tell my clients that whenever they eat any processed carbohydrates, they should take a big spoon of psyllium. This functions as a carbohydrate blocker. So if you are eating white rice, for example, adding psyllium gives it the glycemic profile of brown rice.

At the same time, he also recommends that to counteract the effects of hydrogenated fats or unhealthy oils, flaxseed oil should be a regular part of the diet.

In the morning, you can put it in muesli, oatmeal, or a drink. In the afternoon, drizzle it on an avocado or a hard-boiled egg. And in the evening, mix it into a salad.

Just for Thyroid Patients

For thyroid patients, Dr. Van Lith recommends emphasizing protein in the diet versus carbohydrates. And, according to Dr. Van Lith, thyroid patients do tend to lose weight more slowly on HCG. But he has found that switching to natural desiccated thyroid can help.

For thyroid patients, I only use natural thyroid, because I have found that synthetic T4 inhibits the HCG, and you get better results with natural thyroid. If patients tend to lose 12 kilos [26 pounds] in six weeks, a typical hypothyroid patient might lose 10 kilos [22 pounds]. But once they've started on natural desiccated thyroid, I find they are more likely to lose 11–12 kilos [24–26 pounds] on the next course of HCG.

Should You Try HCG?

Ideally, if you are following an HCG protocol, it should be a medically supervised, prescription HCG program. Do not be tempted by do-it-yourself or over-the-counter HCG programs. That means you should have a consultation with a medical professional before you start, and use a form of HCG prescribed for you.

While some practitioners have told me that they're actually surprised to see that homeopathic HCG has worked with some of their patients, if you want to actually follow the HCG protocol, you should consult with a physician for prescription HCG.

Dr. Rick Ferris, a naturopathic physician and pharmacist, has successfully overseen many patients following the HCG protocol.

There are different forms of prescription HCG—injectable, intranasal spray, topical, sublingual, even nonprescription homeopathic HCG—but I prefer the injectable and sublingual forms. One of the key issues for me is supervision. With the over-the-counter products, you are not being mentored appropriately, and you don't have medical supervision, which can make a key difference.

The injectable HCG seems to be favored by most of the practitioners I interviewed. Dr. Van Lith, who works with both injectable and sublingual prescription HCG, prefers a custom-compounded injectable HCG he formulated. He feels that it may be more effective, and patients won't forget to take a nighttime dose, a problem that can arise with the sublingual HCG.

Dr. Rob Carlson also prefers HCG by injection:

I prefer the injectable approach, using an 0.3 cc syringe and an 8 mm, 31 gauge needle, injected subcutaneously [right underneath the skin] into the tummy fat. These needles are incredibly small, and therefore generate minimal discomfort. I believe another mechanism of why this diet is effective is that if you are going to be committed to injecting yourself daily for twenty-one, twenty-six, or forty-two days, then you are also probably committed to following the diet.

A topical cream form has been developed, but the HCG

molecule is quite large and topical absorption of the HCG is not optimal, and may require high doses several times a day to achieve adequate absorption. There is a sublingual HCG that is sprayed or dropped underneath the tongue. The absorption is, however, variable and a substantially higher dose is required to achieve an adequate dose of the HCG in the bloodstream. Pills are not an option, because HCG cannot survive in the acidic environment of the stomach and be properly metabolized by the liver. A relatively new modality is potentially promising: a rapidly dissolving HCG tablet that is not swallowed but allowed to dissolve in the mouth and absorbed through the venous plexus underneath the tongue. This has a higher absorption than the sublingual spray, and because it is absorbed so well it is only taken once a day.

If you are intimidated by needles, keep in mind that the needles used for HCG injections are usually very small, very thin insulin needles used by diabetics for daily injections. If you've never injected yourself, see a health care practitioner for a lesson in how to safely administer an injection. If you are worried about the pain of an injection, note that if you have any abdominal fat—a "muffin top"—that's a particularly painless place for injections. (I speak from experience!) I can tell you that the injections did not hurt in the slightest. In fact, I barely even felt them. Dr. Van Lith provides his patients who use injectable HCG with a syringe used by children with diabetes. According to Dr. Van Lith, "Most people can't even feel the 3 mm needle, and there is no risk of it going into the abdominal cavity."

Some people should not use the HCG protocol, and different practitioners have different guidelines. Generally, women who are pregnant or nursing should not use HCG. Some practitioners will prescribe HCG for type 2 diabetics but not for insulin-dependent diabetics. Others rule out anyone with heart disease, current cancer, or history of cancer. Some physicians also rule out anyone with gallstones, a history of gout, epilepsy, or kidney disease. Be sure that you provide accurate information about your medical history to the practitioner overseeing your HCG protocol.

More Information

In the Resources section and at my website ThyroidDietRevolution .com, I have more information and links to several reliable and reputable sources who can work with thyroid patients on the HCG protocol.

PRESCRIPTION WEIGHT-LOSS DRUGS

Prescription weight-loss drugs may help jump-start weight loss after a long plateau, but they are not going to return you to a healthy weight and keep you there for life. Ultimately, you still need to figure out how to rebalance your metabolism, optimize your thyroid, incorporate an exercise program, and determine what combination and quantities of protein, carbohydrates, and fats allow you to function your best and maintain a healthy weight.

But if you could benefit from a weight-loss drug, here is a look at the very limited number of prescription drugs available. Note that some of these drugs are being sold online by unscrupulous companies that require minimal health information and no medical examination. You should not purchase diet drugs this way, particularly because there are a variety of potential side effects that can be dangerous. Your health needs to be thoroughly evaluated before you are prescribed diet drugs, and your response to the drugs must be monitored on an ongoing basis by a physician. If you order drugs directly, you are bypassing this important, even lifesaving step.

Orlistat (Xenical, Alli)

Orlistat, made by Roche Laboratories, is known by the brand names Xenical and Alli. Orlistat is a lipase inhibitor—that is, a fat blocker. It has been available by prescription as Xenical in the United States since 1999, and at a lower dose it has been available over the counter under the name Alli since 2007.

Orlistat blocks the absorption of about one-third of the fat ingested in a meal. Absorption is prevented in the small intestine, where orlistat stops the enzyme lipase from digesting fat. The fat then goes through the system undigested. Orlistat's most common side effects are oily discharge from the anus and loose stools, which usually occur when people eat more than 30 grams of fat a day. Orlistat, therefore, trains people to eat a healthier, lower-fat diet because of the looming possibility of intestinal discomfort and oily stools if they stray from the low-fat diet.

Overall, orlistat works in about a third of patients. It appears to help some people lose weight (ten to fifteen pounds, typically over a year or longer), lowers cholesterol levels, and lowers concentrations of glucose and insulin. It can also help people make a lifestyle change to a low-fat diet.

A study of approximately five hundred type 2 diabetes patients treated with the antidiabetes drug metformin and placed on a mildly reduced-calorie diet were also given either orlistat or a placebo. Another study looked at approximately five hundred type 2 diabetic overweight and obese patients receiving insulin on a reduced-calorie diet, who were divided into orlistat and placebo groups. In both studies, patients taking orlistat lost more weight than those taking the placebo. This study also showed that taking orlistat was "associated with a significantly greater improvement in control of blood sugar levels," to the extent that some orlistat participants were able to decrease or discontinue their diabetes medications.

Weight loss is usually temporary if patients go off the drug without further dietary modification. Patients need to follow dietary guidelines on fat intake (less than 30 percent of total daily calories from fat) very carefully to reduce the risk of unpleasant side effects. The fat intake should be divided among three meals. A multivitamin is recommended to counter the loss of some fat-soluble vitamins. Studies showed that levels of vitamins A, D, E, and beta-carotene were lower in patients taking orlistat compared to placebo. More common side effects include an oily spotting on underpants, gas with discharge, an urgent need to have a bowel movement, oily or fatty stools, an increased number of bowel movements, an inability to control bowel movements, orange or brown oil in the stool, and headache. Less common side effects are allergic reactions, which may include an outbreak of hives anywhere on the body, swelling of the throat, shortness of breath, and swelling of the lips and tongue. Menstrual irregularities, back pain, and upper respiratory infections were also mentioned by some participants in clinical trials.

Orlistat should not be taken or should be monitored very carefully among people with difficulty absorbing nutrients from food, gallbladder problems, kidney stones, diabetes, anorexia, bulimia, or sensitivity to any chemical component of orlistat. If people are taking other weight-loss medications or cyclosporine, they may not be able to take orlistat, or their physician may prescribe a lower dose than usual. Orlistat is not to be taken during pregnancy.

Some patients have found that the oily stools and anal leakage side effects are troublesome, particularly in the early weeks, and describe intestinal gas and irritable bowel syndrome, with alternating diarrhea and constipation, as a constant concern while taking the drug.

Orlistat may not be especially suitable for thyroid patients, as it can negatively affect the absorption of thyroid medication. This is a particular concern for thyroid cancer survivors, who need to ensure stable dosage and absorption of thyroid medication as part of their effort to prevent cancer recurrence.

Xenical and Alli tend to be expensive, running from $45 to $375 per month depending on the dose.

Phentermine (Adipex-P, Ionamin, Fastin)

Phentermine is the generic name for an appetite-suppressant drug that goes by the brand names Adipex-P, Ionamin, and Fastin. Phentermine has been on the market in the United States since 1959.

In 1999 phentermine was pulled from the market in the European Union, but it is still available in the United States. Phentermine may sound familiar because it was the "phen" in the huge fen-phen scandal of the late 1990s. The "fen" parts—fenfluramine (Pondimin) and dexfenfluramine (Redux) were pulled from the market after patients taking the fen-phen combination experienced heart valve damage and symptoms of primary pulmonary hypertension, which is sometimes fatal. Lawsuits were filed against the manufacturer of Pondimin and Redux, and the FDA started warning people about the heart condition in the summer of 1997.

Phentermine stimulates the central nervous system like an amphetamine, increasing heart rate and blood pressure and decreasing appetite. Phentermine is intended for short-term use only because the body will grow accustomed to the increased stimulation, and the dose of phentermine will lose effectiveness over time.

Phentermine reportedly does not cause as many jittery feelings as benzphetamine (discussed later). For those with sensitive stomachs who cannot tolerate the Adipex-P immediate-release dose, Ionamin is set in a resin that takes longer to dissolve.

One 2000 review of all placebo-controlled trials since 1960 about antiobesity pharmacotherapy lasting thirty-six to fifty-two weeks found that weight loss attributable to the drug was 8.1 percent, or 17.4 pounds, for those receiving phentermine, which was greater than statistics for sibutramine, orlistat, or diethylpropion (discussed later).

Note, however, that according to the National Institutes of

Health, guidelines now suggest that phentermine not be taken for more than three to six weeks. It's not clear if there is much potential for weight loss in this short a period.

Phentermine can be physically and psychologically addictive. Common side effects include elevated blood pressure, primary pulmonary hypertension, regurgitant cardiac valvular disease, heart palpitations, rapid heart rate, dry mouth, unpleasant taste, diarrhea, constipation, urticaria (hives), impotence, changes in libido, dizziness, blurred vision, difficulty breathing, shortness of breath, restlessness, headache, and insomnia. Less commonly, some people taking phentermine have reported hallucinations, abnormal behavior, and confusion.

Phentermine is not to be taken if moderately high or high blood pressure exists. For diabetics, insulin requirements may need to be altered, and phentermine may decrease the hypotensive effect of guanethidine. Effects of phentermine on cancer, fertility, pregnancy, children, and nursing mothers have not been determined.

Phentermine should not be taken by people who have hardening of the arteries, heart disease, moderate to high blood pressure, hyperthyroidism, known hypersensitivity or idiosyncrasy to the sympathomimetic amines, glaucoma, agitated states, or a history of drug abuse, or during or within fourteen days of the administration of monoamine oxidase inhibitors (hypertensive crisis may result), or if taking a tricyclic antidepressant.

Phentermine is potentially extremely dangerous when used in combination with fenfluramine or dexfenfluramine. This combination may result in primary pulmonary hypertension, which is high blood pressure (caused by the artery getting smaller in diameter) in the main artery of the lungs that carries blood from the heart. The increased pressure within the pulmonary arteries overworks the right side of the heart. The heart then works harder to overcome the increased blood-flow resistance created by the abnormally high pressure in the pulmonary arteries. The right side of the heart can become enlarged, and if the disease progresses, it can result in congestive heart failure. Symptoms of primary pulmonary hypertension include shortness of breath (particularly during exercise), chest pain, and fainting.

While this drug is readily available without prescription on the Internet, it is not advisable to purchase or take this drug unless under a physician's supervision.

Generic phentermine can run from approximately $40 a month up to as much as $75 a month for a brand-name product.

This is the only diet drug I have taken, but only as part of the phen-fen combination in the 1990s, for around four months. While I am lucky to have escaped the permanent damage suffered by some people who took these drugs in combination, I never lost any weight on phen-fen.

There's another reason that thyroid patients probably do not want to take phentermine. Studies have shown that the drug can actually cause a reduction in T3 and an increase in reverse T3. The researchers described it as "a pattern of serum thyroid hormones similar to that observed in resting patients on a total fast."

Benzphetamine (Didrex)

Benzphetamine, one of the first diet drugs on the market, is also known by the brand name Didrex. Benzphetamine is a stimulant that is an anorectic—that is, it acts as an appetite suppressant. The drug has been available in the United States since 1959.

By stimulating the central nervous system, increasing heart rate, and decreasing appetite, the drug has the potential to help with weight loss. Benzphetamine is considered most useful for those who have changed their eating patterns and lost weight but have hit a plateau. It is best given in a long-acting form and requires careful oversight by a physician.

The drug is habit-forming and has considerable potential for addiction. It should only be used short-term (a few weeks at a time) because the body builds up tolerance. Some side effects include heart palpitations, irregular heartbeat, elevated blood pressure, feeling overstimulated, restlessness, insomnia if taken late in the day, tremors, nervousness, sweating, headaches, dizziness, dry mouth, unpleasant taste, nausea, diarrhea, allergic reactions (hives), and changes in libido. Less common side effects include psychological disturbances (hallucinations, confusion), heart damage, depression or withdrawal symptoms after discontinuing benzphetamine, and impotence.

Benzphetamine should not be taken by anyone who has a history of heart disease, hardening of the arterial walls, moderate to severe hypertension, sensitivity to amphetamines, hyperthyroidism, glaucoma, anxiety, or a history of drug abuse, or by those taking monoamine oxidase inhibitors or other central nervous system stimulants. Benzphetamine should not be taken during pregnancy. It should not be taken in combination with guanethidine, tricyclic antidepressants, amphetamines, urinary alkalinizing agents, or urinary acidifying agents.

The typical monthly cost for benzphetamine is approximately $40 to $160 per month.

Diethylpropion (Tenuate)

Diethylpropion—brand name Tenuate—is an appetite-suppressant drug that has been available since the 1960s. The drug is a central nervous system stimulant that curbs appetite and increases heart rate and blood pressure. Diethylpropion has been shown to be effective in helping with weight loss over short periods of time without significant amphetaminelike side effects. Diethylpropion has been on the market a long time with no major problems, although the class of anorectic diet drugs is under more scrutiny now for heart-related problems because of the fen-phen incidents.

Since diethylpropion is an older diet drug, the less expensive generic form is available. Although few long-term studies were done when diethylpropion was first introduced in the late 1960s as a diet drug, there have been no major problems associated with the drug.

Diethylpropion can be habit-forming, so it can only be taken for short periods of time (a few weeks), then the patient must stay off the drug for a few weeks. Side effects may include slightly increased heart rate and blood pressure, sleeplessness, restlessness, dry mouth, nervousness, headache, diarrhea, constipation, and changes in libido. Less common side effects include irregular heartbeat, insomnia, impotence, and allergic reactions.

People with heart disease, high blood pressure, hardening of the arteries, anxiety problems, epilepsy or seizure disorder, or diabetes, or those who have taken monoamine oxidase inhibitors, should be careful taking diethylpropion and need to inform their physician of such conditions. People taking monoamine oxidase inhibitors should not take diethylpropion until they have been off the MAOI for at least fourteen days. Pregnant women should not take diethylpropion. Due to unpredictable episodes of dizziness or restlessness, people should be careful when driving and operating heavy machinery. People taking insulin, guanethidine, and tricyclic antidepressants should inform their doctor because the dosage of these drugs or of diethylpropion may need to be adjusted.

The drug runs approximately $30 a month for the generic, up to $50 for a brand-name prescription.

Phendimetrazine (Bontril, Plegine, Prelu-2)

Phendimetrazine, known by the brand names Bontril, Plegine, and Prelu-2, is an appetite suppressant that has been available in the United States since the late 1960s. It is a central nervous system stimulant that curbs appetite and increases heart rate and blood pressure. Studies have shown that phendimetrazine can be an effective appetite suppressant.

There is potential for abuse or dependence on this drug, since it is related to amphetamines. Tolerance also typically develops in a few weeks, and phendimetrazine is no longer effective at that point.

Side effects may include slightly increased heart rate and blood pressure, sleeplessness, restlessness, dry mouth, nervousness, headache, diarrhea, constipation, increase in urinary frequency, and changes in libido. Less common side effects include irregular heartbeat, insomnia, blurred vision, stomach pain, and impotence.

The drug was pulled from the market in the European Union in 1999. While phendimetrazine is still available in the United States, it carries heavy warnings about heart problems, because, as a stimulant diet drug, there are concerns that it may have serious or even fatal side effects like those seen with the popular but now banned combination of fenfluramine and phentermine (fen-phen).

People with hardening of the arteries, heart disease, moderate to severe pulmonary hypertension, high blood pressure, hyperthyroidism, glaucoma, anxiety, or a history of drug abuse should not take phendimetrazine. Use with other central nervous system stimulants is contraindicated. People with mild hypertension should be cautioned. Diabetics may need to adjust their insulin requirements while taking phendimetrazine.

There is also a danger in a large dosage or overdose, which can cause unusual restlessness, confusion, belligerence, hallucinations, and panic states. Fatigue and depression usually follow the central nervous system stimulation. Cardiovascular effects include arrhythmias, hypertension, or hypotension and circulatory collapse. Gastrointestinal symptoms include nausea, vomiting, diarrhea, and abdominal cramps. Poisoning may result in convulsions, coma, and death.

The drug runs from $20 to $50 a month, depending on brand and dosage.

Topiramate (Topamax)

Topiramate (brand name Topamax) is an antiepileptic drug approved in October 1998. Topiramate helps control seizures by altering chemical impulses in the brain. In 2002, researchers began to publish studies about using topiramate for weight loss.

In one study about the weight changes in patients during clinical trials for topiramate, researchers found that a daily dose of 200 mg resulted in a 5 percent or greater weight loss in 28 percent of the patients; 57 percent of those treated with 800 mg/day lost that amount of weight. The amount of weight lost was proportional to baseline body weight; therefore, the higher the initial body weight, the more weight the patients lost. Interestingly, those who took valproic acid, an anticonvulsant (brand name Depakote), prior to participating in the topiramate clinical trial lost even more weight.

Other studies have shown that topiramate may have applications as a treatment for binge-eating disorders.

The monthly cost for topiramate runs from $60 to $200, depending on dosage.

BUPROPION-NALTREXONE COMBINATION THERAPY

Some physicians are combining the antiaddiction and immune-modulating drug naltrexone with the antidepressant bupropion as an off-label treatment for weight loss. "Off-label" means that the use is not FDA-approved to date. It is legal for physicians to prescribe medications for off-label use. (It is prohibited, however, for drug manufacturers to promote off-label use of medications.)

Naltrexone is sometimes known by the brand name Revia, and bupropion is perhaps best known as Wellbutrin. The combination of the two drugs appears to boost weight loss by changing the workings of the body's central nervous system. Drug manufacturers are studying an experimental medication, Contrave, that combines the two in one pill.

Kent Holtorf, MD, is a physician who has been using these drugs together as an adjunct to weight loss:

> I've found that the antidepressant Wellbutrin (bupropion) does not work well for weight loss. A combination of Wellbutrin and low-dose naltrexone is, however, having some surprisingly good results. Typically, we have the patients on 300 mg of Wellbutrin-SR twice a day, along with an increasing dose of naltrexone, typically 10, up to 20, and then to 30. At a lower dose, for example 4.5 mg daily, it helps as an immune modulator, and at higher doses it seems to help with weight, cravings, and the set point.

While the combination of bupropion and naltrexone is generally well tolerated, some patients complain of sleepiness or nausea. The two medications can run upward of $250 per month.

METFORMIN (GLUCOPHAGE)

Metformin (brand name Glucophage) is an oral drug used to treat type 2 diabetes. Metformin helps decrease the amount of glucose absorbed from food and the amount of glucose produced by the liver. Metformin also increases responsiveness to insulin. It is sold under other trade names as well, including Riomet, Fortamet, Glumetza, Obimet, Dianben, Diabex, and Diaformin.

Several studies have shown that metformin may help nondiabetics lose weight by reducing hunger and by helping sensitize the body to insulin. In one study, about 80 percent of women who took metformin and adhered to a controlled-carbohydrate diet lost 10 percent of their starting weight in a year.

Some physicians suggest that metformin can work best in patients who are closely following a low-glycemic diet that does not spike blood sugar, and when a dosage of metformin is taken three times daily a few minutes before each meal.

Metformin is not recommended in anyone who has kidney, lung, and liver disease, and some forms of heart disease, based on the risk of a rare but serious complication called lactic acidosis.

The main side effects are nausea, upset stomach, and diarrhea, and a risk of hypoglycemic symptoms such as shakiness and dizziness.

While the implications are not clear, thyroid patients should be aware that several studies have shown that metformin suppresses TSH levels. One study found that a number of patients who were hypothyroid and on metformin had suppression of TSH to levels below normal, but without any signs of hyperthyroidism, and no change in free T4 or free T3 indicative of a change in circulating thyroid hormone. Another study found that metformin may be associated with a significant drop in TSH levels. Thyroid patients and practitioners should keep this effect of metformin in mind when evaluating thyroid therapy. It's also another reason why TSH alone can not be considered a reliable gauge for thyroid function, and free T4 and free T3 levels should be run regularly as well.

Metformin in a generic form can run $20 to $40 a month; the brand name drug can run $60 to $100 a month, depending on the dose.

Note that there are anecdotal reports that some patients do not respond to generic metformin, but do respond to the Glucophage brand specifically.

INJECTABLE DIABETES DRUGS

Several drugs used to treat diabetes are now being used by some practitioners as off-label treatments for weight loss and obesity, particularly in patients who are insulin-resistant or leptin-resistant and may be classified as prediabetic.

These drugs typically come as liquid in a prefilled pen that is used to inject under the skin of the abdomen or upper arm, and are usually injected several times daily before or with meals, depending on the drug.

- *Byetta (exenatide).* Byetta helps stimulate the pancreas to secrete insulin when blood sugar levels are high. It also slows the emptying of the stomach and reduces appetite.
- *Symlin (pramlintide).* Symlin is an antihyperglycemic medication that helps slow the movement of food through the stomach, which prevents blood sugar from rising too high after a meal. Symlin may also decrease appetite.
- *Victoza (liraglutide).* Studies suggest that Victoza helps control blood sugar by increasing insulin secretion, delaying gastric stomach emptying, and suppressing the secretion of glucagon.

Risks and Side Effects

These medications can cause side effects, including hypoglycemia (low blood sugar), which can cause shakiness, dizziness, sweating, weakness, pale skin, and even loss of consciousness, among other symptoms. In some cases, elevated blood sugar can occur, and may cause symptoms such as shortness of breath, breath that smells fruity, and unconsciousness. These symptoms require immediate medical intervention.

There have been problems with Byetta in people who have any kidney problems or history of pancreatitis. The FDA has also indicated that there may be concerns about an increased risk of thyroid cancer in Byetta and Victoza, and while the link hasn't been clearly established in humans, animal studies have shown a connection.

Byetta is more associated with general side effects than the other medications. While all these drugs have been reported to produce some stomach upset and other associated symptoms, users of Byetta typically report more of the gastrointestinal side effects, including acid stomach, diarrhea, indigestion, nausea, and vomiting, especially when first starting the medication.

Dr. Kent Holtorf prescribes these medications for weight loss as part of his practice:

> The biggest side effect is nausea, which occurs in about 25 percent of patients. Most of the time it is mild and diminishes with continued use, but a few patients will not be able to tolerate it. For Byetta, I recommend starting with a 5 mcg injection before meals. Some patients start with half a shot for the first few days (only pushing the plunger halfway). The nausea in some people can be due to an increased production of stomach acid, so Zantac (ranitidine) or a proton pump inhibitor drug—like Prilosec (omeprazole), Prevacid (lansoprazole), or Nexium (esomeprazole) for example—can be helpful. Nausea is less commonly a side effect of Symlin compared to Byetta, so it's preferable for some patients. For Symlin, the optimal dose is 120 mcg three times per day.

Should You Consider an Injectable Diabetes Medication?

Whether or not to use one of these medications for weight loss is a decision you and your practitioner will need to make. Here are some considerations.

First, will it work for you? According to Dr. Holtorf, you are more likely to have better results if you have demonstrable leptin or insulin resistance, as evidenced by elevated leptin levels or elevated fasting glucose levels.

While none of these drugs are approved by the FDA for weight loss, Symlin in particular is being studied in people without diabetes.

One six-week trial of Symlin reported in the *American Journal of Physiology—Endocrinology and Metabolism* found that obese patients who injected Symlin three times daily before each meal lost an average of four and a half pounds, compared to a control group that injected placebo and lost no weight. The study subjects also reported feeling full despite eating less.

I've talked with several thyroid patients who have lost twenty to thirty pounds in several months taking Byetta or Symlin. Kelly had an excellent experience:

> Nothing I was doing was working weightwise, and I have a history of diabetes in my family, so at 190 pounds, I was terrified that I was on my way to being diabetic. I was a bit freaked out at the idea of injecting myself, but the little pen actually is easy and I barely felt it. I felt kind of green the first few days, but I was able to tolerate it, and it was, truly, the first time in years that the scale started to move. I was able to lose twenty-five pounds in three months, and I continue to lose a few pounds a month while eating a healthy diet. This is phenomenal for me, as usually I have to suffer for weeks just to lose a pound. Even better, my blood sugar level is now normal. At some point, my doctor will wean me off the Symlin, and hopefully my blood sugar and weight will stabilize at a lower weight.

Joanne tried Byetta for weight loss but had a different experience.

> I have high leptin levels and am slightly insulin-resistant, so my doctor and I thought a trial of the Byetta would be reasonable. I started at the lowest dose and was very committed to making this work. But I wasn't able to tolerate the side effects at all. I felt exhausted all the time I was on it. I was nauseous every single day while on Byetta, and I threw up so much, I felt like the drug was making me a drug-induced bulimic, to be honest. I put up

with this for two months, and despite being really careful on my diet and constant vomiting, I couldn't believe that I only lost four pounds. It wasn't worth it to me to stay on the medication.

While an occasional patient like Kelly has reported dramatic weight loss, and some have significant side effects like Joanne, those who tolerate these medications should not expect dramatic weight loss. Many patients using them off-label are reporting modest weight loss at best.

Second, what about the inconvenience of injections? Says Dr. Holtorf:

Taking a subcutaneous shot several times a day can be problematic, but when patients have great results it is worth it for most. Some people are concerned that the medications require refrigeration, but it's usually not necessary, as these medications are very stable at normal daytime temperatures. So it's not a problem to keep it in your purse or in the desk drawer.

Third, there is the issue of side effects and risks. These medications do frequently have side effects that can range from temporarily uncomfortable to thoroughly intolerable. It's also important to keep in mind the increasing concerns on the part of regulators regarding the potential thyroid risks posed by Byetta and Victoza.

Finally, a key consideration is cost. Symlin, Byetta, and Victoza are quite expensive, and when prescribed off-label are usually not reimbursed by insurance companies. A thirty-day supply of these drugs can run $250 to $400 or more, depending on the dosage.

For some patients, however, one of these medications may be the key to breaking a plateau or starting a successful effort to finally lose weight gained after a period of hormonal imbalance. The objective is not to remain on these medications forever, but rather, to lose weight, help lower the leptin and insulin resistance, and then go off the medication at a point where the weight, metabolism, and hormonal balance will make it easier to maintain the weight loss or allow for continued weight loss.

WEIGHT-LOSS DRUGS IN DEVELOPMENT

One thing to be encouraged about is that since there are so many overweight, frustrated people in the world, finding solutions has become a major priority for the scientific community. Tremendous research efforts are looking at various weight-loss drugs and approaches, and many new developments and drugs are in the works. Here is a brief look at some of the things you're likely to hear about in the future.

Contrave

Contrave was mentioned earlier, and is the manufactured drug that combines naltrexone (Revia) and bupropion (Wellbutrin). In preliminary studies, the combination drug has helped users drop an average of 5 percent of body weight over a yearlong clinical trial. In the study, half of those who took the highest dose of naltrexone lost 5 percent of their weight or more, compared to only 16 percent of those taking placebos. Contrave does have side effects, however. One in three participants had nausea, and participants complained of other side effects including headache, constipation, dizziness, vomiting, and dry mouth. Half of the study participants dropped out before completing a year of treatment.

Empatic

Empatic is an experimental drug that combines the antidepressant bupropion with the anticonvulsant drug zonisamide. It is in the process of testing but has shown a fairly substantial weight-loss effect. One study found that participants who took the drug daily for sixteen weeks lost an average of nearly thirteen pounds, compared with about two pounds in patients taking placebo pills.

Nastech PYY Nasal Spray

Another product that is in the testing phase is a nasal spray that delivers peptide YY (PYY) for the treatment of obesity. PYY is a hormone naturally produced by the stomach in relation to the calorie content of a meal. According to results from various studies, obese or nonobese patients given a ninety-minute intravenous infusion of PYY consumed on average 30 percent fewer calories. All the people studied experienced a significant decrease in their overall twenty-four-hour calorie intake. Furthermore, obese patients were observed to have lower levels of circulating PYY. Therefore, increasing levels of PYY may be an effective therapeutic strategy in treating obesity, and the nasal formula has been shown to deliver sufficient amounts of PYY for therapeutic value. Studies are still ongoing.

WEIGHT-LOSS SURGERY

There are a number of surgical procedures currently being performed as treatments for obesity in those who are significantly overweight. In the last decade, bariatric surgery has become the second most common abdominal operation in the United States.

In this section, you'll find a review of some of the more common procedures as well as the newer approaches gaining popularity. We'll also take a look at the pros and cons, and the relevance and safety for thyroid patients.

Gastric Bypass (Roux-en-Y) Surgery

Gastric bypass is also known as Roux-en-Y (pronounced "roo-on-why") or Roux-en-Y gastric bypass (RYGB). RYGB surgery can be done in two ways: via an open incision, or laparoscopically, meaning that the surgeon inserts the surgical instruments, including a light and tiny camera, through a small incision. In RYGB surgery, the stomach is divided—often using staples—and only a small pouch, initially capable of holding only a small amount of food, about one ounce, is left to connect to the small intestine. Because the stomach is smaller, one feels full on far less food, and since food bypasses the duodenum, fat absorption is also reduced.

Gastric Sleeve Surgery

Gastric sleeve surgery is also called a sleeve gastrectomy and vertical sleeve gastrectomy. In this surgery, the stomach is divided into a smaller section—typically about 20 percent of its total volume—and that section is then separated from the rest (often with staples) and left connected to the small intestine. This procedure can be done via open incision or laparoscopy. When compared to traditional gastric bypass, studies show that patients tend to be more satisfied and lose more weight with the Roux-en-Y procedure versus gastric sleeve, though both are generally considered similarly effective.

A new variation on gastric sleeve surgery, known as trans-oral gastroplasty (TOGa), is in clinical trials, but will likely become a popular option. TOGa surgery is performed endoscopically, through the mouth, and does not involve an incision. A flexible endoscopic tube is inserted so the surgeon can see the procedure, and a small, remote-control surgical device is also inserted, which can push certain parts of the stomach out of the way, suck certain parts of the stomach into itself with a vacuum method, and staple sections together to form the "sleeve" that limits the amount of food that can enter the stomach at any one time. The rest of the stomach is still present.

Gastric Banding or Laparoscopic Gastric Banding (Lap-Band)

Gastric banding involves the placement of an adjustable silicone band near the top (esophagus end) of the stomach, creating a smaller stomach pouch and a narrow passage into the larger remaining portion of the stomach. In this procedure, the food intake is restricted, but the normal digestive process is not changed. The small passage delays the emptying of food from the pouch and causes a feeling of fullness. A port is placed on the outside of the patient's abdomen for the surgeon to use in adjusting the size of the band, which can be tightened or loosened over time to change the size of the passage; initially the pouch holds about 1 ounce of food and later expands to 2 to 3 ounces. The surgery is done with an open incision, or in some cases is done laparoscopically, in which case it's called laparoscopic gastric banding (LAGB, or lap-band surgery). Gastric banding is sometimes used as a follow-up surgery when patients fail to lose weight after a traditional gastric bypass.

A note about laparoscopy: For any weight-loss surgeries, while laparoscopy is often preferred due to faster recuperation time, surgeons may choose not to use this technique for patients who have had abdominal surgery in the past and therefore have scar tissue that can interfere with the surgery. In some cases, surgeons also may choose open incision versus laparoscopy for patients who have severe heart and lung disease, and for those who weigh more than 350 pounds.

Other Procedures

Less commonly performed are surgical procedures that reduce nutrient absorption by bypassing larger portions of the digestive tract. These include:

- Bileopancreatic diversion, in which a considerable portion of the stomach is removed, and the small section remaining is connected to the final section of the small intestine, bypassing most of the small intestine. Weight is lost because most of the calories and nutrients are directed into the colon and not absorbed.
- Bileopancreatic diversion with duodenal switch, in which a larger portion of the stomach is left intact, including the pyloric valve, and the duodenum and small intestine are both divided near this valve. This form of surgery is sometimes used in patients who have a very high body mass index, over 50—a level referred to as "super-obese"—as those patients have a failure rate of some 40 percent after traditional Roux-en-Y surgery.

Who is Eligible for Bariatric Surgery?

Typically, according to the National Institutes of Health, the American Medical Association, and bariatric physicians, bariatric surgical procedures are only considered for people who are considered severely obese. This is defined as being one hundred pounds overweight or having a body mass index greater than 40. In some cases, a patient may be considered eligible for bariatric surgery if he or she has a BMI of 35 or more and is experiencing serious obesity-related health conditions, such as high blood pressure, heart disease, diabetes, sleep apnea, or degenerative joint disease.

Effectiveness

The popularity of bariatric surgery has grown because the surgery, and in particular the RYGB surgery, has demonstrable results, including:

- Average excess weight loss that is usually higher than with purely restrictive dietary procedures

- One year after surgery, a typical weight loss averaging approximately 75 percent of excess body weight
- Continued weight loss, as studies have shown that as long as ten years postsurgery, a large majority of patients maintain 50 to 60 percent of excess body weight loss
- Improvement or resolution of major health conditions, including back pain, sleep apnea, high blood pressure, diabetes, and depression, in almost all patients

Generally, studies have shown that patients tend to be most satisfied and lose the most weight with the traditional RYGB procedure. It has the longest history and is the most studied, and many bariatric surgeons consider it to be the basic, most reliable surgical method for weight loss. RYGB is the most frequently performed bariatric surgery in the United States.

In terms of effectiveness, there are many studies that show that the body weight lost at one year postsurgery is considerably greater for RYGB versus gastric banding. One study showed that approximately 75 percent of excess body weight is typically lost after RYGB and diabetes fully resolved in 78 percent of patients, versus 48 percent of excess weight lost and 50 percent resolution of diabetes after laparoscopic adjustable gastric banding.

In one pilot study of the TOGa procedure, forty-seven people who weighed on average 120 pounds more than their ideal body weight had the procedure, and after six months, the subjects had lost more than a third of their excess body weight. By twelve months, their excess weight loss averaged almost 40 percent. This is less than the traditional gastric bypass, but the TOGa endoscopic procedure—as compared to laparoscopic or open surgery—is associated with quicker recovery, shortened hospital stay, decreased complications, and no incision or scarring.

Research has shown that patients who have an extremely high

body mass index (over 70) do best with an open incision gastric bypass versus laparoscopy.

Complications and Problems

No weight-loss surgery should be undertaken lightly, and the decision to have bariatric surgery is one that a patient needs to make in conjunction with a knowledgeable bariatric expert. It generally should be a decision that is made only after a comprehensive nonsurgical effort to lose weight has been unsuccessful.

All bariatric surgeries have risks, and rare but serious complications of any surgery include bleeding, infection, reactions to the anesthesia, and blood clots in the legs.

The most serious problems, however, including infection and even death, are most common after RYGB surgery compared to the other surgeries. Substantially fewer immediate complications in the short term are associated with sleeve gastrectomy, laparoscopic band procedures, and endoscopic procedures.

One serious complication is gastric leakage, in which there is a leak at the staple line and stomach contents leak into the abdomen. This is dangerous because the acid can eat away other organs; an additional surgery may be required to correct the problem, along with a lengthy recuperation. Gastric leakage is more common after sleeve gastrectomy than other procedures.

Another complication is "dumping syndrome," whereby stomach contents are passed rapidly into the small intestine. This can be triggered by too much sugar or larger amounts of food. Dumping syndrome can cause malnutrition, and is also very uncomfortable, causing nausea, vomiting, weakness, sweating, faintness, and diarrhea.

Almost a third of patients develop nutritional deficiencies after bariatric surgery, because the body is less able to absorb iron, calcium, and other nutrients efficiently. Nutritional deficiencies can specifically lead to iron deficiency anemia, chronic anemia, osteoporosis, and other bone problems stemming from low calcium.

While gastric banding surgery tends to have a lower complication rate than gastric bypass—with shorter hospitalization and faster recovery—it does carry with it a longer-term risk for band erosion or migration, which can cause infection or ineffectiveness and require additional surgery to reposition, revise, replace, or remove the gastric band entirely. Some experts estimate that as many as half of all patients ultimately require subsequent surgeries.

There are other possible complications as well:

- The success of the procedure can be reduced substantially if even slightly increased amounts of food are eaten and the stomach pouch is stretched. This requires another surgery to repair it.
- The opening between the stomach pouch and the small intestine may get narrower, which can require corrective surgery.
- Gallstones and gallbladder attacks, which occur more often when you lose weight quickly. It's estimated that up to 30 percent of patients develop gallstones after bariatric surgery.
- An incisional hernia (a bulging of tissue through the site of the incision). This is more common when an open procedure is done.
- Kidney stones.
- Gastritis (inflamed stomach lining) or heartburn.
- Ulcers, including bleeding stomach ulcers.
- Vomiting from eating more than the stomach pouch can hold.
- Breakdown of staple lines (band and staples fall apart, reversing the procedure).
- Low blood sugar (hypoglycemia).
- Chronic dehydration.

The Future of Bariatric Surgery

A number of newer procedures are being tested or on the horizon in the area of bariatric surgery, including:

- *Natural orifice transluminal endoscopic surgery (NOTES).* Besides the TOGa procedure, we can expect to see more use of the mouth and other orifices for incisionless gastric surgery.
- *Restorative obesity surgery, endolumenal (ROSE).* If stomach stretching has resulted in weight gain after gastric bypass, this incisionless endoscopic surgery can restore the stomach pouch back to its original postsurgery proportions.
- *Intragastric balloon.* This is a balloon that is implanted endoscopically in the stomach area to reduce the size of the stomach and therefore create a sensation of fullness. Some balloons are fixed in size, but the more recent development is an adjustable valve that allows doctors to increase or decrease the balloon's size with saline or air through an endoscopy procedure on an as-needed basis. At present, the balloons being tested are only left in for six months, but some studies are being done on balloons being left in for as long as a year or more. In one study that lasted for fifteen months, patients lost 10 percent or more of their body weight in a four-to-six-month period with the balloon.
- *Intragastric injection of botulinum toxin.* This slows the emptying of the stomach and creates a feeling of fullness.
- *Gastrointestinal neuromodulation.* The idea is that some kind of microchip or device would be implanted to stimulate the vagus nerve, mimicking a feeling of fullness and suppressing appetite.

Especially for Thyroid Patients

In consulting with a number of bariatric surgeons, there do not appear to be any specific warnings against any bariatric surgery techniques for thyroid patients. Most agreed, however, that no patient should undergo *any* weight-loss surgery until the thyroid hormone level is normal. Bariatric surgery should only be performed after normalization of thyroid levels if weight remains a problem and the patient meets the criteria for a bariatric surgical intervention.

Some surgeons have indicated that Crohn's disease, an autoimmune condition, is a contraindication for bariatric surgery. Also, anyone who has a history of chronic, long-term steroid use may not be eligible for bariatric procedures.

There are few studies that look at the results of bariatric surgery in patients with hypothyroidism, or autoimmune Hashimoto's disease specifically, though more studies in this vein would be helpful to have as part of the decision-making process for patients. One study did look at the results of RYGB surgery in twenty morbidly obese hypothyroid patients. Among those studied, one patient died as a result of the surgery, and four others had serious complications. The remaining fifteen patients experienced weight loss as well as what is referred to as "improvement in thyroid function."

Another study looked at eighty-six patients who underwent gastric bypass or adjustable gastric banding. The patients were not on thyroid treatment—though their mean TSH level was measured at 4.5, a level considered subclinically hypothyroid by some physicians. The mean body mass index of the patients went from 49 to 32 after surgery, and this was associated with a mean reduction in the TSH level from 4.5 to 1.9.

Interestingly, one 2008 study from the journal *Obesity Surgery* looked at twenty morbidly obese women with hypothyroidism who were on thyroid replacement therapy. After RYGB surgery, the hypothyroidism resolved in 25 percent of the women, improved in 10 percent of the patients, was unchanged in 40 percent, and worsened in 25 percent of the patients; the ones whose hypothyroidism worsened all had autoimmune Hashimoto's disease. The researchers have concluded that hypothyroidism appears to improve in the majority of morbidly obese patients who undergo RYGB surgery, except for those whose thyroid disease is autoimmune in nature. Bariatric experts consulted were not concerned regarding this one small study, however, suggesting that a worsening of hypothyroidism—as defined by a need for an increased dosage of medication—may be due to poor absorption of the medication and is likely to be offset by the benefits of the weight loss.

Feedback from thyroid patients who have had bariatric surgery suggests that their results tend to mirror the success and complication rates of the general population. However, some patients' comments indicated that their weight-loss postsurgery was slower than that of others who did not have a thyroid condition, or that their loss plateaued earlier and at a point when a smaller overall percentage of body weight had been lost.

Keep in mind that if you have any sort of bariatric surgery, you should:

1. Ensure that your thyroid function is optimized before surgery.
2. Be sure that you will be allowed to take your thyroid medication while hospitalized. (Some patients find that it's easier—and less expensive—to bring their own medication from home.)
3. Get thyroid levels retested frequently after surgery, to evaluate any changes in your absorption or thyroid requirements. If you have substantial weight loss, your need for thyroid medication may drop, so retesting is especially important.

Choosing a Surgeon and Hospital

If you decide to investigate bariatric surgery, keep in mind that a number of research studies have shown that the best results are likely with surgeons and hospitals that do substantial numbers of bariatric surgeries a year. Some guidelines suggest that you choose only hospitals that do at least one hundred weight-loss surgeries a year. One study found that low-volume surgeons and hospitals have double the complication rate compared to surgeons and hospitals that do a high volume of bariatric surgeries. Also make sure that your surgeon is a board-certified bariatric surgeon.

For additional reference, a list of some of the top bariatric surgeons and hospitals is online at the website for the book, ThyroidDietRevolution.com.

LIPOSUCTION

The liposuction technique was invented by Italian surgeons in 1974. In recent years, liposuction has not been used in attempts to remove large amounts of fat but rather to "sculpt" body parts. Liposuction is usually performed in patients who have lost all the weight they can, or who have areas of the body that are especially resistant to fat loss. Areas such as thighs, buttocks, and the abdomen are common for liposuction.

Long-term weight loss is never a goal or result of liposuction. But I'm including it here because thyroid patients regularly ask if liposuction is safe for them, and some patients who have already lost weight are interested in spot reduction of stubborn areas.

Certain preexisting conditions need to be specifically evaluated before any of the several types of liposuction is performed, and may make a patient ineligible for liposuction. These include:

- History of heart problems (heart attack)
- High blood pressure
- Diabetes
- Allergic reactions to medications
- Pulmonary problems (shortness of breath, air pockets in bloodstream)
- Allergies (antibiotics, asthma, surgical prep)
- Smoking, alcohol, or drug use

Tumescent Liposuction (Fluid Injection)

Tumescent liposuction is the most common type of liposuction. It involves injecting a large amount of medicated solution into the areas before the fat is removed. The fluid is a mixture of local anesthetic, a drug that contracts blood vessels (epinephrine), and a salt solution. The lidocaine in the mixture helps to numb the area during and after surgery, and may be the only anesthesia needed for the procedure. The epinephrine in the solution helps reduce the loss of blood, the amount of bruising, and the amount of swelling from the surgery. The salt solution allows the fat to be removed more easily, and it is suctioned out along with the fat. This type of liposuction generally takes longer to perform than other types.

Super-Wet Technique

The super-wet technique is similar to tumescent liposuction, except that less fluid is used during the surgery. This technique takes less time; however, it often requires intravenous sedation or general anesthesia.

Ultrasound-Assisted Liposuction

Ultrasound-assisted liposuction (UAL) is a technique used in the United States since 1996. In UAL, ultrasonic vibrations are used to liquefy fat cells. After the cells are liquefied, they can be vacuumed out. UAL can be done in two ways: externally (above the surface of the skin with a special emitter) or internally (below the surface of the skin with a small heated cannula). This technique may help remove fat from denser, more fibrous areas of the body, such as the upper back. UAL is often used together with the tumescent technique, in follow-up (secondary) procedures, or for greater precision.

Laser Liposuction

Laser liposuction is a newer technique and is done as an outpa-
tient procedure, often under local anesthesia (or light sedation if
more fat removal is involved). In laser liposuction, the fat, heated
by lasers, becomes softer and easier to remove. Fluid—a mixture
of saline and local anesthetic—is then inserted under the skin
in the area to be treated. Proponents of laser liposuction claim
that the heat of the laser stimulates the production of collagen,
which improves appearance of the skin and results in less bruising. Critics say that the procedure has all the risks of traditional
liposuction plus the additional risk of skin burns from the laser
and added cost.

Risks and Side Effects

As with any surgery, liposuction has risks from anesthesia, pulmonary embolism, infection, organ damage, and, for UAL surgery,
burns. There are various reports that put the risk of death from
liposuction at about 3 deaths for every 100,000 liposuction procedures.

One of the key downsides to liposuction is that up to 20 percent
of liposuction patients wind up with lumps, texture changes, and
asymmetry (referred to as fat fibrosis and necrosis) after the procedure. In some cases, additional surgery is required to address these
issues.

Some patients have brown discoloration of skin in the area that
has had the liposuction procedure. Up to 6 percent of patients report
problems with nerves—resulting in a pins-and-needles feeling and
other neurological symptoms—as a result of liposuction.

Ultimately, when fat cells are removed by liposuction, they do not
grow back. But if you gain weight, the fat goes to remaining fat cells,
which can result in asymmetrical distribution of fat.

Plastic surgeons consulted did not have any particular concerns regarding liposuction in general for thyroid patients. Some experts have suggested that laser liposuction techniques may be less effective for people with hypothyroidism, due to a slowdown in the body's ability to process the liquefied fat.

PART 4

STARTING YOUR

OWN REVOLUTION!

CHAPTER 11

The Mind and Body Connection

I speak two languages, Body and English.

—MAE WEST

One key challenge to weight loss is the fact that stress, and your own thought patterns, can get in the way on so many levels. Part of a successful weight-loss effort means that you need to address stress on many different levels.

Jena la Flamme, weight-loss coach and cofounder of the Weight Loss Pleasure Camp, explains:

> No matter how sensible it appears to the mind, any weight-loss strategies that are stressful to implement—for example, portion control, dieting, punishing exercise regimes—are counterproductive by nature. Simply put, stressful weight-loss strategies trigger the body's self-protection instinct, inhibiting the very thing they set out to accomplish—lasting weight loss.

MIND-BODY COMMUNICATION

We often hear about the "mind-body connection"—but that's an overused phrase in many ways. The mind and body are always connected. But the real issue, and the one that has a very definite impact on your ability to have success in reaching a healthier weight, is whether your mind and body are effectively communicating with each other.

To that end, one of the most important things I hope you can take away from this book is how crucial it is for you to facilitate clear and open communication between your mind and body regarding the issue of getting to a healthy weight. I realize that for some readers this may sound rather far out, but bear with me while I explain.

It's easy to forget that while they are always together, mind and body can operate at times as two competing entities, speaking very different languages. The conscious mind speaks in the language of words and thoughts. But the body speaks in the language of feelings, symptoms, hormones—and in some cases, health conditions.

Dr. Steven Gurgevich is one of the nation's leading experts on mind-body medicine, and author of the bestselling book and CD *The Self-Hypnosis Diet*. He explains a bit more about this concept:

> Body and mind are always connected—they are inseparable. I use the term *functional dualism*, meaning that one doesn't function without the other. But the message each one is holding—the intention each one is holding—become different. They are always connected, and always talking. Neither misses what's going on with the other—everything that happens with the body has a parallel with the nervous system and brain. And everything with the brain has a parallel in the body. What derails people from weight loss and healing is that the intention held in the mind is different from the intention held in the body. For example, the mind may be saying, "I want to lose weight, I want to be thin, I want to

exercise." But the body is saying, "I need to protect you," or "You don't love me. You've been telling me how fat I am—how can I be told every day I'm too fat, and now you expect me to become thin? I just follow orders."

One challenge is that many people who are overweight go around berating themselves, thinking, "I'm fat, I'm unattractive, I have a terrible metabolism, I'm never going to lose weight, I hate exercise." How we think and what we tell ourselves has a very real effect on our stress level and our body's ability to lose weight. According to Marc David, nutritional psychologist, author of *The Slow Down Diet*, and cofounder of the Weight Loss Pleasure Camp:

> Any guilt about food, shame about the body, or judgment about health are considered stressors by the brain and are immediately transduced into their electrochemical equivalents in the body. . . . Our thoughts also directly impact some of the most powerful metabolic chemicals we know of—hormones.

In some cases, the negative self-talk also turns into anger, which is stressful and counterproductive. Dr. Gurgevich explains:

> When we are angry with our body we are doing more harm than we can see. If you had a child who wasn't behaving, the more angry you get and the more you punish them, the less results you get. It's the same with the body. A starting point for recovery and weight loss is to acknowledge the anger, move through it, and then start taking positive steps to start turning around to love your body.

Jena la Flamme has a metaphor for this relationship. She says that we need to realize that the body is an animal.

By forgetting to take into consideration that the body is a "living, breathing, feeling, decision-making animal," the overweight body assumes the status of "lesser than" beside the mind, and something tragic occurs—listening stops. When listening stops, even if your body is speaking out loud and clear (which it usually does), you can't hear what's being said! True listening only happens in the company of equals, and unless the mind holds the body as its equal, listening is out of the question. If you brand your body as unlovable as it is right now, deem it "not good enough," or call it an overweight loser that needs to be "fixed," then all messages your body communicates to you will necessarily fall on deaf ears. Your mind will miss out on your body's wisdom. This invaluable natural resource—the body's instinctive know-how for natural weight loss—will be left untapped. When it puffs itself up as "better than," the mind squanders its intimate access to the cues and guidance that your body, your beloved animal, is trying to give you all day long.

FACILITATING BETTER MIND-BODY COMMUNICATION

There are a number of ways to help facilitate better mind-body communication.

Change Your Terminology

Jena la Flamme recommends a technique that I think is a particularly effective way to learn how to better tune in to and really hear your body's signals. She recommends that we should refer to our bodies by gender, as in "she" or "he," but not "it."

Linguistically, it's a departure from conventional grammar, but we're using it for a reason. Think about any living creature to which you're emotionally connected . . . if you're connected, you'll say "she" or "he." An example: you wouldn't call a beloved family cat or dog "it." By referring to our bodies as "she" or "he," we remind ourselves that our body is a living, breathing animal that deserves to be listened to and treated with compassion, not neglect.

Be Kind to Your Animal

By recognizing that your body is an animal, you will also realize that there are times when you are not listening to him or her. La Flamme believes that weight gain, like other symptoms, is in part a sign of rebellion and anger from a body that is not being listened to.

The body is talking all day long, but it speaks in signs and symptoms: hunger, fatigue, gastrointestinal issues, weight gain. If they're heeded early enough, they're messages. For example, your body tells you she is thirsty. But if you say, "Tough luck, I'm busy, I'm not getting up, because I have to finish this e-mail," that's just cruel! We want to take a step out and really understand that the body is a being, a life, the life you've been given, the one and only life you've been given, and realize that she deserves consideration and treatment, not neglect. Any animal that is told, "No, you can't have water, no, you can't sleep even if you're tired, no, you can't eat even if you're hungry," well, the poor neglected creature is eventually going to rebel. And weight gain, well, it's a red flag, saying "Hello, I'm here, and I'm changing!" It certainly gets your attention. And at some point you're going to have to pay attention if you don't fit in your pants.

La Flamme has also suggested that we realize that at times the body can behave like a petulant toddler or a whiny pet. In those cases, realizing that your body is an animal unto herself may also help you when she's whining for something that simply isn't good for her. We all know that chocolate isn't good for dogs, and candy isn't good for children. So imagine your dog is whining and begging for a piece of chocolate, or your three-year-old is threatening a tantrum to get her favorite candy. You have three choices. One is to give in to the whining, begging, and tantrums. But that's not good for either a dog or a child, and so it's clearly not a kind or caring thing to do. The second thing you do is smile, give a big sympathetic hug, and say no. And the third thing you can do is pull out a healthy treat and use a bait-and-switch approach. Think about it the same way when your body is whining inappropriately for something that not's good for her. Will you give in? Or will you sympathetically refuse, or offer an appropriate alternative?

Embodiment and Pleasure

One mind-body approach that is very important for anyone who wants to take better care of his or her health, and in particular for thyroid dieters, is the concept of embodiment—truly feeling inside your body and allowing yourself to feel pleasure. Jena la Flamme explains:

> Some people are in so much internal pain that numbing themselves—making themselves comatose with sugar, for example—actually stops them from feeling their pain. That's where instead of numbing that pain, we need to listen, and do something to cope with the pain and emotions locked in the body.

How do you get embodied? Some common ways toward embodiment, according to Jena and other experts, include:

- Breathwork
- Yoga
- Dance

- Taking a nap
- Sex
- A hot bath
- Gardening
- Walking in nature

Whatever it is, to achieve embodiment, it must be something you enjoy and that gives you pleasure.

Pleasure is increasingly being understood as an important aspect of a successful weight-loss program. La Flamme explains:

> It's a subtle yet profound shift. How could you make weight loss as fun for your body as it will be for you? Starting from this perspective—holding curiosity and respect for your body's likes and dislikes—uncovers all kinds of wonderful information. Paradoxically, despite fears that too much pleasure will be our downfall when it comes to weight loss, pleasure is a direct catalyst for the body's "relaxation response," the state in which fat burning occurs. Unlike the stress response, where weight is hoarded for protection, the relaxation response allows the body to feel safe and at peace, and therefore metabolically able to let go of the stored weight that previously was maintained as protection.

Develop Your Emotional Padding

One thing you definitely need to explore is how extra weight has served you and protected you. Says Jena la Flamme:

> Although it's easy for the mind to perceive unwanted weight on your body as a barrier and an obstacle to what you want, from the body's perspective weight is a well-intended protection mechanism! Excess weight is literally padding. It's a shield that insulates us from stressors, making us bigger and more resilient to

danger. Extra weight can serve a "natural" or "wise" function for the body and psyche. Weight can protect us from physical harm; it can protect us sexually by keeping men away; it can protect us emotionally by keeping others distant from us. It can numb us to uncomfortable feelings and past hurts, lower expectations placed upon us, and pull our attention away from important issues at work or in our intimate relationships. So if you're indeed carrying some extra pounds, what purpose might those extra pounds serve? How have you needed them to feel safe or comfortable?

La Flamme recommends journaling or writing about what role weight may be serving and what it may be protecting you from.

Once you've written down some brief words or thought about this, then ask yourself, "Am I ready to let go of using weight for protection, or comfort, or security, or numbing out? And how else can I protect myself in life—in a positive way—without needing extra weight?"

Fill the Real Voids

Life, health, and wellness coach Rebecca Elia, MD, says that we need to look closely at what role food and weight are serving in our life, and find other ways to fill the void.

The emotional component of food is often about unfulfilled needs. If you are not getting what you need, then there's a void, an empty space. If you are not conscious about how you are going to get these needs met, if you don't have a plan, then you're going to use the first convenient thing that comes along to fill the void—and it may be food. When you reach for food, ask, "Am I hungry?" If the answer is no, then ask, "What am I feeling?" and "What do I need, in this moment, that I am not getting?" This is a clue about what needs you are trying to meet through the act of eating. Many women in particular place their own needs last, so a multitude of needs go unfulfilled, and we end up searching for a quick and easy way to get these needs met. Enter addictive behaviors. If we can come up with healthy ways to get our needs met and give ourselves permission to fulfill our needs, then we have come a long way in combating unconscious behavior and addictions. Everyone has needs. We deserve to have our needs met in healthy, conscious ways. Food is one of the wonderful ways in which we nurture our bodies. Respect your body by feeding it consciously and joyfully.

Jena la Flamme has similar advice:

Every time you eat something, stop and say to yourself, "How is what I'm eating now going to make me feel in a few minutes? How will I feel in an hour? How will I feel in a few hours? How will I feel in a day? A few days? A month? Is this what she or he truly wants and needs?"

THE STRESS CONNECTION

It's important to understand that we have two different aspects to our nervous system. The sympathetic nervous system is the part of our nervous system that mobilizes the body's resources under stress. The sympathetic nervous system is continually active in order to maintain balance in the body. In extreme situations, however, it generates what's known as the "fight-or-flight response," in which:

• Blood flow is diverted away from the digestion and toward muscles and lungs
• The heart rate increases
• Coronary arteries dilate

By contrast, the parasympathetic nervous system is the part of the nervous system that controls smooth muscle contractions, regulates your heart muscle, and stimulates or inhibits your glands. Sometimes the parasympathetic nervous system is summarized as "rest and digest." Among many functions of the parasympathetic nervous system, it:

- Promotes calming of nerves and enhances digestion after a fight-or-flight response
- Dilates blood vessels leading to the gastrointestinal tract to increase blood flow after eating
- Stimulates your salivary gland secretions, aids in digestion, and helps with absorption of nutrients from food
- Causes the blood pressure and heart rate to decrease

Generally, the sympathetic nervous system is a stress response, and the parasympathetic nervous system is a relaxation response.

Many of us, however, are living, eating, and going about our daily lives primarily in a sympathetic mode, under chronic stress. We may not be in any imminent danger, but because we are constantly exposed to all sorts of stressors, our body doesn't really know the difference anymore, and chronic stress becomes the norm.

When you are under chronic stress, you flood your body with cortisol—a hormone that stimulates appetite. At the same time, the increased adrenaline raises fatty acid and blood sugar levels, stimulating the body to store those extra calories primarily as fat in the deep abdominal area—from a health standpoint, the worst place to gain weight. The abdominal fat makes you more insulin-resistant and produces various inflammatory markers that increase your risk of diabetes and heart disease.

Whether it's your own thoughts and negative perceptions, the stress of overexercising, lack of sleep, a jam-packed schedule, or poor-quality food, there is no shortage of stressors, and stress has a negative effect on your ability to lose weight.

One of the most important aspects of your own Thyroid Diet Revolution will be to determine what sort of physiologic stress reduction approaches are most effective for you, and make them a regular practice.

While we might describe many activities—such as reading or watching television—as relaxing, they are not necessary stress-reducing. When we're talking about physiologic stress reduction, we're talking about activities that demonstrably lower the heart rate, lower respiration, balance stress hormones, and have a physiologic effect on your body and your health.

Typically, these therapies fall into two categories: physical therapies, such as energy work, and mental therapies, such as biofeedback. There are therapies that combine aspects of both, such as yoga or tai chi. Mind-body work also includes imagery, hypnosis, Transcendental Meditation, psychotherapy, prayer or spiritual healing, music therapy, art therapy, breathing exercises, humor therapy, and other forms of relaxation.

Sometimes the success of these therapies is written off as due to the placebo effect, but that overlooks their effectiveness. If we believe that unconscious thoughts—general stress, for example, or negative self-talk—can cause illness, why wouldn't we think that conscious, positive thought could help ward off illness or heal the body? Rather than simply serving as a placebo, mind-body therapy also has a strong medical basis. The field of psychoneuroimmunology is showing us more every day about how the mind can communicate with the nervous system, the immune system, and our endocrine system via substances called neurotransmitters. Various chemical and hormonal releases can then affect health and physical function as a result of conscious thought.

Research shows that mind-body techniques are particularly useful in stress reduction. They are also empowering, involving you in your own health as an active participant. I would like to mention several approaches that, based on my own experience, I feel are particularly effective.

Yoga and Pranayama

Yoga is an important way to relieve stress and can be particularly helpful for thyroid patients. When you think of yoga, you may assume it means stretching or sitting in a cross-legged lotus position. But yoga is actually an ancient science that focuses on putting the whole body, mind, and intellect in harmony with the universe. Some of the many health benefits of yoga have been conventionally tested and proven, and are even discussed in Western medical journals. For example, certain forms of yoga have been found to have a strong antidepressant effect. Yoga has also been found to improve lung function and breathing.

In addition to gentle stretching and postures, yoga also includes the practice of pranayama, breathing exercises that help to cleanse and harmonize the energy pathways. The most basic technique of all is deep abdominal breathing. To try it yourself, lie flat on your back, or stand. Put your hand on your abdomen and take a deep breath, filling your belly with air so that your hand rises, then exhale. Start the basic pranayama practice by simply doing this for ten or fifteen minutes each day, and you'll be surprised at how much more relaxed yet energetic you'll feel.

More and more interest is also now focusing on specialized yoga breathing techniques that have the ability to change the nervous system in various ways. For example, one study looked at three different pranayamas. One group did breathing in and out of the right nostril (the other nostril is pressed closed with a finger), one group did breathing in and out of the left nostril, and a third group did alternate nostril breathing. Yoga experts believe that these types of breathing help balance the metabolism, generate increased energy, concentration, and mood, and help to balance endocrine disorders in particular. In the study, these practices were carried out as twenty-seven respiratory cycles, and repeated four times a day over the course of a month. At the end of the month-long practice, the right-nostril pranayama group showed a 37 percent increase over their baseline oxygen consumption. The left-nostril group showed a 24 percent increase, and the alternate-nostril group showed an 18 percent increase. The increase in oxygen consumption can help make the metabolism more efficient.

Here are brief guidelines on how to do nostril breathing:

- Sit on the floor in lotus position with legs comfortably crossed, or on a couch or chair, making sure your spine and head are straight.
- Rest your right hand on your right knee or in your lap.
- Place the index and middle fingers of your left hand at the center of your eyebrows.
- Keep the right nostril open and close the left nostril with the thumb.
- Inhale slowly and deeply through the right nostril to the count of four.
- Hold the breath for the count of two.
- Exhale to the count of four.

That is one cycle of nostril breathing. Repeat the cycles, starting with one to two minutes, and working up to several sessions of ten minutes a day.

There is also a specific breathing exercise that is designed to help the thyroid. Breathe in through your nose, focusing the inhalation toward the back of your throat. Your throat should feel slightly "closed" or "blocked" while you perform this breathing exercise. Mentally, you should try to feel as if you are taking in the air through the front of your throat. Do this several times a day, but not for long periods, as it might make you dizzy.

Finally, there is a specific asana or pose that is thought to be of great benefit to the thyroid. The half shoulder stand (*viparit karani mudra*) and shoulder stand (*sarvangasan*) positions both invert and stimulate the thyroid. In a shoulder stand, you lie flat on your back and, keeping your legs together, raise them up until they are at a right angle to your shoulders and neck, perpendicular to the floor, chin tucked into your chest, resting the weight of your body on your shoulders and elbows, arms supporting your hips. Work up to a daily session of a full two minutes by starting with two or three shorter sessions. If you can't get into a shoulder stand position, simply lying on the floor with your feet elevated and propped up against a chair or the wall can also provide similar benefits.

Breathing

Whatever you call it, a program of deep breathing exercises that is designed to take in more oxygen and release more carbon dioxide with each breath seem to help people with hypothyroidism to lose weight.

We know that hypothyroidism affects the strength of the respiratory muscles. Hypothyroidism is also known to increase reactivity of the bronchial passages, even if you don't have asthma. Even when treated, a substantial percentage of people with hypothyroidism report shortness of breath, feeling like they're not getting enough oxygen, or even needing to yawn to get more air as continuing symptoms.

For many of us, the ability to take in and process oxygen may be forever changed once hypothyroidism sets in. Even when we are fully treated, I suspect that most of us still don't take in and process oxygen fully. That is why specific attention to breathing seems to help some people with hypothyroidism. And learning how to breathe is about as inexpensive as it can be. All you need is some air and a pair of lungs to start. And no one can say that learning to breathe better isn't good for you, thyroid problem or not.

Breathing experts point to numerous health benefits of systematic breathing practice, including increased oxygen delivery to the cells, which helps provide sufficient energy to fuel metabolism, improve digestion, decrease fatigue, and create more energy.

Breathing is also an important way to help reduce our stress while we eat. Nutritional psychologist Marc David says, "The royal road to shortcut the physiologic stress response and bring you to relaxed, slow eating is conscious breathing." He suggests that before any meal or snack, we should take five deep breaths into the midsection. And he also recommends stopping to take several deep breaths while eating.

Jena la Flamme explains further:

> The apparently innocent offense—forgetting to breathe as you eat—is our number one common weight-loss downfall. Just as wood in a fire requires oxygen to burn, so our bodies literally need oxygen to "burn" the food we put in our stomachs. The simple combination of oxygen plus food is what makes up 95 percent of the energy your body generates. When you eat food without the oxygen your body needs to accompany it, digestion is sluggish and calories are stored as fat rather than burned off as energy. In other words, low oxygen intake leads to poor digestion, which leads to weight gain.
>
> Here's how to do it: Before you eat, stop and breathe. Without picking up the fork, breathe for as long as it takes you to reach a slow, deep breathing rhythm. If you are already relaxed, three breaths may be enough. If you are feeling highly strung, it may take a few more. Give yourself those breaths no matter what. Rest assured you deserve it. As you breathe you'll start to smell the food, which is also good for your digestive power, giving your digestive juices a moment to prepare.
>
> Then, as you begin to eat, continue to breathe mindfully. Breathe through your nose, as your mouth will be busy chewing your food! It's as simple as that.

In addition to incorporating regular breathing into our daily life around our meals and snacks, I also highly recommend a particular mind-body focused breathing technique called Transformational

Breathing. Created by Dr. Judith Kravitz and taught in workshops by trained facilitators, Transformational Breathing is a unique conscious breathing technique that is designed to help improve oxygenation, reduce stress, achieve balance and peace, and gain greater physical, mental, and spiritual health. Learning Transformational Breathing typically requires several sessions with a facilitator, but it quickly becomes a powerful technique that may help you not only relieve stress but also get rid of psychological blockages that are getting in the way of healthy weight loss. It's a practice that I use regularly, several times a week, to help keep mind, body, and spirit in balance.

Meditation

An effective way to reduce stress and foster mind-body communication is meditation. According to the Center of Integrative Medicine at Thomas Jefferson University Hospital in Philadelphia, meditation training can provide an improved sense of well-being, reduce body tension, and increase clearness of thinking—all effects that help you better cope with stress. Meditation has also been able to lower blood pressure, help clear up skin problems, and increase melatonin levels. By using magnetic resonance imaging, researchers have also established that meditation actually activates certain structures in the brain that control the autonomic nervous system.

I have found a variety of meditation approaches incredibly helpful in my own efforts to foster spirituality. In particular, I like the following audio programs:

- *Meditation for Beginners*, by Jack Kornfield
- *How to Meditate*, with Pema Chodron
- *Meditation in a New York Minute*, by Mark Thornton

Another wonderful tool to aid in learning and practicing meditation and relaxation breathing is a fantastic product called Relaxing

Rhythms, from Wild Divine. Relaxing Rhythms is an inexpensive biofeedback program and system that easily attaches to your home computer or laptop and .offers interactive training on how to use your body's own signals—heart rate, for example—to monitor physical and emotional reactions to stress. Relaxing Rhythms features three prominent mind-body experts—Deepak Chopra, Dean Ornish, and Andrew Weil—who teach you using more than thirty different breathing and meditation exercises.

You can boost energy, reduce stress, reduce anxiety and depression, and surprisingly, improve specific symptoms such as interrupted sleep and insomnia, urinary incontinence, headaches, and high blood pressure.

The way it works is that by providing you with physiological information—such as heart rate, or body temperature—that you might not normally be aware of, you learn which types of activities—certain breathing, relaxation and meditation patterns—can bring about specific and measurable changes in your physical response.

Guided Imagery

According to the nation's leading guided imagery expert, therapist Belleruth Naparstek, your brain doesn't know the difference between something you actually see and something you imagine. So your body responds as strongly to an image as to the real thing.

I am a devoted fan of Naparstek's excellent series of guided imagery health programs. One of my favorites is her program for weight loss, which you can get on CD or online as an MP3 download. I frequently listen to it when I'm on the treadmill, and it is very relaxing and inspiring. It motivates me to keep going!

Naparstek told *Prevention* magazine that guided imagery helps you "get in under your mind's radar" so that you can persuade your body to do something. "It may be to increase brain chemicals that make you feel calm and centered, decrease hormones that make you hungry, change the levels of biochemical components in your blood-stream that affect blood sugar, even build more immune system cells to fight everything from cancer to the common cold."

Cognitive Behavioral Therapy

Cognitive behavioral therapy is not about sitting on a therapist's couch for years exploring early childhood experiences. It is practical and solution-oriented, with the goal of helping you to rework the way you think about and therefore react to different situations. It is particularly helpful for people who are attempting to lose weight or maintain weight loss. There are a number of specific behavioral strategies you can learn and practice with the aid of a therapist or support group. These include:

- *Tracking.* The self-monitoring of your eating habits and physical activity in an objective way through observation and recording is an important part of cognitive behavioral therapy. You can keep track of the amount and types of food you eat, calories, and nutrient composition, as well as frequency, intensity, and type of physical activities. For even more insight, keep track of feelings and motivations to eat and exercise. Reviewing these records will help you gain insight into your own eating and exercise patterns and habits. You may also be able to identify particular situations such as boredom or frustration that trigger your worst episodes of unhealthy eating.

- *Stimulus control.* Identifying situations that may encourage you to eat poorly enables you to limit your exposure to high-risk situations. Examples of stimulus control strategies include learning to shop carefully for healthy foods, keeping high-calorie foods out of the house, limiting the times and places of eating, and consciously avoiding situations where you are likely to overeat.

- *Problem solving.* This involves looking at problem areas you have in terms of eating and physical activity, brainstorming possible solutions, and evaluating outcomes of possible changes in behavior. For example, some people who used to be inveterate snackers while watching television have taken up new habits, keeping manicure supplies, needlework, or crossword puzzles handy to replace snacking.
- *Rewards.* You can help change your own behavior by using rewards for specific actions, such as rewarding yourself for increased time spent exercising or for cutting consumption of particular foods. Self-rewards can be monetary (e.g., putting aside money for a special item or buying yourself something you've wanted) or social (e.g., going to the movies).
- *Cognitive restructuring.* You may have unrealistic goals or inaccurate beliefs about weight loss and body image, such as "I can lose ten pounds in two weeks," "I'm not attractive unless I'm a size 6," or "Women don't think men are sexy unless they have a six-pack." If so, you need to change the self-defeating thoughts and feelings that undermine weight-loss efforts. Cognitive behavioral therapy helps you come up with rational responses to replace negative thoughts. For example, you could replace "I blew my diet this morning by eating that doughnut; I may as well eat what I like for the rest of the day" with "Well, I ate the doughnut this morning, but I can still eat in a healthy manner at lunch and dinner."

Healing Touch (Somatic Experiencing)

Another approach that some people find effective is energy work, and in particular, techniques such as Healing Touch. Daphne White, a thyroid patient herself, is a Kensington, Maryland–based practitioner of Healing Touch and Somatic Experiencing:

> Healing Touch is a form of energy medicine: it uses a warm and gentle flow of energy from the healer's hands to stimulate

the energy flow within a client's body. It's like acupuncture in many ways, but without needles. Healing Touch is thought to work with the body's electromagnetic field and helps bring balance and coherence to all the body's systems. So, for example, when the thyroid works in a coordinated and coherent way with other glands and organs, hormonal levels are more likely to stabilize at an optimal level. Healing Touch provides an energetic tune-up to the entire body: it stimulates the spontaneous healing and relaxation response. In a culture as stress-filled as ours, energy medicine helps restore a more natural rhythm and flow to our entire body.

MINDFUL EATING

Finally, one of the most important things you can start doing right away as part of your own Thyroid Diet Revolution is focusing on more mindful eating. But what *is* mindful eating?

Have you ever sat in a darkened movie theater, totally absorbed in a film, and munched away unthinkingly at the food in your lap, only to realize after the film is over that you've had a huge bucket of popcorn, a giant soft drink, and other high-calorie treats—and you barely even realized that you were eating, let alone how much you ate? And on top of it all, even if you feel sort of queasy after eating all that junk food, you might still be hungry!

That's the power of mindless eating. Eating without looking at what you're eating, without paying attention to what you're eating, or while distracted by something else is a recipe for overeating, for bad food choices, and for being hungry after eating. And it's definitely a factor that will prevent weight loss.

Mindful eating means that you approach the process of eating thoughtfully and allow yourself time to look at your food and truly taste it. Along with eating slowly, mindful eating is an essential part of any weight-loss effort, and while it may sound New Age-y, it actually is rooted in practical, hormonal factors.

According to Marc David, you want to look at and smell the food you are about to eat, carefully and thoroughly. He explains:

> You know how your mouth waters when you smell something delicious? Or your stomach starts to churn when you think about lunch? These signals are actually the beginning of your body's digestive response, before the food even passes your lips. It's called the cephalic phase digestive response (CPDR), a fancy term for the pleasures of taste, aroma, satisfaction, and the visual stimulation of a meal. In other words, it's the "head phase" of digestion, when we engage our senses and turn on our awareness with food. The power of CPDR to catalyze nutrient assimilation, digestion, and calorie-burning ability is astounding. In fact, researchers have estimated that as much as 30 to 40 percent of the total digestive response to any meal is due to CPDR. Really smelling, seeing, and tasting our food initiates a chain of reactions to prepare our body for incoming food and metabolize it efficiently.
>
> Unfortunately, many of us skip out on this powerful phase of digestion. Eating has become a prime multitasking opportunity in our society, and it often occurs without awareness. As a result, we could be metabolizing our meal at only 60–70 percent efficiency.

Besides looking at and smelling your food, you also want to eat it slowly. Eating slowly is an essential part of mindful eating, and an important weight-loss strategy. According to a study published in the *Journal of Clinical Endocrinology and Metabolism*, eating a meal quickly, as compared to slowly, curtails the release of hormones that induce feelings of being full. The decreased release of these appetite-regulating hormones can often lead to overeating.

Part of eating slowly is also chewing your food thoroughly. When you chew thoroughly, you let the digestive juices in your mouth and throat do their work to properly break down and begin digesting your food. At the same time, you extend the time you're actually eating, giving your brain more time to receive the "I feel full" feeling, which doesn't get generated until about ten minutes after you start eating.

Weight-loss coach Jena la Flamme says that multitasking is not conducive to mindful eating. La Flamme says that it's a straight-forward diet and weight-loss rule, and should be easy to follow—but often isn't. When you are eating, you should not be:

- Talking on the phone
- Watching a television screen
- Texting
- Reading a computer monitor
- Driving
- Walking
- Reading—including the newspaper, a book, a magazine, or the cereal box

La Flamme also says that you should not eat while standing up. "You are not at a gas station to 'fill up'—so no standing while you eat. Standing tells your body that she's not even important enough for you to sit down with for a meal."

Another way to encourage mindful eating is presentation. If you regularly eat alone, or get takeout or fast food, you may be tempted to simply eat things out of foam containers or paper wrappings, but what sort of impression are you making on your body? You are telling your body that she deserves disposable food in disposable containers. If you wouldn't do it for an honored guest, try to make it a habit not to do it for yourself. It's not hard to put down a placemat and use a real plate, a real glass, and regular utensils instead of disposable tableware. It's all part of being mindful when you eat.

Some people complain that they feel lonely when they eat if they aren't reading, talking, or otherwise busy doing something else. Says la Flamme:

> Imagine if you went on a dinner date but spent the whole date reading or talking on your phone. How will you get to know your date? It's the same with food and our body. How can you get to know your body if you can't even pay attention to how it feels when you're eating?

Mindfulness is also useful in evaluating how you feel—what your response is to the foods you eat. You can gauge how effectively you are eating by stopping to ask yourself the following questions around two or three hours after eating:

- Was I hungry or dissatisfied soon after eating?
- Am I having any cravings for sweets?
- Do I feel the need to snack before my next meal?
- Am I still feeling tired after I last ate?
- Is my thinking fuzzy?
- Am I feeling hyper, jittery, shaky, nervous, or speedy?
- Is my pulse racing?
- Am I feeling sleepy or spaced out?
- Am I feeling depressed or sad?

The more yes answers you have, the more likely it is that you did not eat the right foods for you and your body. If you eat a meal that's right for you, you'll feel full, satisfied, energetic, and free of cravings, and you won't be hungry again until it's time to eat your next meal.

THE POWER OF SELF-HYPNOSIS

I've talked about why we want to create more effective mind-body communication, reduce stress, and eat mindfully, along with various techniques that can help you achieve those objectives. But one of the most important tools to help you launch your own successful Thyroid Diet Revolution, in my experience, is self-hypnosis.

Self-hypnosis helps us understand that what we are thinking about—and what we think we may want—may not always be communicated effectively to the body.

Says Dr. Steven Gurgevich: "You can walk around all day repeating a mantra or affirmation—delivering the message multiple times—but the question is, is your subconscious accepting it? Because when the subconscious accepts an idea, it acts upon it as real and true."

The subconscious is where we can directly communicate to our body in a language that she or he understands. We want to ensure that what we are consciously thinking—for example, "I want to eat a healthier diet"—gets through to our body as a clear, unequivocal message. And by carefully observing and listening to the body's signals, we will be able to recognize in our conscious mind the messages our body is delivering.

I know self-hypnosis may sound a bit out there, but it's a straightforward idea. What if you could take your thoughts and desires, translate them into a language the body truly understands, and deliver the message clearly and effectively? That's what self-hypnosis does.

In his *Self-Healing* newsletter, Andrew Weil, MD, one of the nation's leading holistic physicians, dispelled some common misunderstandings about self-hypnosis:

> For some people who have never tried it, the idea of going into a hypnotic trance may seem weird or scary. But the fact is that we've all experienced trance states in everyday life—whether

daydreaming, watching a movie, driving home on autopilot, or practicing meditation or other relaxation techniques. Essentially, trance is an altered state of consciousness marked by decreased scope and increased intensity of awareness. What distinguishes hypnotherapy is that it involves a deliberate choice to enter this state of consciousness for a goal beyond relaxation: to focus your concentration and use suggestion to promote healing. It can be done in person with a hypnotherapist or you can do it yourself, called self-hypnosis.

There are many self-hypnosis weight-loss CDs out there, and I've reviewed many of them. I can tell you that most of them are not worth the time or money.

But Dr. Steven Gurgevich has written a superb book, *The Self-Hypnosis Diet*, which has an accompanying CD that features the guided trancework, and it's truly a powerful tool for dieters. The book explains specific techniques that help you increase willpower, change unhealthy eating patterns, and create new and lasting healthy behaviors, and the CD actually helps you put those techniques into action for yourself.

You learn in the book that we should never go around saying, for example, "I have a slow metabolism. I just look at a donut and I gain weight" because it actually delivers a message to our body to fulfill our beliefs! He refers to studies showing that people who went around saying "I have a high metabolism, I burn things up the minute I eat them" actually have a comparatively higher metabolic response to food, and when they ate more calories than usual, they would speed up metabolically (as well as with digestion and elimination) to burn them off more quickly. *The Self-Hypnosis Diet* helps you deliver the message to your subconscious that your thyroid, body, and metabolism actually do know how to work effectively.

In my own case, I notice that when I regularly listen to *The Self-Hypnosis Diet*'s guided sessions, it shuts down any negative self-talk.

I find that I sleep better, have increased energy, and, surprisingly for me, crave vegetables. (I like vegetables, but I normally don't crave them!) My appetite decreases, and it makes it much easier to eat well, get physical activity, and have a positive self-image.

One of my friends tried listening to *The Self-Hypnosis Diet* for a few weeks to help curb her cravings for chocolate. Four weeks later, she was definitely craving less chocolate. She told me she also had a totally unexpected side effect: she stopped smoking—something she had been thinking about doing for years! Clearly, for some people, *The Self-Hypnosis Diet* helps your body hear, understand and act upon your conscious mind's best intentions.

CHAPTER 12

Your Thyroid Diet Revolution: Making It Happen

The greatest revolution of our generation is the discovery that human beings, by changing the inner attitudes of their minds, can change the outer aspects of their lives.

—WILLIAM JAMES

So now you know about the foods, the mind-set, the activity—everything you need to help you start your own Thyroid Diet Revolution. Here are some additional tips, dos and don'ts, and lifestyle guidelines that can help you make your revolution a success.

MEASURE, WEIGH, AND TEST YOURSELF REGULARLY

I frequently hear people advise that you should never get on a scale. And in a perfect world, I'd agree. We should know what to eat and what not to eat, know what's working for our body. But when you are trying to lose weight and maintain weight loss, many studies show that weighing every day is actually a very valuable feedback tool. In fact, one University of Minnesota study shared that daily weighing helps dieters achieve greater weight loss, and maintain that loss over time.

One study found that dieters who weighed themselves every day lost two times the weight of people who weighed themselves once a week. They say this is because the scale helped the dieters who weighed themselves daily to focus on their weight-loss goal and that tracking weight can actually improve mood by giving you a sense of control.

Rena Wing, PhD, director of the Weight Control and Diabetes Research Center at Brown Medical School, was part of a study that taught successful dieters "self-regulation," which basically meant that participants weighed themselves daily, and if weight went outside a five-pound range around their target weight, they adjusted diet and exercise to ensure that they returned back to that range. The method worked, and fewer participants regained five or more pounds during the eighteen-month study.

Weigh yourself at the same time every day to get a clearer picture of your true weight—which can fluctuate during the day depending on type of food and drink you've consumed, as well as whether you've had a bowel movement. It is also important to put the scale in the same place for consistency, since the type of floor can change the reading by a few pounds. Flat surfaces are best because bath mats and carpet can give you an inaccurately low reading. (Wondering if your scale is accurate? A dumbbell can be used to check.)

Hopping on a scale to keep track of weight loss is also important because as you're losing weight, it provides specific feedback regarding how your body responds to different foods and activity levels. Do you gain several pounds seemingly overnight after you've eaten bread or had dairy products? This may be a clue to a sensitivity that is affecting your ability to lose weight. Do you find that you lose a bit more weight after you've had a few days of good hydration? This is another clue about how you lose weight that you'll want to take note of and incorporate into your ongoing program.

Body measurements are also important, especially your waist measurement, because it gives a picture of cardiovascular and diabetes risk and is a marker for insulin and leptin resistance. Particularly for thyroid patients, who may have more early results in building muscle than in losing pounds, keeping track of measurements can provide important feedback and may even provide incentive on those days or weeks when you don't see much movement on the scale.

Finally, don't forget to have periodic thyroid blood tests. You will probably be adding fiber to your diet, so your thyroid levels should be retested about six to eight weeks after you stabilize at a new level of fiber intake, because you may need a change in your dosage of thyroid hormone replacement. Remember also that if you lose more than 10 percent of your body weight, that is also a time to get retested, because you may need an adjustment to your dosage.

If your insurance covers retesting, that's terrific. But if your doctor's office will not retest as often as you need to while you're on a weight-loss program, or if the retesting is expensive and you'll have to pay for it out of pocket, consider ordering your own thyroid tests via a self-testing service such as MyMedLab. Information on self-testing with MyMedLab is in the Resources section.

KEEP TRACK OF WHAT YOU EAT

It's essential to make healthy eating a habit. This is where tools for planning and tracking, as well as support from other people on the journey, can make or break your efforts. Whatever program you're following or however you are eating, research shows that writing down what you eat, tracking calories and nutrition, helps make any diet more successful.

The explosion of online tracking programs and apps for smart-phones make it very easy to keep track of data related to your diet and fitness, including foods eaten, calories, nutritional composi-tion of your daily and weekly diet, intake of carbs and fat, water intake, minutes or hours of activity, calories burned, hours slept, and other details.

The tool you choose depends on whether you're participating in a particular diet program. If you're following the South Beach Diet or Weight Watchers, for example, membership includes access to their Internet-based tools. DukeDiet.com has a personalized meal planner, shopping list tool, nutrition guide, weight tracker, exercise video library, food log and journal, calorie and fitness calculators, and more, for people who access their online program.

There are also a number of free online services that provide a combination of tracking tools and support communities. These in-clude CalorieCount, FitDay, and SparkPeople. SparkPeople, for in-stance, allows you to develop a personalized diet and fitness plan, and includes calorie counters, workout trackers, recipes, exercise demos and videos, and active communities for dieters, organized around geography, specific diseases, and other unique interests. SparkPeople also has apps for the iPhone, BlackBerry, and other mobile devices that allow you to access it on the go. Other popu-lar mobile trackers include MyFitnessPlan, LoseIt, and dozens more calorie, diet, and fitness tracking apps.

Jojo, a hypothyroid woman in her mid-forties, said that she used an iPhone application—LoseIt—to help with her successful diet:

> The app makes it easy to look up calories and to track them. I lost twenty pounds in three and a half months, and I've been able to maintain that. What I found was that I learned quite a bit about my eating habits, and by logging what I ate every day, it really made this more of a lifestyle change than a diet. Now, if I want a donut, I get the one with the least calories, and I adjust what I've eaten the

rest of the day. And it keeps track of calories by the week as well. So, over time, a great day followed by a bad day can balance each other out, so I never end up saying, "I blew my diet—I give up!" I even use the app to plan what I'll get *before* I go to a restaurant, so I don't have to even open the menu and get tempted. I'm too easily distracted by cheese and carbs to trust myself!

One of my favorite tools is an especially powerful software program called DietPower. Company president Terry Dunkle created this diet software in 1998 in response to his own health problems. DietPower software costs around $35 but is available for a free trial to test the program. Central to DietPower is an innovative calorie counter that tracks thirty-three nutrients, monitors your metabolism, and recommends foods you like that are best for your nutrition. It takes about five minutes a day to track your food intake with the program. Personally, in terms of providing detailed nutritional information, I think DietPower is the best of all the tracking tools. You can get information about how to download a free trial of DietPower, and links and information to all the tools mentioned, among others, at the book's website at ThyroidDietRevolution.com.

EAT SMART WHEN YOU EAT OUT

In general, Americans are eating out more than ever before. And this may be contributing to expanding waistlines.

A large coffee drink can have as many calories as a McDonald's Big Mac. A blueberry muffin at your favorite coffee spot can have 500 calories. An order of kung pao chicken at your favorite Chinese restaurant can have 1,600 calories. Fettuccine Alfredo will set you back 1,500 calories. And one of those batter-dipped, deep-fried whole onions served with dipping sauce? You're talking about more than 2,000 calories and 163 grams of fat.

Restaurant food tends to be high-calorie, loaded with simple carbohydrates, and served in huge portions. Some restaurants now have healthier options on the menu, and at most restaurants you can get a salad, dressing on the side, and some grilled chicken, beef, fish, or shrimp. Skip the bread, rice, pasta, and dessert. One technique I like to use is to ask for a takeaway container right from the start. I put half or more of my meal away immediately, which removes the temptation to overeat.

If you have to eat at a burger place, get a burger or chicken sandwich, take off half or all of the bun, get a side salad without dressing, and definitely skip the fries! One 6-ounce order of fast-food fries typically has as much as 600 calories and 30 grams of fat.

FOLLOW THE 95/5 OR 99/1 RULE

When you're starting out on an effort to lose weight, it's impossible to be "perfect." That's why it's useful to adopt the 80/20 or 90/10 rule, basically aiming to follow your guidelines 80 or 90 percent of the time. But if you're not losing weight on a sound diet, or when you have a thyroid problem that is making your metabolism less efficient, you may want to eventually move toward a 95/5 or even 99/1 rule. When you are trying to rehabilitate and repair your metabolism, you really can't afford much in the way of splurges, treats, cheat days, or multiple "just this once" occasions.

In particular, pay attention to weekends. We have a tendency to want to give ourselves the weekend off from dieting, but consistency is going to be important for you. One study found that most Americans consume more calories, fat, and alcohol Friday through Sunday compared with the rest of the week—sometimes as much as 100 calories more a day. If you do this every Friday, Saturday, and Sunday, those extra weekend calories could slow down or stall your weight-loss efforts. If you're in maintenance, it could result in weight gain.

GET SUPPORT FROM OTHERS

When it comes to weight loss, some of us are social animals and do better when we're in a support group. One study looked at more than five hundred people, half of whom were doing a self-help weight-loss program and half of whom were doing a commercial weight-loss program. After two years, about 150 people from each group were still continuing. The self-help group lost about three pounds in a year on average, then gained it back during the second year. In contrast, the commercial group—those going to Weight Watchers—maintained a weight loss of around ten pounds in the first year and after the second year concluded they were still an average of six pounds lighter than when they started. Those who went to more Weight Watchers sessions did better than those who attended fewer sessions.

If you find in-person support and camaraderie essential, consider joining a group like Weight Watchers or Overeaters Anonymous. Local hospitals also frequently offer weight-loss support groups, and many companies even encourage employees to organize weight-loss groups or lunchtime walking programs for weight loss.

If group support is not your style, you may prefer more of a one-on-one counseling approach. You have several options. You can work with a dietitian, nutritionist, or therapist who has a style and philosophy compatible with your own. This may sound expensive, but in the long run it's comparable to what you'd end up paying for some of the more costly commercial weight-loss centers that offer one-on-one counseling, and you won't have the pressure to buy products and supplements. Plus you'll have much more customized support from highly trained experts, rather than a canned diet program and support from folks who typically are not experts in physiology, nutrition, weight loss, or cognitive behavioral therapy, although they are trained to help you implement their company's program.

Finally, more and more people are turning to online support communities to help with weight loss. There are thousands of interactive forums, bulletin boards, chats, listservs, and other interactive online support activities available twenty-four hours a day. The key is to find the community that has the types of support you need when you need it. You may want to participate in a community at a paid online program such as South Beach Diet or Weight Watchers, join a free weight-loss and diet message group such as those found at CalorieCount or SparkPeople, or participate in the specialized thyroid diet and weight-loss support groups we have at ThyroidDiet Revolution.com and on Facebook.

BE WILLING TO TRY SOMETHING NEW

One way to make healthy eating more exciting—and flavorful—is to try new foods. For example, whenever I mention the grain quinoa, eyes start glazing over. (I know, because before I ate it, mine did too.) You probably don't even know how to pronounce quinoa (it's "keen-wah"), much less cook it, so it's not likely that it will end up on your grocery list. But why not? Quinoa, which resembles couscous and has a delicious, slightly nutty flavor, is gluten-free, high in fiber, high in protein, and lower in carbohydrates than most grains, making it a healthy food in general, and one that can be especially helpful for thyroid patients who are trying to eat healthy and lose weight. You can find quinoa in most grocery stores in the rice or pasta aisle, or you can get it in bulk at stores such as Whole Foods.

If you want to start using quinoa, the best thing to do is cook up a batch of it at the start of the week. It's really easy to cook—trust me! Just rinse the quinoa in a strainer under the tap until water runs clear. Then put it in a saucepan, and whatever amount of quinoa you have, add double the amount of water. Bring to a boil. Reduce the heat to a simmer, cover, and cook until all the water is absorbed, usually ten to fifteen minutes. When quinoa is cooked, it will appear translucent. That's it. After cooking, you can store your quinoa for up to a week in an airtight container in the refrigerator.

I love quinoa as a breakfast cereal—I add plain yogurt and some fresh berries and mix it all up to make a cold, fruity breakfast "porridge" of sorts. It's delicious! For an on-the-go lunch, take some cooked quinoa, add chopped tomatoes and onions, goat cheese or feta cheese crumbles, some seeds or nuts, and a vinaigrette dressing, and you have a healthy, filling, high-protein salad. You can even add some chicken, shrimp, or beans for extra-filling protein. Or you can toss in some garlic and parsley and heat to serve it as a side dish. Cooked quinoa is also a great substitute for rice or pasta as a base for chili or stews.

Karilee Shames, PhD, RN, a holistic health expert and therapist who herself has a thyroid problem, is sensitive to dairy products. Says Karilee:

> One thing that really works for me, since I had to give up cow's milk cheeses years ago, is sheep's milk or goat cheese. I find I can digest it easily. I sometimes make a sandwich with goat cheese, sprouts, whatever greens I have (I love basil and arugula). So it's like an open-faced sandwich-salad. I sometimes put tomato and avocado on it, then drizzle with olive oil and lemon. It's like a full salad that is also a sandwich, giving plenty of aminos, minerals, and protein.

Karilee is also a fan of smoothies:

> I like to start the day with a shake that really helps get me going in the morning. It's a breakfast salad! I like to use hazelnut, rice, or a similar nut milk, add my omega oils, then put my salad greens in there and whip it up. The milks have protein, but you can always add your favorite protein powders from health food

stores. Most blenders will mix up greens, but I find the Vitamix is the best gift we can give ourselves. You can put anything in there with any liquid and blend it into a drink or soup.

IDENTIFY YOUR TRIGGER FOODS

While there are guidelines, we all have foods that we know we need to particularly avoid, even if they haven't been identified as common allergens. So think about your own personal "hit list" of trigger foods that you should limit or even avoid. These would include foods and drinks that:

- Cause an allergic reaction
- Give you diarrhea, stomach cramps, or abdominal pain
- Cause you to feel shaky, sweaty, dizzy, or light-headed
- Make your pulse go up
- Make you hungrier than before
- Make you feel tired
- Make you feel bloated
- Make your skin break out
- You can't control—as in you just can't eat one, so you eat the whole box, bag, or carton

A weight-loss journal, food diary, or tracking system, along with daily weigh-ins (if you can stand it), can really be a help. After a few weeks of tracking, you'll start to see patterns that reveal some of the unique aspects of your own physiology and way of eating, and how you respond to particular foods.

I can't tell you which foods will be on your personal list, because that list will be unique. Some people can drink a cup or two of coffee; other people find that it makes them shaky and messes up their blood sugar for the day. Some people can use dairy products, whereas others find that dairy gives them a stomachache, bloats them up for a day or two, and stalls weight loss. In my own case, here are a few examples:

- I'm very allergic to raw tree fruits (apples, pears, peaches, plums, cherries) and tree nuts (walnuts, pecans, etc.).
- I cannot eat just one Butterfinger, so I don't eat any.
- Drinking fruit juice (like orange juice) makes me shaky and incredibly hungry.
- I seem to have some intolerance to milk products, so I avoid drinking milk—but I can eat yogurt.

So it's going to be up to you to determine which foods maximize your metabolism, help you to feel your best, and help you to lose weight most effectively while not feeling hungry, bloated, constipated, and so on.

AVOID HIDDEN PERSUADERS

There are many "hidden persuaders" built into our economy and society—these are factors, products, and situations that subtly encourage you to eat more than you realize. These include:

- *Extra-large and "supersize" containers.* Studies show that you are very likely to eat more from a larger container than a smaller one.
- *All-you-can-eat buffets, "unlimited pasta bowls," etc.* People rarely will limit their intake to a healthy amount when they are in a situation with unlimited food.
- *Store sales.* Studies show that people tend to buy more of a food item if the sign says it's "3 for $6" than if it says "$2 each."

Do your best to avoid all-you-can-eat and buffet-type restaurants, and when they ask you if you want to supersize, well, you know the answer!

GET ENOUGH SLEEP

If you want to lose weight, you are going to have to get enough sleep. According to the National Sleep Foundation, most adults need from seven to nine hours a night, yet the average American gets only six and a half hours of sleep per night, and two out of every ten Americans sleep less than six hours a night.

What happens if you don't get enough sleep? Insufficient sleep may:

- Reduce basal metabolic rate
- Cause more cortisol to be released, increasing stress and hunger
- Reduce non-exercise-associated thermogenesis—the involuntary activity, such as fidgeting, that burns excess calories during the day
- Interfere with the body's ability to metabolize carbohydrates, causing high blood levels of glucose, which leads to higher insulin levels and greater fat storage
- Drive down leptin levels, which causes the body to crave carbohydrates
- Reduce levels of growth hormone, which helps regulate the body's proportions of fat and muscle
- Lead to insulin resistance and contribute to increased risk of diabetes
- Increase blood pressure
- Increase the risk of heart disease

A study of nearly seventy thousand women found that those who sleep five hours or less per night are 32 percent more likely to experience major weight gain—defined as an increase of thirty-three pounds or more—over a sixteen-year period and 15 percent more likely to become obese, compared to those who slept seven hours a night. Even six hours wasn't quite enough—the women who slept six hours per night were still 12 percent more likely to have major weight gain and 6 percent more likely to become obese, compared to the women getting seven hours of sleep per night. (Note that they tried to see if sleep was connected to activity level, but there was no correlation between exercise levels or physical activity and sleep. What they did find is that the women who were getting less sleep were actually eating less, yet gaining more weight.)

Even in young, healthy people, a sleep deficit of three to four hours a night over the course of a week has a triple-whammy effect on metabolism. Just this limited amount of sleep deficit interfered with the ability to process carbohydrates, manage stress, and maintain a proper balance of hormones. In one sleep-restricted week, study participants had a significant loss in their ability to process glucose and an accompanying rise in insulin. Insulin levels were so high, in fact, that the men were considered to be in a prediabetic state.

How much sleep do you need? Target seven hours or more a night of actual sleep. You might try adding an additional fifteen minutes per night each week, until you get to a point where you are waking refreshed and are not exhausted during the day. You'll also want to make sure that the sleep you're getting is of good quality. That means no light in your bedroom—turn off the television, the lights, and your cell phone, and use room-darkening curtains or shades, because ambient light can disturb sleep and interfere with the normal nightly melatonin and growth hormone cycles. Avoid disturbing television or books in the hour or two before bedtime. Don't bring work, bills, studies, or your telephone to bed; avoid caffeinated products after midafternoon; and consider taking a warm bath or shower before bedtime.

A Few More Tips

- Regular exercise can help, but try to avoid exercise within three hours of bedtime because it can jazz you up too much.
- Avoid caffeine, nicotine, and alcohol in the late afternoon and evening.
- If you have trouble sleeping at night, don't nap during the day.

- If you can't sleep, don't stay in bed. After thirty minutes, go to another room and do something else that is relaxing until you feel sleepy.
- Try melatonin. For some people, 1 to 3 mg at night, an hour before bedtime, can help them fall asleep and have more restorative sleep.

GET MOVING

Don't forget that you have to move. Weight-bearing exercise is critical to raising metabolism. I'm not suggesting that you have to live in the gym or take up step aerobics, but you'll need to move. Gentle exercise helps lower insulin resistance, increase growth hormone, and build muscle, without increasing appetite.

Some diets and weight-loss programs tell you that you can lose weight without any exercise. That may be true for some people and some programs. But it's not likely to be true for most thyroid patients. And what those diet programs don't tell you is that most people who are not exercising will eventually regain the weight over time. Even if you're not a big fan of physical activity, you'll have to accept it: moving your body is not optional. I talk about this more in chapter 9.

CONSIDER A SPECIAL DETOX, CLEANSE, OR JUMP START

Some dieters find that starting off a new way of eating with a detoxification program, a cleanse, or even a short fast can ease your shift into healthier eating and help jump-start the weight-loss process.

Therese, a thyroid patient, said that she always loses weight and feels great when she visits a vegan health spa.

Daily exercise, vegan food (including raw food and sprouts), wheatgrass juice two times daily, walks outside daily, a sauna two to three times a week, three meals a day and nothing in between except for herb teas and water. After ten days I feel totally energized and have lost weight (usually seven to nine pounds), and symptoms like joint pain and stiffness vanish.

Two-Week Jump Start: Smoothie Shakedown

As I mentioned earlier, I especially like Dr. Ann Louise Gittleman's Fat Flush Body Protein, a protein powder for smoothies. I also like her Fat Flush Kit, a combination of three separate supplements—a multivitamin, gamma-linolenic acid, and a weight-loss formula that includes chromium and acetyl-L-carnitine. The Fat Flush Body Protein and supplements are combined in a two-week jump-start program created by Dr. Gittleman called the Smoothie Shakedown. If you are looking for a gently detoxifying way to jump-start your own weight loss, I think the Smoothie Shakedown can be a good choice for thyroid patients.

Basically, it involves having a Fat Flush Smoothie for breakfast and lunch. The smoothie is made with the Body Protein, plus some low-glycemic fruit, a small spoonful of flaxseed oil, some ground flaxseed or chia seeds, and water. Then dinner is 4 to 6 ounces of grilled or broiled lean protein, unlimited veggies, a large salad, and a dressing of either lemon juice or apple cider vinegar.

In addition, Dr. Gittleman recommends drinking half your body weight (in pounds) in ounces of water (so if you weigh 150 pounds, you'd drink 75 ounces of water), and using the Fat Flush Kit supplements if possible.

While I frequently use the Fat Flush Body Protein to make breakfast smoothies, I've also followed the Smoothie Shakedown program, and when I'm on it for those two weeks, I feel energetic and usually lose at least four or five pounds. Some thyroid patients have reported losing as much as ten pounds.

Websites: www.unikeyhealth.com/shakedown, www.annlouise forum.com/fat-flush-smoothie-shakedown, www.smoothieshake down.com

GO TO "WEIGHT LOSS PLEASURE CAMP"

As you may have noticed, I have frequently quoted nutritional psychologist Marc David, author of *The Slow Down Diet: Eating for Pleasure, Energy, and Weight Loss*, and weight-loss expert Jena la Flamme, founder of New York City's popular Jena Wellness Center. David is the founder and director of the Institute for the Psychology of Eating and a pioneer in the psychology of eating. Both are graduates of the prestigious Institute of Integrative Nutrition in New York.

Marc and Jena are knowledgeable nutritionists who have a very mind-body approach to weight loss, and they have joined forces to create an online workshop called Weight Loss Pleasure Camp.

Weight Loss Pleasure Camp is not a diet, but rather a way of applying the key principles outlined in *The Slow Down Diet* and in Jena's successful weight loss and wellness coaching. The premise of their approach is that when you experience the pleasure of food, you are able to maximize metabolism and fat-burning power.

In *The Slow Down Diet* Marc David says:

> We can only achieve and sustain optimum metabolism when we eat, exercise, and live under an optimum emotional state. Our frame of mind directly impacts metabolism to such a degree that what we think and feel profoundly influences how we digest a meal. Metabolic power is not only about what you eat but who you are when you're eating.

The Weight Loss Pleasure Camp program helps you learn how to eat, exercise, and live under an optimum emotional state, and how to harness the power of mind, emotions, and hormones to aid in metabolism.

Their four-week telecoaching program focuses on providing step-by-step training in their unique weight-loss principles, tools, ideas and strategies, which focus not on dieting, deprivation, food restriction, portion control, self-control, calorie reduction, diet pills, and exercise, but instead on relaxation, pleasure, sensuality, curiosity, nourishment, and nurturance as foundations for weight loss.

Sessions focus on how to use pleasure as a catalyst for lasting weight loss, shifting away from deprivation-based dieting methods, how men and women lose weight differently, how to base a weight-loss approach on pleasure-based strategies, how to join forces with body wisdom, using intimacy with your body to fuel fat burning, techniques for achieving emotional satisfaction with food, and ways to sustain weight loss and stay on track.

I highly recommend Weight Loss Pleasure Camp as a unique and effective way to start off any new way of eating.

Website: www.weightlosspleasurecamp.com

CHAPTER 13

Keeping the Faith

I've been on a constant diet for the last two decades. I've lost a total of 789 pounds. By all accounts, I should be hanging from a charm bracelet.

—Erma Bombeck

How do you keep the faith—maintain the hope that you will be able to find the right approach, stick with it, lose the weight, and keep it off? It requires a combination of time, the right attitude, and a bit of forward thinking. I've put together some suggestions on how to keep the faith, even when the weight-loss process can seem frustrating.

TROUBLESHOOTING FRUSTRATIONS AND PLATEAUS

One of the key ways you'll be working with your diet is to adjust your plan to make sure it fits you perfectly and helps you lose weight. For example, you may find that you are losing weight, but extremely slowly. If that's the case, don't abandon the plan and start a different one, hoping you'll lose pounds more quickly! Instead, recognize that you're on the right track, and consider making some modifications to your plan to see if you respond with slightly increased weight loss.

Keep in mind, though, that it takes time to make adjustments, so give yourself a week or two after you make a modification before you decide to abandon it, adopt it permanently, or try something else. Also, don't make multiple modifications and adjustments at the same time, because if you do, you won't know which change is working.

But if the time comes where you hit a plateau, or things just don't seem to be working, what next?

Here are some foods to consider eliminating from your diet to help you get past a plateau or help trigger successful weight loss. Keep in mind that you don't have to commit to a lifetime without these items. Rather, you're doing a trial, typically a few weeks to a month or two, to see if eliminating this food from the diet may be the key to more successful weight loss.

Cut Coffee

If you are still drinking coffee, eliminate it. Some people find that even if they're eating well, just one cup a day of coffee derails their weight. It's not clear what mechanism may be in play, but if you are a coffee drinker and your diet is stalled or not working, try eliminating coffee for just a few weeks and see if that gets things moving in the right direction.

Cut Gluten

Some people who still eat wheat or gluten products find that despite their best efforts, they get stalled or are not having success with weight loss. For some of these patients, removing all gluten from the diet seems to be a useful tactic. Even if they do not have celiac disease, some low-level intolerance or sensitivity to gluten may be a factor that is causing inflammation, which then blocks weight loss. Going gluten-free can sometimes be a successful approach.

Even though she wasn't diagnosed with celiac disease, Ellyn tried eliminating gluten from her diet.

I thought it was the middle-age curse. I had gained about fifteen pounds over a three-year period. I had read about cutting
out glutens from my diet, so I tried it. I substituted salads for
sandwiches at lunchtime and replaced wheat with other grains
like rice. Within a very short time I lost the weight and felt so
much better.

Cut All Starchy Carbohydrates

If you are following a plan that allows for some starchy carbohydrates, you may need to cut them out completely in order to lose
weight. Thyroid patient Mari said that the biggest mistake in her
diet was trying to eat low-fat and low-calorie but with a lot of simple
carbohydrates.

This did not work for me, but I didn't understand why. I gave
up sugar, bread, potatoes, and pasta. I find that I can eat more
calories in protein, complex carbs, and fat than I can in simple
carbs. I notice how my body reacts to what I eat, and avoid foods
that give me a hypoglycemic response. By doing this, I avoid the
afternoon slump and the extreme hunger I used to get at three in
the afternoon.

Reduce Saturated Fat

If you are freely eating animal protein, you may need to cut back
on the saturated fat in your diet in order to lose weight. This means
passing on the beef, pork, lamb, and full-fat dairy products and
eating primarily fish, nuts, chicken, vegetables, and low-fat dairy.
Says Dr. Ron Rosedale:

My take on fat is that if I am treating a patient who is generally hyperinsulinemic or overweight, I want them on a diet low in

saturated fat. Most of the fat they are storing is saturated fat, and when their insulin goes down and they are able to start releasing triglycerides to burn as fat, what they are going to be releasing mostly is saturated fat. So you don't want to take any more orally.

Increase Your Water Intake

Up your water intake—your body needs a constant, steady source of water in order to flush out toxins and fat, and to keep metabolism functioning smoothly. So if you're drinking 64 ounces a day, try adding three to five more 8-ounce glasses, for a total of 88 to 104 ounces of water. And if you're already drinking more than 100 ounces a day, try working your way up to drinking your body weight (in pounds) in ounces of water.

Cut Calories

If you're on the calorie-sensitive plan, cut 50 calories daily. It may mean the difference between staying where you are and starting to lose weight.

Drop Snacks

If you're a regular snacker, consider dropping your snacks. Try focusing on eating a larger breakfast and a slightly larger lunch.

Eliminate Alcohol

Alcohol puts stress on your liver, which not only slows down the ability to clear toxins and burn fat but may also interfere with your body's ability to convert T4 to T3. Alcohol, at 7 calories per gram, is also entirely empty calories, with no nutritional value. Consider eliminating it.

PUT YOURSELF FIRST

Whatever new way of eating you choose, you are going to have to push yourself up higher on your priority list. I know that I am much more likely to do just about anything—work, favors for friends, answering e-mails, playing with my children—than jump on my treadmill, because everything else seems so much more urgent.

But how much more important and urgent are everyone else's needs versus your own health and self-esteem? So make time for yourself—time to plan what you'll eat, shop for healthy foods, cook meals, exercise, reduce your stress. And don't be so quick to donate your valuable time to everyone and everything else when one of the most worthy causes of all is looking at you in the mirror!

TRUST YOURSELF AND YOUR OWN INSTINCTS

It's important that, whatever plan you choose to follow, you listen to yourself and trust your own instincts. Health and beauty expert Kat James, in *The Truth About Beauty*, says:

> Relying on cultural or commercial cues for our choices is what causes us to stray from our better instincts in the first place. If you start sentences with "My doctor has me taking this" or "My trainer has me doing that," stop yourself. Only you have yourself doing whatever it is you choose to do. Stop following and start setting your own course.

DON'T PUT YOUR LIFE ON HOLD

Don't put your life on hold simply because you want to lose weight. Many of us make weight loss into some sort of oasis in the desert that we are traveling toward.

- When I lose weight, I'll start going to the beach again.
- When I lose weight, I'll reunite with my old friend.
- When I lose weight, I'll make an effort to find a new romance.
- When I lose weight, we'll finally schedule the wedding.
- When I lose weight, I'll finally try to get a new job.

And so on . . .

Life is too short to keep putting everyone and everything on hold until some day in the future when you achieve your "perfect" weight. Give yourself permission to live, and do the things you enjoy today!

PRAISE YOURSELF

Even if you're overweight and frustrated, find a part of your body that you do like and regularly praise yourself. Maybe you have terrific-looking feet, really great eyes, or the best-shaped calves in town. Just pick one part of your body and continually tell yourself how terrific that part is. If you like even one part of yourself, it's a start.

PHRASE YOUR GOALS POSITIVELY

Think about your goals positively. Phrase them in your mind without using a negative word. In yoga, a resolution is called a *shankalpa*. In yoga practice, you must always phrase your *shankalpa* positively in order for success. So instead of "I need to lose weight," focus on "I will eat more healthfully and get more exercise so that I can get to a better weight for me."

I don't know why this works, but it does. Perhaps instead of challenging your body to a duel and telling it you are going to take away something, you are saying that you will be adding good things to it, improving it, and making it better.

Patricia is going into her weight-loss efforts with the right attitude:

> I'm working with the diet, and with the changes I've made (and even though I've made some mistakes), I am feeling more "clear," and it seems my hunger is more satisfied, if you know what I mean. When I'm hungry, it's as if I have control over the hunger rather than feeling as if I have to eat now. I'm looking forward to feeling better, even if I don't lose weight. If the weight— fifty pounds—comes off as well, what a plus that will be!

REALIZE THAT IT'S NOT A DIET—IT'S LIFE!

Don't view your change in eating habits as a diet that you can go on and off. This is life. This is hypothyroidism. This is not where you lose the extra couple of pounds, then it'll be easy to keep it off. You're on a journey and you may arrive at a target weight, but that's not your destination, because you need to change your way of eating and step up your physical activity—consistently, and for life.

Leanne Ely, a radio host and bestselling author of the book *Body Clutter:*

> I lost over fifty pounds and kept it off. What I learned is that weight loss with a thyroid condition isn't impossible, it's just hard. Consistency is what finally made the weight drop off. It was a long

process, but I learned a ton about food, supplements, what worked for me, and the amazing power of exercise.

SET SMALL GOALS, AND TAKE IT SLOW

British thyroid advocate and weight-loss coach Ali Jagger went from a size 10 to a size 20 in six months as she endured misdiagnosis by her doctors. Once she was finally correctly diagnosed and treated for her hypothyroidism, she turned her attention to losing the hundred pounds she had gained. Her first step: joining a gym to start swimming.

> The bravest thing I ever did was put on a swimming costume and not cry when I saw my reflection! I didn't recognize that person—she was so huge! I couldn't work at the time as I was more or less unemployable, got colds, was often ill, so I tried to go to the gym and swim. I lost on average about fourteen pounds a year, but it was a really hard slog. The goal to lose all the weight was so huge I sometimes gave up—it was very slow progress. I set small goals and was determined to get better.

Over time, Ali went on to lose a total of a hundred pounds, and then she turned her energy toward an effort to help others. In addition to speaking as a thyroid advocate in British newspapers and on television programs, Ali trained as a life coach, and now she helps thyroid patients and others struggling with weight problems to have a healthier lifestyle and lose weight. Says Ali:

> I made a pact with myself that I would get better and really get my story out there! During my long journey back to good health and my subsequent fight for the correct medication, I was determined to make sure that no one ever went through what I went

through. I remember feeling very isolated, lonely, and desperate, and I never wanted anyone else to feel that way if I could help it. I wanted to get back to good health so I could fight for others who were going through what I did. I remember all too well the agony I was in, having gained fifty-five pounds in just a few short months. I kept thinking, "If I could just be thin again, things would be perfect." I was able to lose the weight, and I think there are several important steps.

First, you must be thyroid-well before you can achieve any weight-loss goals. You need to give your body the time it needs to hormonally heal.

Next, you need to learn your body and where your thyroid hormones need to be for you. Track your symptoms so that you know when your treatment is working its absolute best. If you think you are not being properly treated or if you're not in thyroid treatment at all, don't surrender to "I'm just overweight and I don't feel well." Get a second opinion.

Finally, once your thyroid is optimized, you can start to regain the energy you need to lose the weight. Go back to the absolute basics of good eating, and make healthy lifestyle changes that will increase your vitality and get you back in shape. It can be done, and you're worth the time. Take it slow and make it your goal to live thyroid-well and be thin once again.

TRY NEW THINGS

Kathy, a papillary thyroid cancer survivor, had her thyroid completely removed.

I was already overweight from my thyroid not working. I have had my Synthroid changed many times, and working out did not help at all. I was put on the antidepressant Zoloft, which made me gain twenty pounds in two weeks. I had my endocrinologist check my T3 levels, and they were extremely low. We added T3, I was changed from Zoloft to Wellbutrin XL, and I have started eating low-carb. The weight is slowly starting to come off. It seems like a combination of the right medications along with eating things my body can burn is what works better for me. I still have twenty-five pounds to go, but I am a cancer survivor, I feel great, and I know I can lose more weight with the right tools.

DEFEAT NEGATIVE THINKING

Therapist Dr. Dave Junno feels that negative thinking can really put a damper on efforts to lose weight. According to Junno, many of us go around saying, "I can never give up the foods I love," or "I can't do an exercise program." Or if we tried to change our diet or tried to exercise more and were not successful, then we might say, "I tried that and it hasn't worked," or "I don't have the discipline or the willpower."

According to Junno, this creates a self-defeating cycle. Our negative thinking leads to inaction, which leads to no results, which confirms and reinforces the negative thinking. "It is like we have given ourselves a life sentence without parole," says Junno. His suggestion is to introduce one word into your vocabulary when you talk about your weight-loss efforts: *yet*.

- "I haven't been able to give up the foods I love . . . yet."
- "I can't do an exercise program . . . yet."
- "I tried that and it hasn't worked . . . yet."
- "I don't have the discipline or willpower . . . yet."

Dr. Junno says it may sound like a small step, but it opens up big possibilities.

It introduces the potential for success, which can help keep us motivated to continue trying. In the future all things are possible. Anyway, how do we know we can never stay with a diet or exercise program? Where is it written that this is impossible? Others have made these changes. Why can't we? Sure, it may take work, but that doesn't mean it can't be done. Just because we haven't done it so far doesn't mean we won't be able to eventually. Many people who succeed at making healthy lifestyle changes at first experienced some failures.

Junno also suggests that we keep in mind the many things we were unsuccessful at doing the first time we tried but were eventually able to master. "Remember riding a bike? Did you ride perfectly the first time? Probably not. Chances are you needed to practice a number of times, or build up your confidence, or just be in the right frame of mind to be willing to try."

I love the idea of holding on to the power of the word *yet*. I was a smoker from my late teens until my early thirties, and I must have stopped smoking a dozen times. I finally decided that all my attempts weren't failures. Instead, I was practicing, and eventually I would get so good at it that I would successfully stop smoking forever. And I did! I didn't use a smoking cessation program. I just went on straight willpower, along with a number of things I'd learned about myself in all my previous attempts. I have viewed my weight-loss efforts in a similar way. I'm learning what works and what doesn't work in my own efforts to optimize my thyroid and maintain a healthy weight. And the times that things haven't worked—well, those weren't failures, they were practice! Weight loss is a process, and while I may not have everything figured out yet, I will get there eventually. And you can, too!

BELIEVE IT CAN BE DONE!

For more than a decade, the National Weight Control Registry, a collaboration between the University of Colorado and the University of Pittsburgh, has maintained a database of more than two thousand people who have successfully lost at least thirty pounds and kept it off. The registry has found that:

- The most popular form of exercise for people who have successfully taken off weight is walking.
- More than 50 percent of those in the database did not participate in a formal weight-loss program. Instead, they employed a lot of personal discipline.
- The average registrant has lost sixty pounds and kept it off for five years.

Don't buy into the gloom-and-doom statistics about weight loss or thyroid disease. It's hard to lose weight, but it's not impossible. You can do it, and *The Thyroid Diet Revolution* will help!

Perhaps the best thing is for you to hear the inspirational words of your fellow thyroid patients. Kelli had to call around to interview doctors to find the right one to help her diagnose her thyroid problem.

You were right! It's tough to find the right one. But I found one in my area. And I think she is learning from the information I have shared with her. I was strong in my approach. The blood tests came back clearly indicating that I was hypothyroid, and I asked to be put on Armour, which is working wonders. I asked for follow-up blood tests just this last week, after being on the medication for only six weeks, and it is working! My joints no longer are painful, I am starting to lose weight, and my depression is lifting. It's like a miracle.

Until being diagnosed with thyroid cancer, Karenna was, as she describes herself, a "size 6 with bundles of energy."

I didn't exercise, but could run up four flights of stairs without missing a beat. After the removal, my weight ballooned from 130 to 175 pounds. It took three years to take off twenty pounds. Currently I have reduced my carb intake. I did not do a full-scale low-carb, high-fat diet. I eat protein for breakfast, salad for lunch, and protein with a light salad or fruit for dinner. I steer clear of all sugar, flour, etc. It seems to work for me. I now weigh around 155 pounds. I have more energy and seem to fit proportionately in my clothes better. People notice that I have lost weight and look healthier. It is a constant struggle. My former thyroid doc told me I was depressed, and I should eat a more balanced diet and exercise more. How to exercise when you can hardly lift your head off the pillow is beyond me. My new thyroid doc (love him!) added Cytomel to my Synthroid and understands that losing weight isn't easy. He even tells me I look great the way I am!

Some readers have found their own way to weight loss. For example, Mandy has found that Weight Watchers is helping her.

I've lost almost twenty pounds in nine weeks, and it has been a very comfortable process. I only needed to lose about fifteen pounds to begin with. It is a very healthy way to lose weight. You can eat anything, so there are no cravings. One simply has to be mindful of healthy choices and proportions.

Susan found the low-glycemic approach helpful:

I have been on a low-glycemic-index diet, and it has been a miracle. Nothing else worked since I was diagnosed with hypothyroidism fifteen years ago, and because I haven't broken this diet once in three years, my earlier failed attempts were obviously not due to a lack of willpower! I lost sixty pounds over the course of fifteen months, and while I did gain ten pounds back, I have stabilized at a size 12 as opposed to an 18.

Jane said she had tried different eating plans, and nothing had worked.

Until now, that is. I've lost ten pounds in about two months since starting your diet. I'm also working out at Curves (for the past six months) and have reduced twenty inches but wasn't dropping real weight. The weight wouldn't come off for anything until I started this diet. It's perfect for my thyroid disorder, which started out as Graves' disease. I was very sick until I was finally diagnosed. Eventually I took the radioactive iodine and since '89 I had gained 110 pounds. I am fifty years old now and had been prepared to gain some weight with my age, but that was just too much. Before I couldn't lose more than eight pounds and always gained it back. Six months ago I was at 240; now I'm 229.5. I know the resistance exercise at Curves has helped me in many ways, but the weight loss is definitely from this diet. Believe me, I've learned enough about my own body to know what is and isn't going to work.

Linda has found the secret to her success:

It seems that if I religiously walk and stretch, watch my diet, take time for myself, I have gone from 200 pounds to 180 pounds. My symptoms seem much better as long as I follow my schedule, which I am happy with. Although I've come to accept some days my symptoms will come and go, it's nothing like it used to be! I still read anything I can get my hands on about thyroid and receive Mary Shomon's thyroid newsletter every month to keep up with new research. No matter what any doctors tell me, I trust in myself and how I feel, and do my own research. Then I go to the doctors and tell them I want to try something new!

Phyllis is sixty years old, five feet tall, and a comfortable 114 pounds. She exercises five to six times a week. She says that once she got in touch with the emotional reasons why she ate, she was much more conscious about everything. For two years she has maintained her weight on a low-calorie food plan she devised herself that emphasizes lean protein and vegetables.

I feel great at this weight. I have also been told I look great. This motivates me to keep watching what I eat. I am now down to a size 6 and am consistently happy. I might also add, I do fine when I go out to eat. Whether lunch or dinner, I maintain by eating a chicken salad. When I go to McDonald's, I select a chicken salad, and I even am able to have an ice cream cone. This combination is very satisfying, and I look at it as a treat.

Anna lost thirty-seven pounds when she became hyperthyroid but gained it back, plus some, under treatment.

They gave me radiation and then I quit smoking and got fat, gaining more than fifty pounds. My doctor said no diet would help me. I have tried all the wrong things—till I found *The Thyroid Diet*. I want to thank you for giving me hope. I feel so good about myself again. I have lost nineteen pounds in seventy-five days— I've dropped a few sizes already—and I have to thank you.

Marie went from 185 to 154 pounds and is still dropping more.

I used to be a size 1X and am five feet tall. I now weigh 154 and can wear clothes that I couldn't wear before, and everyone including neighbors are asking me why I look so good!

Roberta read about and started following my approach to weight loss for thyroid patients six months ago.

After reading your diet guide, I was amazed with the information that my doctors did not tell me regarding hypothyroidism. I wanted to let you know that since I started taking the advice in your book, I have lost thirty-five pounds.

On other diets, Barb would lose five pounds, then hit a permanent plateau.

On the diet you recommend, I've lost twelve pounds in three months. I lost a pound a week for the first nine pounds, and then have slowed down to a pound every two weeks or so. I'm five foot three and weighed 138 pounds when I started the diet. I plan to follow the outlines of your diet for the rest of my life.

Jill offers an encouraging success story:

I purchased your book *The Thyroid Diet* and read it cover to cover several times. The book in and of itself helped relieve the hopeless feeling that there was nothing I could do to change. I learned so much from your book—it certainly was the best purchase I have ever made. Since then I have continued to do much research on my own as well, mostly reading your articles and such. I began by experimenting with the supplements and vitamins you suggested that help thyroid health and metabolism. It has been a very, very long twenty months, with much trial and error and many setbacks. I began the journey at five feet five inches tall and 144 pounds. This morning I weighed 116 pounds, and I cannot thank you enough. In the beginning I used everything you suggested. From there I worked with different combinations as I noticed that I would lose a pound or two or gained weight. Additionally, I started walking on a treadmill once or twice a day for thirty minutes each session. Slowly but steadily I finally began to lose weight. I eat real food but I am conscious of what I eat and how it will affect my thyroid, again thanks to your book. I just want any woman out there who feels as hopeless as I did to know *you can do it*, and this book is the starting block.

MOLLY'S STORY

I want to leave you with Molly's story. Molly is a thyroid patient and blogger who spent her teens in great shape, never having to worry about her weight, and even, as she said, wondering how other people could let themselves become overweight. After having radioactive iodine for Graves' disease, however, Molly's body seemingly turned on her, and she ended up gaining two hundred pounds.

> I was always used to having a perfect body. So once I started gaining weight it was really hard for me. I was in college, and while my family thought I was overeating, I wasn't. I was eating cereal twice a day and a meal, working out regularly, and the weight was just pouring on. I kept going on diets, and would lose ten to twenty pounds, and then gain it back. Or I'd actually gain weight on a diet.
>
> Over time, I didn't think about it, until I got the pictures back from my wedding, and I was bawling—it was the most heartbreaking thing. My husband was so sorry to see me crying about pictures of what was supposed to be a happy day. Over the next six months, I gained even more. That was when I realized that I had to make one last effort to lose weight.
>
> That's when I found out about *The Thyroid Diet*. And it has been the best thing for me. I jumped in, started doing the diet, and I knew there was something different in the first three days—I was losing weight, about two pounds a day, and I felt good while I was doing it. I loved the foods I was eating, not feeling deprived,

my body felt amazing. The foods made me feel good, and I was losing weight at an incredible rate.

After she started working with *The Thyroid Diet*, Molly also started a blog to chronicle her weight-loss experience. She ended up connecting with hundreds of thyroid patients around the world.

> I'd never met anyone with my problems, and now I have people talking to me from India, Australia—everywhere, really. I've never felt so normal, so accepted, and so part of something that's been going on, because no one else I'm friends with has had to deal with this. Hearing their stories are heartbreaking, and I've cried with every story, but at the same time, it's an incredible feeling that there are people who are changing their lives and who are inspired by my blog.

I was so inspired by Molly's effort and her willingness to share her journey with others that I offered to help Molly with telephone coaching sessions as well. Molly and I talked several times a month to focus on how she could get the most out of the suggestions in *The Thyroid Diet*. Along the way, I recommended that Molly start the T-Tapp More program, and she found it was a helpful addition.

> I don't have to do T-Tapp every day to really feel the results. I'm working all the parts of my body, and truly, anybody can do it. When you do some workout DVDs, all you see are these good-looking people with rocking bodies, and that's already a blow to self-esteem. The mix of real people in Teresa's T-Tapp DVDs tells me that everybody can do it. I have bad balance, and since starting T-Tapp, my balance is much better, and I am definitely building strength in my legs and arms. T-Tapp kicks my butt, but when I finish a session, I still think, "Wow, I'm already done." That's what I love about it. And Teresa is so fun on the DVDs! Every time she says, "Yes you can," I say, "Yeah, I know I can, so let's go!"

In several months, Molly had already lost over forty pounds and was feeling stronger, healthier, and much more in control of her life and her health.

> The thyroid diet was a last chance, a final straw for me. I had so many failures before. Knowing that I have showed doctors they are wrong, shown everyone they're wrong, that I have taken my life back, has been giving me drive. I'm taking control when everyone else said it was impossible!

Molly says that, like many husbands, hers doesn't say a lot about her efforts, but she knows he's proud of her, and he has been supportive of her efforts.

> But I have to say, I was just blown away the other day. We were getting dressed to go out to dinner. I put on some new, smaller-size clothes, and he said, "Molly, you need to come over here." "Why?" I asked. "Because you look incredible, and you need to come look at yourself in the mirror!"

So, like Molly, have faith, don't give up, and don't forget—you're never alone.

I invite you to connect with me, Molly, and hundreds of other thyroid patients at the Thyroid Diet website, ThyroidDietRevolution. com. I predict that someday soon you'll be sharing the story of your own successful Thyroid Diet Revolution!

You can write to me at mshomon@thyroid-info.com, or by mail at

Mary Shomon
PO Box 565
Kensington, MD 20895-0565

APPENDICES

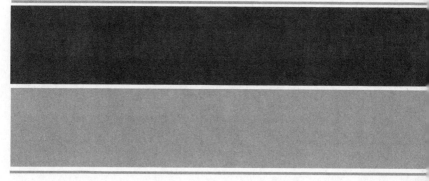

RESOURCES

THE THYROID DIET WEBSITE

Thyroid Diet Revolution
www.thyroiddietrevolution.com

This site is the home page for this book, and a source for ongoing information about thyroid and weight loss, including the Weight Off My Mind e-mail newsletter, the Thyroid Diet blog, the latest news on metabolism, hormones, thyroid, and weight loss, our Thyroid Diet Community, a bookstore, and the online Thyroid Diet Revolution program you can join. It's an online starting point for successful weight loss.

MARY SHOMON'S SUPPORT, BOOKS, AND E-BOOKS

Thyroid Coaching Sessions with Mary Shomon
www.thyroidcoaching.com
888-810-9471, 301-493-6109
E-mail: coaching@thyroid-info.com
PO Box 565, Kensington, MD 20895

Thyroid coaching with Mary Shomon is an ongoing, action-oriented relationship designed to help transform your health and provide you with the information and tools you need to live and feel well. Telephone coaching includes a comprehensive assessment of your thyroid and other health questions, plus an introduction to new information, treatment options, practitioners, and approaches. You'll have time to share your successes and frustrations, to brainstorm, and to get feedback. Advanced coaching helps to prepare you for doctor's visits, identify new approaches, and outline actions and steps to take, with specific recommendations and action items.

Thyroid Menopause Solution: Overcoming Menopause by Solving Your Hidden Thyroid Problems, HarperCollins, 2009
www.menopausethyroid.com

Women over forty will appreciate this integrative investigation into the association between thyroid function and the imbalances of female hormones that characterize the forties and fifties—the years of perimenopause and menopause. In recognizing the symptoms of a thyroid problem versus those of perimenopause, learn how to get your problems properly diagnosed and treated. Lifestyle changes, diet, and exercise are essential for good health to improve metabolism, lose weight, and increase energy. Included is a chapter featuring the T-Tapp exercise routine by exercise physiologist Teresa Tapp. Key resources list books, websites, and support forums, as well as pharmaceutical and practitioner resources. This book is essential for women interested in integrative approaches to living well with thyroid disease, perimenopause, and menopause.

Thyroid Guide to Hair Loss, 2008
www.thyroid-info.com/hair

Millions of Americans are suffering from hair loss due to undiagnosed or poorly treated thyroid disease, and thyroid patients with continuing hair loss problems need practical solutions to resolve their hair issues. This 100-page guide helps hair loss sufferers understand the problem, get proper thyroid diagnosis and treatment, and slow, stop, or even reverse thyroid-related hair loss. This must-have guide is available as a book or e-book.

The Thyroid Hormone Breakthrough: Overcoming Sexual and Hormonal Problems at Every Age, HarperCollins, 2006
www.thyroidbreakthrough.com

An integrative look at diagnosing and treating thyroid problems in conjunction with all aspects of hormonal health, including puberty, PMS, the menstrual cycle, fertility, pregnancy, postpartum, breastfeeding, libido, sexual function, and menopause. This book is especially helpful for women with thyroid disease who are trying to conceive, who have suffered recurrent miscarriages, or who want to ensure a healthy pregnancy and postpartum period for themselves and their babies.

Living Well with Hypothyroidism: What Your Doctor Doesn't Tell You . . . That You Need to Know, second edition, HarperCollins, 2005
www.thyroid-info.com/book.htm

This bestselling book, first published in 2000, was updated for the second edition in 2005. It features conventional and alternative information on every aspect of hypothyroidism, from getting diagnosed to treatment alternatives, residual symptoms such as fatigue, and weight gain. Special issues such as pregnancy, depression, and life after thyroid cancer are explored.

Living Well with Graves' Disease and Hyperthyroidism: What Your Doctor Doesn't Tell You . . . That You Need to Know, HarperCollins, 2005
www.thyroid-info.com/graves

This book is a comprehensive look at the conventional and alternative approaches to Graves' disease and hyperthyroidism, including the first detailed protocol for natural management of an overactive thyroid. It evaluates the pros and cons of the key treatments, including antithyroid drugs, radioactive iodine, surgery, and natural approaches, and explores nutritional approaches and long-term management.

Living Well with Chronic Fatigue Syndrome and Fibromyalgia: What Your Doctor Doesn't Tell You . . . That You Need to Know, HarperCollins, 2004
www.cfsfibromyalgia.com

An integrative approach to diagnosis and treatment of chronic fatigue syndrome and fibromyalgia, two conditions that are more common in thyroid patients and which share similar symptoms. While most books promote one particular theory and treatment approach, *Living Well with Chronic Fatigue Syndrome and Fibromyalgia* looks at the bigger picture, exploring a myriad of theories and treatment options from conventional therapies such as medication and vitamins to alternative approaches including yoga and massage.

Living Well with Autoimmune Disease: What Your Doctor Doesn't Tell You . . . That You Need to Know, HarperCollins, 2002
www.autoimmunebook.com

After numerous printings, *Living Well with Autoimmune Disease* has established itself as the definitive guide to understanding mysterious and often difficult-to-pinpoint autoimmune disorders such as thyroid disease, Hashimoto's thyroiditis, Graves' disease, multiple sclerosis, rheumatoid arthritis, Sjogren's syndrome, lupus, alopecia, irritable bowel syndrome, psoriasis, Raynaud's, and many others. It offers a road map to finding conventional and alternative diagnosis, treatment, recovery, and in some cases even prevention or cure! *Alternative Medicine* magazine said, "*Living Well with Autoimmune Disease* should not only prove inspirational for those afflicted with these mysterious conditions, but also offers solid, practical advice for getting your health back on track."

MARY SHOMON'S HEALTH AND THYROID WEBSITES

Mary Shomon's Thyroid-Info
www.thyroid-info.com

Thyroid-Info has been the Internet's most popular thyroid patient website since 1997, featuring articles, forums, books, newsletters, and the latest news on all facets of thyroid disease, including both conventional and alternative approaches to diagnosis and treatment.

Thyroid Top Doctors Directory
www.thyroid-info.com/topdrs

A directory of patient-recommended top thyroid practitioners from around the country and the world, organized by location.

Thyroid Site at About.com
thyroid.about.com

Managed by Mary J. Shomon since 1997, the Thyroid Site at About.com, part of the New York Times Company, features hundreds of articles, links to top sites on the Net, a weekly newsletter, an active support community, and more.

The Thyroid Blog: Thyroid and Health News, Information, and Opinion
www.thyroidblog.com

This blog brings you up-to-date thyroid news and is packed with information on all aspects of thyroid disease.

Thyroid Menopause Solution
www.menopausethyroid.com

Featuring detailed resources links and information, articles, newsletters, support groups, and more for women interested in integrative approaches to living well with thyroid disease, perimenopause, and menopause.

MARY SHOMON ON SOCIAL MEDIA

Mary J. Shomon: Thyroid Advocate on Facebook
www.facebook.com/thyroidsupport

Mary exchanges news, information, and the latest thyroid ideas with an active community of more than five thousand Facebook friends who are interested in thyroid disease and health.

Thyroid Diet on Facebook
www.facebook.com/thyroiddiet
 A Facebook home page for thyroid dieters.

ThyroidMary on Twitter
www.twitter.com/thyroidmary
 On Twitter, Mary shares the latest thyroid news, information, and support with an active community.

MARY SHOMON'S COMMUNITY SUPPORT FORUMS

Visit a variety of thyroid-specific online forums and bulletin boards, where you are welcome to participate, share information, and find support and camaraderie from your fellow patients and several key facilitators and experts.

About.com Thyroid Support and Information
forums.about.com/ab-thyroid

The Thyroid Diet Community
ThyroidDietRevolution.com
 Interact with other thyroid dieters at the Thyroid Diet Community, moderated by Mary Shomon.

Thyroid Support Listserv at Yahoo
groups.yahoo.com/group/thyroid

NEWSLETTERS

Sticking Out Our Necks: The Thyroid Patient Newsletter
www.thyroid-info.com/subscribe.htm
888-810-9471
E-mail newsletter: www.thyroid-info.com/newsletters.htm
Sticking Out Our Necks/Thyroid-Info, PO Box 565, Kensington, MD 20895-0565
 Sticking Out Our Necks is Mary Shomon's newsletter, designed to keep thyroid patients up to date on important thyroid-related and health news,

both conventional and alternative. *Sticking Out Our Necks* has no affiliations with any pharmaceutical companies or patient groups, leaving it free to present honest information about thyroid drugs, treatments, and pharmaceutical company politics that have an impact on *your* quality of life. The 12-page print newsletter is published every other month, available by subscription and sent by regular mail. The e-mail edition is a brief summary of news and goes out monthly online.

A Weight Off My Mind Newsletter
www.thyroid-info.com/dietnews/index.htm
diet@thyroid-info.com

This e-mail newsletter features key thyroid-related news, developments, links, interviews, and more.

THYROID AND ENDOCRINOLOGY ORGANIZATIONS

Coalition for Better Thyroid Care
www.betterthyroidcare.org
www.facebook.com/betterthyroidcare

The Coalition for Better Thyroid Care, a patient-driven organization newly created in 2010, promotes improvements in thyroid care. As millions of thyroid patients have found, the road to feeling well again can be a long and winding one. Contrary to popular myth, thyroid disease is not always easy to treat, nor are there one-size-fits-all solutions. Our goal is a world where every health care professional has a big tool kit, with the resources to meet the individual needs of thyroid patients. We aim to do all we can to make sure that the full range of tests and treatment options are well known, understood, accepted, and utilized.

American Autoimmune Related Diseases Association
www.aarda.org
586-776-3900
E-mail: aarda@aol.com
22100 Gratiot Avenue, East Detroit, MI 48021

AARDA provides information about more than fifty different autoimmune disorders, including Hashimoto's disease and Graves' disease.

American Association of Clinical Endocrinologists
www.aace.com
904-353-7878
245 Riverside Avenue, Suite 200, Jacksonville, FL 32202

The American Association of Clinical Endocrinologists (AACE) is a professional medical organization devoted to clinical endocrinology. They sponsor an online Specialist Search Page at www.aace.com/directory, which allows you to identify AACE members by geographic location, including international options. A unique feature of this page is the ability to select by subspecialty.

American Thyroid Association
www.thyroid.org
Patient Information Line: 800-THYROID (800-849-7643)
703-998-8890, fax 703-998-8893
6066 Leesburg Pike, Suite 550, Falls Church, VA 22041

Founded in 1923, ATA promotes scientific and public understanding of the biology of the thyroid gland and its disorders, so as to improve methods for prevention, diagnosis, and management of thyroid disease.

The Broda O. Barnes, M.D. Research Foundation
www.brodabarnes.org
203-261-2101, fax 203-261-3017
info@BrodaBarnes.org
P.O. Box 110098, Trumbull, CT 06611

The Barnes Foundation focuses on promoting knowledge about thyroid and adrenal disorders, honoring the work of the late Dr. Broda Barnes. The group maintains lists of practitioners knowledgeable about diagnosing thyroid and adrenal disorders and those willing to treat with natural and physiological hormone replacement.

Thyroid Foundation of Canada/La Fondation Canadienne de la Thyroide
www.thyroid.ca
800-267-8822
263 MCG Building, Labrosse Avenue, Pointe-Claire, Quebec, H9R 1A3, Canada

Established in 1980, Thyroid Foundation of Canada was the first thyroid patient organization in the world. The volunteer-run foundation offers information in English and French for thyroid patients and interested practitioners.

The Endocrine Society
www.endo-society.org
301-941-0200
8401 Connecticut Avenue, Suite 900, Chevy Chase, MD 20815

A group with a mission promoting the understanding of hormones and endocrinology, and the impact of this knowledge on preventing, diagnosing, and treating disease, including thyroid disease and obesity. The group publishes a number of journals and maintains an informational website. *Journal of Clinical Endocrinology and Metabolism* is available at http://jcem.endo journals.org.

Hormone Foundation
www.hormone.org
800-HORMONE (800-467-6663)
8401 Connecticut Avenue, Suite 900, Chevy Chase, MD 20815-5817

The Hormone Foundation, the public education affiliate of the Endocrine Society, is a leading source of hormone-related health information for the public, physicians, allied health professionals, and the media.

Thyroid UK
www.thyroiduk.org
01255 820407
32, Darcy Road, St. Osyth, Clacton on Sea, Essex UK CO16 8QF

Lyn Mynott is the chair and chief executive of this patient-oriented organization helping raise awareness of thyroid issues and improve the level of thyroid care in the United Kingdom.

TESTING LABORATORIES

MyMedLab
www.thyroid-info.com/thyroidtests.htm
888-MYMEDLAB (888-696-3352)

Through MyMedLab, you can order almost any thyroid or hormone blood test without a doctor's prescription, at low costs with no markup. Have your blood drawn at one of thousands of LabCorp and other collection laboratories around the country, and get the results sent directly to you by mail and online.

ZRT Laboratory
www.salivatest.com
866-600-1636
8605 SW Creekside Place, Beaverton, OR 97008

Diagnos-Techs, Inc.
www.diagnostechs.com
800-878-3787
Clinical and Research Laboratory, 19110 66th Avenue S., Bldg. G, Kent, WA 98032

The Canary Club
www.canaryclub.org

Free membership in the Canary Club, an Internet-based consumer group, offers discount-priced access to ZRT and Diagnos-Techs test kits.

Hakala Research
www.hakalalabs.com
877-238-1779, 303-763-6242
883 Parfet Street, Suite C, Lakewood, CO 80215

Urinary iodine clearance testing.

TISSUE MINERAL ANALYSIS TESTING AND INTERPRETATION

Trace Elements.com
www.traceelements.com
800-824-2314 or 972-250-6410, fax 972-248-4896
4501 Sunbelt Drive, Addison, TX 75001

Uni Key Health Systems, Inc., with Dr. Ann Louise Gittleman
www.annlouise.com
www.unikeyhealth.com
800-888-4353, Service: 208-762-6833, fax 208-762-9395
181 West Commerce Drive, PO Box 2287, Hayden Lake, ID 83835

OTHER TESTING

Genova Diagnostics
www.genovadiagnostics.com
800-522-4762, 828-253-0621
63 Zillicoa Street, Asheville, NC 28801

Saliva hormone testing for estradiol, estrone, estriol, progesterone, and testosterone, in a variety of panels. Only available through your health care provider.

CELIAC, ALLERGY, AND FOOD SENSITIVITY TESTING

Better Control of Health/York Allergy
www.bettercontrolofhealth.com
786-953-4945
info@bettercontrolofhealth.com

THYROID DRUGS AND THEIR MANUFACTURERS

Levoxyl, Cytomel, Tapazole

Levoxyl is a levothyroxine product. Cytomel is liothyronine, the synthetic form of triiodothyronine (T3). Tapazole is the brand name for the antithyroid drug methimazole. Levoxyl, Cytomel, and Tapazole were made until recently by King Pharmaceuticals, until the company was purchased by Pfizer.

Pfizer
www.pfizer.com
212-733-2323
235 East 42nd Street, New York, NY 10017

Levoxyl
www.levoxyl.com

ARMOUR THYROID, THYROLAR, LEVOTHROID

Armour Thyroid is a natural thyroid hormone replacement product. Thyrolar is the brand name for liotrix, a synthetic T4/T3 levothyroxine/liothyronine combination drug. Levothroid is a levothyroxine drug.

Forest Pharmaceuticals
www.forestpharm.com
800-678-1605, ext. 66297
13600 Shoreline Drive, St. Louis, MO 63045

Armour Thyroid
www.armourthyroid.com

Thyrolar
www.thyrolar.com

Levothroid
www.levothroid.com

Unithroid
215-333-9000

A brand of levothyroxine. Distributed by Lannett Pharmaceuticals, 13200 Townsend Road, Philadelphia, PA 19154.

Nature-Throid, Westhroid

Nature-Throid and Westhroid are prescription desiccated thyroid drugs. Westhroid is a cornstarch-bound natural thyroid hormone product. Nature-Throid is bound with microcrystalline cellulose and is hypoallergenic.

RLC Laboratories
www.rlclabs.com
877-797-7997
28248 N. Tatum Boulevard, Suite B1-629, Cave Creek, AZ 85331

Nature-Throid
www.nature-throid.com

Westhroid
www.wes-throid.com

Synthroid
www.synthroid.com
www.abbott.com
800-255-5162
Abbott Laboratories, 100 Abbott Park Rd., Abbott Park, IL 60064-3500

Synthroid is the top-selling levothyroxine drug.

Erfa Natural Desiccated Thyroid
www.thyroid.erfa.net
514-931-3133
8250 Boulevard Decarie, bur. 110, Montreal, Quebec H4P 2P5, Canada

Thyrogen
www.thyrogen.com
617-252-7500
Genzyme Therapeutics, 500 Kendall Street, Cambridge, MA 02142

Thyrogen is a drug that, when used along with tests to detect recurrent or leftover thyroid cancer, can prevent the need to become hypothyroid as part of that testing.

Tirosint
Akrimax Pharmaceuticals, LLC
www.tirosintgelcaps.com
908-372-0506
11 Commerce Drive, 1st Floor, Suite #100, Cranford, NJ 07016

Tirosint is a gel capsule form of levothyroxine.

HERBS AND SUPPLEMENT INFORMATION

iHerb
www.iherb.com

An excellent website for a variety of diet foods, low carb products, and supplements.

ConsumerLab
www.consumerlab.com

This site is a great resource for people interested in taking herbal supplements. ConsumerLab offers independent testing of popular herbs to help consumers evaluate the safety of vitamins, minerals, herbal products, and more.

Drug Digest
www.drugdigest.org

This comprehensive site has a section that provides detailed information about drugs, herbs, and supplements. Also includes interactions with medications and information about specific conditions.

FDA: Overview of Dietary Supplements
www.fda.gov/food/dietarysupplements/consumerinformation/ucm110417.htm

This Food and Drug Administration article offers basic information about what dietary supplements are, how to read labels, and more.

WEIGHT-LOSS DRUG INFORMATION

Obesity Meds and Research
www.obesity-news.com/newdrugs.htm

Obesity News and Research for health care professionals and interested patients. Subscription is $104 a year.

Medscape Drug Info
search.medscape.com/drug-reference-search

Search page at Medscape for information about all drugs and drug interactions.

FITNESS AND EXERCISE INFORMATION

Exercise at About.com
exercise.about.com

This about.com site provides comprehensive information about all aspects of exercise including cardio, strength training, apparel, gear, and more. Includes exercise articles, support forum, newsletter, free workouts, and product reviews.

ExRx Exercise Information
www.exrx.net

ExRx is an excellent website offering basic information about getting started with exercise. Articles cover fitness components, injury prevention, motor development, and more.

Fitness Online
www.fitnessonline.com

Fitness Online contains a variety of information about fitness and exercise including getting fit, eating healthy, building muscle, and losing weight. Includes online calculators, expert advice, and instructional workouts.

IDEAfit.com
www.ideafit.com

The IDEA Health and Fitness Association provides news as well as 5,000+ articles and fitness facts covering all aspects of exercise for fitness enthusiasts. Pilates and professional-grade courses are here as well. Memberships access low-cost medical insurance and cost $99 to $199 a year with a thirty-day free trial.

Internet Fitness
www.internetfitness.com

Internet Fitness provides information about exercise, walking, running, motivation, strength training, home fitness, and more. An authority in his or her field moderates each category. Get in shape with the experts.

Workout.com
www.workout.com

Workout.com offers fourteen professionally developed exercise video demonstrations by Tony Thomas.

OTHER PRODUCTS OF INTEREST

T-Tapp
www.t-tapp.com
800-342-0717

Teresa Tapp's exercise program has taken the world by storm. Innovative and successful, the exercises rely upon a creative approach to bending, stretching, isometrics, and careful standing and walking postures. The program is available on DVDs and is designed to be done anywhere: home, office, or workplace. Teresa's media has now diversified. Clients can purchase the book *Fit and Fabulous in 15 Minutes* which includes a free DVD ($16.95). DVDs ($16.95 and up) offer specialized instruction, and a Total System DVD set is available ($140).

Belleruth Naparstek's Weight-Loss Guided Visualization Audio/CD/ DVDs
belleruthnaparstek.com/guided-imagery/index.php

Guided imagery accesses the imagination and creative daydreaming, and may well alter serotonin levels in the brain. Weight loss, fitness, and emotional eating are addressed with several DVD, CD, and MP3 products. Pricing for these packages ranges from $9.99 to $51.99.

Paraliminal Ideal Weight Audio CD by Paul Scheele
www.learningstrategies.com

An audio session designed to help activate the mind to make transformations related to diet, weight loss, stress reduction, and balance.

DietPower Software
www.dietpower.com

Company president Terry Dunkle created this special diet in 1998 in response to his own health problems. DietPower sells a Diet Software CD for around $50 with a fifteen-day free trial. Central to DietPower is an innovative calorie counter that tracks 33 nutrients and monitors your metabolism, yet only requires a five-minute daily time commitment. DietPower coaches the user to follow any diet program, or no diet at all, to achieve lasting weight-loss success with a food log, calorie bank, and nutrient summary.

Fatigued to Fantastic! Energy Revitalization System, formulated by Jacob Teitelbaum, MD
www.enzymatictherapy.com

Fat Flush Body Protein, and Fat Flush Kit, formulated by Dr. Ann Louise Gittleman
www.unikeyhealth.com
800-888-4353

Dr. Levine's Ultimate Weight-Loss Formula
www.thindoctor.com
800-641-2907

Transformational Breathing
www.transformationalbreathing.com
866-515-4040 or 603-286-8333, fax 603-286-8118
Transformational Breath Foundation, PO Box 248, Tilton, NH 03276
   Book: *Breathe Deep, Laugh Loudly*, by Judith Kravitz

WEIGHT-LOSS INFORMATION, SUPPORT AND TOOLS

Calorie King
www.calorieking.com
   Founded by clinical dietician Allan Borushek, Calorie King features the Food and Calorie Diary that integrates 70,000 foods into an innovative recipe, diet, and meal planning system. Online community forum and blog are there to share experiences and tips. There is a seven-day free trial, after which monthly cost is $12. Calorie King Nutrition and Exercise software is $45 after a seven-day free trial, and is available for PCs, Macs, and some mobile devices.

FitDay
www.fitday.com
   FitDay is an online tracking system that offers a personal journal to track the foods you eat and daily activities. FitDay analyzes your diet and exercise and offers reports on calories, nutrients, weight loss, and more. A subscription is free.

WebMD
www.webmd.com/diet/default.htm
   WebMD is on everyone's list of the top ten diet and weight-loss websites. WebMD has encyclopedic coverage of every aspect of health and nutrition and is famous for depth of information on every listed topic. One of their six priority areas is Healthy Eating and Diet. No-cost tools include Diet Evaluator, BMI/Plus Calculator, Food/Fitness Planner, and Portion Size Plate. Calculate your indices, plan meals and learn from the extensive information.

Weight Loss at About.com
weightloss.about.com

Extensive database of articles and resources on weight loss, including well-known diets such as South Beach, Atkins, and Weight Watchers; information on the latest diet trends and weight-loss options; and tips on creating a healthy lifestyle. The About.com Weight Loss Forum offers support if you are trying to lose weight and maintain the loss. Register for free, post questions, learn from others' experiences, and search through the forum for specific information about diets, nutrition, diet buddies, obesity, and other popular topics.

Low Carb Forum at About.com
lowcarbdiets.about.com

The About.com Low Carb Forum offers support if you are trying to lose weight and maintain the loss. The focus is on using low-glycemic foods to keep blood sugar stable. Glucose tolerance problems such as insulin resistance and diabetes are discussed regularly. Register for free, post questions, learn from others' experiences, and search through the forum for specific information about diets, nutrition, diet buddies, obesity, and other popular topics.

DietTalk.com
www.diettalk.com

"Desire, Dedication, Determination and Discipline = Success" for any diet. Through forums and chat, develop your motivation and commitment to pick the best diet for your individual needs. Since 1996, DietTalk.com has been a place to meet and discuss diet issues with others, with twenty-four-hour daily support to help you achieve your weight-loss goals.

My Diet Buddy
www.mydietbuddy.com

The support of two or more people can tremendously boost your motivation and will power. Now you can find good diet buddies who will provide mutual support through e-mail exchanges. It's a great way to connect with others and share encouragement, recipes, tips, and ideas.

iPhone/Smartphone Apps/Tools
- My Fitness Pal—www.myfitnesspal.com
- iPhone app—www.myfitnesspal.com/mobile
- LoseIt—www.loseit.com

HCG PROTOCOL PROGRAMS

Dirk Van Lith, MD
www.W8drops.com
   Integrative physician, medical weight loss and HCG support.

HCG Protocols for Thyroid Patients
www.hcgturnaround.com

OTHER FEATURED DIET/WEIGHT-LOSS RESOURCES

Weight Loss Pleasure Camp—www.weightlosspleasurecamp.com
Weight Watchers—www.weightwatchers.com, 800-651-6000
Take Off Pounds Sensibly (TOPS)—www.tops.org, 414-482-4620
Overeaters Anonymous—www.oa.org, 505-891-2664
Rosedale Diet—www.drrosedale.com
Physicians Weight Loss Centers—www.pwlc.com
Diet Center—www.dietcenter.com
Jenny Craig—www.jennycraig.com
Nutrisystem—www.nutrisystem.com
Optifast—www.optifast.com
Lindora—www.lindora.com
Medifast—www.medifast1.com
LA to Your Door—www.latoyourdoor.com
Jillian Michaels—www.jillianmichaels.com
Zone Diet—www.zonediet.com
In the Zone Delivery—www.inthezonedelivery.com
Eat Right for Your Type/Blood Type Diet—www.dadamo.com
Sanford Siegal, MD's Cookie Diet—www.cookiediet.com
Smart for Life Cookie Diet—www.smartforlife.com

MEAL DELIVERY SERVICES

Diet-to-Go—diettogo.com, 800-743-SLIM
eDiets—www.ediets.com, 800-650-9052
BistroMD—www.bistromd.com, 1-866-401-DIET
Freshology—www.freshology.com, 1-877-89FRESH

BOOKS MENTIONED AND RECOMMENDED

21 Life Lessons from Livin' La Vida Low-Carb: How the Healthy Low-Carb Lifestyle Changed Everything I Thought I Knew, by Jimmy Moore

Beat Sugar Addiction Now, by Jacob Teitelbaum, MD

Before the Change by Ann Louise Gittleman, PhD, CNS

Breathe Deep, Laugh Loudly by Judith Kravitz, PhD

Eat Right 4 Your Type: The Individualized Diet Solution to Staying Healthy, Living Longer, and Achieving Your Ideal Weight, by Peter J. D'Adamo, MD

The Fat Flush Diet, by Ann Louise Gittleman, PhD, CNS

Fats That Heal, Fats That Kill, by Udo Erasmus, PhD

Feeling Fat, Fuzzy and Frazzled, by Richard Shames, MD, and Karilee Halo Shames, PhD, RN

Fit and Fabulous in 15 Minutes by Teresa Tapp

From Fatigued to Fantastic, by Jacob Teitelbaum, MD

Good Calories, Bad Calories: Fats, Carbs, and the Controversial Science of Diet and Health by Gary Taubes

Guess What Came to Dinner? Parasites and Your Health, by Ann Louise Gittleman, PhD, CNS

The Gut Flush Diet by Ann Louise Gittleman, PhD, CNS

The Healing Miracles of Coconut Oil, by Bruce Fife, ND

How to Meditate, with Pema Chodron

Iodine: Why You Need It, Why You Can't Live Without It, by David Brownstein, MD

Livin' La Vida Low-Carb: My Journey from Flabby Fat to Sensationally Skinny in One Year, by Jimmy Moore

Mastering Leptin, by Byron Richards, CCN

Meditation for Beginners, by Jack Kornfield

Meditation in a New York Minute, by Mark Thornton

The Miracle of Natural Hormones, by David Brownstein, MD

Natural Highs, by Hyla Cass, MD

New Atkins for a New You: The Ultimate Diet for Shedding Weight and Feeling Great, by Eric Westman, MD

Overcoming Thyroid Disorders, by David Brownstein, MD

The Paleo Diet: Lose Weight and Get Healthy by Eating the Food You Were Designed to Eat by Loren Cordain

The Perricone Weight-Loss Diet: A Simple 3-Part Plan to Lose the Fat, the Wrinkles, and the Years by Nicholas Perricone, MD

The Primal Blueprint: Reprogram Your Genes for Effortless Weight Loss, Vibrant Health, and Boundless Energy by Mark Sisson

The Rosedale Diet, by Ron Rosedale, MD

The Self-Hypnosis Diet, by Steven Gurgevich, PhD

The Slow Down Diet: Eating for Pleasure, Energy, and Weight Loss, by Marc David

Solved: The Riddle of Illness, by Stephen Langer, MD

The South Beach Diet Supercharged, by Arthur Agatston, MD

Thyroid Power, by Richard Shames, MD, and Karilee Halo Shames, PhD, RN

The Truth About Beauty: Transform Your Looks and Your Life from the Inside Out, by Kat James

Turn Up the Heat, by Philip L. Goglia

Ultrametabolism: The Simple Plan for Automatic Weight Loss, by Mark Hyman, MD

The UltraSimple Diet: Kick-Start Your Metabolism and Safely Lose Up to 10 Pounds in 7 Days, by Mark Hyman, MD

Why Am I Always So Tired? by Ann Louise Gittleman, PhD, CNS

Zapped: Why Your Cell Phone Shouldn't Be Your Alarm Clock and 1,268 Ways to Outsmart the Hazards of Electronic Pollution by Ann Louise Gittleman, ND, PhD

The Zone Diet, by Barry Sears

FEATURED IN THE BOOK

David Brownstein, MD
www.drbrownstein.com
248-851-1600
info@drbrownstein.com
The Center for Holistic Medicine, 5821 W. Maple Road, Suite 192,
West Bloomfield, MI 48322
Books: *The Miracle of Natural Hormones; Drugs That Don't Work and Natural Therapies That Do; Overcoming Arthritis; Overcoming Thyroid Disorders; Iodine: Why You Need It, Why You Can't Live Without It*

Board-certified family physician and practitioner of holistic medicine. Medical director of the Center for Holistic Medicine in West Bloomfield, Michigan.

Robert G. Carlson, MD, FACS
www.andlos.com
941-955-1815
2914 Bee Ridge Road, Sarasota, FL 34239

Cardiac surgeon, hormone expert, and antiaging integrative physician, founder of Andlos Institute.

Hyla Cass, MD
www.cassmd.com
> Integrative and holistic physician and psychiatrist
> Books: *Natural Highs, Supplement Your Prescription*

Adrienne Clamp, MD
Well Being–Being Well
www.dradrienneclamp.com
703-635-2158
6862 Elm Street, Suite 720, McLean, VA 22101
> Integrative physician with expertise in hormone balance and thyroid treatment. Cofounder of Wellbeing–Being Well.

Marc David, MA
www.psychologyofeating.com
www.weightlosspleasurecamp.com
303-440-7642
Book: *The Slow Down Diet: Eating for Pleasure, Energy, and Weight Loss*
> Nutritional psychologist, founder and director of the Institute for the Psychology of Eating, health and nutrition consultant, author, coach, cofounder of the Weight Loss Pleasure Camp

Rebecca Elia, MD
Health/Wellness Life Coach
www.creatingfemininehealth.com
510-250-2474
info@creatingfemininehealth.com

Udo Erasmus, PhD
Nutritionist, researcher, founder of Udo's Oils, consultant
www.udoerasmus.com
Book: *Fats That Heal, Fats That Kill*

Rick Ferris, PhD, ND
Doctor of naturopathy, clinical pharmacist
Drugcrafters
877-378-4272
www.drugcrafters.com

Bruce Fife, ND
Nutritionist, naturopathic physician, expert on coconut oil
www.coconutresearchcenter.org
719-550-9887
contact@coconutresearchcenter.org
Coconut Research Center, P.O. Box 25203, Colorado Springs, CO 80936
Books: *The Healing Miracles of Coconut Oil*; *Eat Fat, Look Thin*

Ann Louise Gittleman, PhD, CNS,
Integrative nutritionist, naturopath, author, weight-loss expert
www.annlouise.com
800-888-4353, 413-525-0044
Uni Key Health Systems,181 West Commerce Drive, PO Box 2287,
Hayden Lake, ID 83835
Books: *Before the Change, Fat Flush Diet, Gut Flush Diet,* and others

Sara Gottfried, MD
Integrative gynecologist, hormone expert, founder and medical director of
the Gottfried Center
www.gottfriedcenter.com
twitter.com/DrGottfried
drgottfried.blogspot.com
510-893-3907
Gottfried Center for Integrative Medicine, 300 Lakeside Drive, Suite 202,
Oakland, CA 94612

Steven Gurgevich, PhD
Medical hypnotist, mind-body expert, clinical assistant professor of medi-
cine in Dr. Andrew Weil's Arizona Center for Integrative Medicine
www.tranceformation.com
www.healingwithhypnosis.com
Book: *The Self-Hypnosis Diet*
CD: *Relax Rx*
DVD: *Hypnosis Housecall*

Joy Gurgevich
Behavioral nutritionist
www.behavioral-nutrition.com

Kent Holtorf, MD
Hormone, thyroid and weight-loss expert, founder of the Holtorf Medical Group
www.holtorfmed.com
877-508-1177
23456 Hawthorne Boulevard, Suite 160, Torrance, CA 90505
1241 East Hillsdale Boulevard, Suite 150, Foster City, CA 94404

Nicolet (Nikki) Hundt-Prohaska
Advocate and leader for thyroid patients
www.medhelp.org/personal_pages/user/393685
www.medhelp.org/forums/Thyroid-Disorders/show/73

Ali Jagger
Personal wellness and weight-loss coach
www.elitelifecoaching.org
info@elitelifecoaching.org
21 Claremont Road, West Kirby Wirral CH48 5EA

Kat James
Autoimmune disease and eating disorder survivor, holistic health and
beauty expert, author, Total Transformation Program creator, radio host
www.informedbeauty.com
www.totaltransformation.com
www.thekatjamesshow.com
Program: Total Transformation Program
Book: *The Truth About Beauty: Transform Your Looks and Your Life from the Inside Out*

David Junno, PsyD
Psychologist, coach, and author
www.drjunno.com
413-586-7559, fax 413-586-7560
drjunno@drjunno.com
51 Locust Street, Northampton, MA 01060
380 Union Street, Suite 17, West Springfield, MA 01089
Book: *Lowering High Cholesterol and Reducing Your Risk of Heart Disease–
Ready or Not!*

Karta Purkh Singh Khalsa, DN-C, RH
Herbalist, coauthor of *Herbal Defense*
www.kpkhalsa.com

Jena la Flamme
Weight-loss coach, founder of Jena Wellness, cofounder of Weight Loss Pleasure
Camp
www.jenawellness.com
www.weightlosspleasurecamp.com
212-260-6064
1133 Broadway, Suite 1107, New York, NY 10010

Stephen Langer, MD
Holistic physician, thyroid and hormone specialist
510-548-7384
3031 Telegraph Avenue, Suite 230, Berkeley, CA 94705-2051
Books: *Solved: The Riddle of Illness* and others

Kate Lemmerman, MD
Integrative physician with expertise in hormone balance and thyroid treatment. Cofounder of Wellbeing–Being Well.
www.drkatelemmerman.com
703-635-2158
Well Being–Being Well, 6862 Elm Street, Suite 720, McLean, VA 22101

Scott Levine, MD
Board-certified internist in private practice, creator of Dr. Levine's Ultimate
Weight Loss Formula
www.thindoctor.com
407-363-1515
Mid Florida Medical Specialists, 7350 Sandlake Commons Boulevard,
Suite 2215, Orlando, FL 32819

Jimmy Moore
Professional health blogger, low-carb diet expert, Founder of Livin' La Vida
Low-Carb, author
livinlavidalowcarb.com
lowcarbdoctors.blogspot.com

Byron Richards, CCN
Expert in clinical nutrition, private practice and consulting
www.masteringleptin.com
800-717-9355
7155 Amundson Avenue, Minneapolis, MN 55416
Book: *Mastering Leptin*

Marie Savard, MD
Women's health advocate, ABC television and *Good Morning America* medical contributor, author
www.drsavard.com
eileen@drsavard.com
Books: *Ask Dr. Marie: Straight Talk and Reassuring Answers to Your Most Private Questions; How to Save Your Own Life: The Savard System for Managing–and Controlling–Your Health Care;* and *The Savard Health Record: A Six-Step System for Managing Your Health Care.*

Katie Schwartz
Patient advocate, founder of DearThyroid
www.dearthyroid.org

Richard Shames, MD, and Karilee Halo Shames, PhD, RN
Holistic, integrative health practice; telephone consulting; office practice; authors
www.thyroidpower.com
415-472-2343, fax 415-472-7636
teamshames@thryoidpower.com
PO Box 2466, Sebastopol CA 95473
Books: *Thyroid Power; Feeling Fat, Fuzzy and Frazzled; Thyroid Mind Power*

Teresa Tapp
Physiotherapist, trainer, creator of T-Tapp program, author of *Fit and Fabulous in Fifteen Minutes.*
www.t-tapp.com
800-342-0717, 727-724-0123
T-Tapp, 1450 10th Street South, Safety Harbor, FL 34695

Jacob Teitelbaum, MD
Internal medicine specialist, chronic fatigue, fibromyalgia and hormone expert, medical director of the Fibromyalgia and Fatigue Centers
www.endfatigue.com
www.fibroandfatigue.com
Books: *From Fatigued to Fantastic; Beat Sugar Addiction Now*

Dirk Van Lith, MD, MPH
Integrative physician, medical weight loss and HCG support for the European community
www.W8drops.com
www.gewichtsverlies.nl
Amsterdam, Netherlands

Paige Waehner
www.exercise.about.com

Along with being a certified personal trainer for more than twelve years, Paige is author of the *About.com Guide to Getting in Shape*, coauthor of *The Buzz on Exercise and Fitness*, and author of the e-book *Guide to Become a Personal Trainer*. Paige has written articles for *Desert Paradise, Pregnancy Magazine, Runner's World*, and many other websites, newsletters, and magazines.

Daphne White
Healing Touch, Somatic Experiencing Practitioner
www.daphnewhite.com
301-949-0378
Kensington, MD

REFERENCES

Abbott Laboratories. "Meridia (sibutramine hydrochloride monohydrate) product information." May 2002. www.rxabbott.com/pdf/meridia.pdf.

"Absorption and transportation of nutrients." NutriStrategy (from National Institutes of Health National Institute of Diabetes and Digestive Kidney Diseases). 2001. www.nutristrategy.com/digestion.htm.

Abu Abeid S et al. "Treatment of intra gastric band migration following laparoscopic banding: safety and feasibility of simultaneous laparoscopic band removal and replacement." *Obes Surg.* 2005; 15(6): 849–852.

Alpor CM. "Effects of chronic peanut consumption on energy balance and hedonics." *International Journal of Obesity.* 2002; 26(8): 1,129–1,137.

Anderson RA. "Cinnamon, glucose tolerance and diabetes." Agricultural Research Service. United States Department of Agriculture. November 17, 2006.

Anoja S et al. "Antidiabetic effects of Panax ginseng berry extract and the identification of an effective component." *Diabetes.* 2002; 51: 1,851–1,858.

Arnot R. *Dr. Bob Arnot's Revolutionary Weight Control Program.* Little, Brown; 1997.

Astrup A et al. "Randomized controlled trials of the D1/D5 antagonist ecopipam for weight loss in obese subjects." *Obesity* (Silver Spring). 2007; 15(7): 1,717–1,731.

Atkins RC. *Dr. Atkins' New Diet Revolution.* Avon Books; 2002.

Backgrounder: why sleep matters. National Sleep Foundation. March 2002. www.sleepfoundation.org/nsaw/pk_background.html.

Balsiger BM et al. "Ten and more years after vertical banded gastroplasty as primary operation for morbid obesity." *Journal of the American Medical Association.* 1999; 282(16): 1,530–1,538.

Barclay L. "Topiramate useful for binge eating disorder in obesity." *American Journal of Psychiatry.* 2003; 160: 255–261.

Barkeling B et al. "Short-term effects of sibutramine (Reductil) on appetite and eating behavior and the long-term therapeutic outcome." *International Journal of Obesity.* 2003; 27(6): 693–700.

Batterham RL, Cohen MA, Ellis SM, Le Roux CR, Withers DJ, Frost GS, Ghatei M, Bloom SR. "Inhibition of food intake in obese subject by peptide YY3-36." *New England Journal of Medicine.* 2003; 349: 941–948.

Batterham RL, Cowley MA, Small CJ, Herzog H, Cohen MA, Dakin C, Wren AM, Brynes A, Low M, Ghatei M, Cone R, Bloom SR. "Gut hormone PYY3-36 physiologically inhibits food intake." *Nature.* 2002; 418: 650–654.

Behavior Risk Factor Surveillance System. Trends data, 2001. Centers for Disease Control and Prevention, National Center for Chronic Disease Prevention and Health Promotion, Division of Adult and Community Health. February 18, 2003. www.cdc.gov/brfss/index.htm.

Benzphetamine. RXlist.com. www.rxlist.com/frame/display.cgi?drug=DIDREX.

Blackburn GL, Bevis LC. "The obesity epidemic: prevention and treatment of the metabolic syndrome CME." Medscape. www.medscape.com/viewprogram/2015 _index.

Blankson H et al. "Conjugated linoleic acid reduces body fat mass in overweight and obese humans." *Journal of Nutrition.* 2000; 130: 2,943–2,948.

BMI for Adults, Body Mass Index Formula. Centers for Disease Control and Prevention, National Center for Chronic Disease Prevention and Health Promotion, Division of Nutrition and Physical Activity. April 21, 2003. www.cdc.gov/nccdphp /dnpa/bmi/bmi-adult-formula.htm.

Body Mass Index (BMI) Table. Centers for Disease Control and Prevention, National Center for Chronic Disease Prevention and Health Promotion, Division of Nutrition and Physical Activity. April 21, 2003. www.cdc.gov/nccdphp/dnpa/bmi/00binaries/bmi-adults.pdf.

Bosch B et al. "Human chorionic gonadotrophin and weight loss. A double-blind, placebo-controlled trial." *S Afr Med J.* February 17, 1990; 77(4): 185–189.

Boza C et al. "Laparoscopic adjustable gastric banding (LAGB): surgical results and 5-year follow-up." *Surg Endosc.* July 22, 2010.

Brain M. "How food works." HowStuffWorks.com. home.howstuffworks.com/food.htm/printable.

Bray GA et al. "A six-month randomized, placebo controlled, dose-ranging trial of topiramate for weight loss in obesity." *Obesity Research.* 2003; 11: 722–733.

Brownstein D. *The Miracle of Natural Hormones.* Medical Alternative Press; 1999.

Brownstein D. *Overcoming Arthritis.* Medical Alternatives Press; 2001.

Brownstein D. *Overcoming Thyroid Disorders.* Medical Alternatives Press; 2002.

Brunova J et al. "Hyperthyroidism therapy and weight gain." [Abstract.] 84th annual meeting of the Endocrine Society. June 2002.

Bupropion. RXList.com. www.rxlist.com/frame/display.cgi?drug=Wellbutrin.

Cabot S. *The Liver Cleansing Diet.* SCB International; 1996.

Carney DE, Tweddell ED. "Double blind evaluation of long acting diethylpropion hydrochloride in obese patients from a general practice." *Medical Journal Australia.* 1975; 1(1): 13–15.

Cass H, Holford P. *Natural Highs.* Avery; 2002.

Chapman AE et al. "Laparoscopic adjustable gastric banding in the treatment of obesity: a systematic literature review." *Surgery.* March 2004; 135(3): 326–351.

Chiellini C et al. "Study of the effects of transoral gastroplasty on insulin sensitivity and secretion in obese subjects." *Nutr Metab Cardiovasc Dis.* March 2010; 20(3): 202–207.

Chikunguwo S et al. "Influence of obesity and surgical weight loss on thyroid hormone levels." *Surg Obes Relat Dis.* November–December 2007; 3(6): 631–635.

Clinical guidelines on the identification, evaluation, and treatment of overweight and obesity in adults: the evidence report. National Institutes of Health; National Heart, Lung, and Blood Institute; and National Institute of Diabetes, and Digestive and Kidney Diseases. NIH Publication Number 98-4083. September 1998. www.nhlbi.nih.gov/guidelines/obesity/ob_gdlns.htm.

Closset J et al. "Laparoscopic gastric bypass as a revision procedure after transoral gastroplasty." *Obes Surg.* December 10, 2009.

Cohen P. Understanding insulin signaling. July 12, 2000. www.wellcome.ac.uk /en/1/awtpubnwswlkbcksp3inssig.html.

Committee for Proprietary Medicinal Products. Opinion: following an Article 31 referral: sibutramine. European Agency for the Evaluation of Medicinal Products Postauthorization Evaluation of Medicines for Human Use. December 2, 2002. www.emea.eu.int/pdfs/human/referral/451402en.pdf.

Complications of obesity. WebMD. 2003. www.medscape.com/viewarticle/4579 26_10.

Coté GA et al. "Emerging technology: endoluminal treatment of obesity." *Gastrointest Endosc.* November 2009; 70(5): 991–999.

Craddock D. "Anorectic drugs: use in general practice." *Drugs.* 1976; 11(5): 378–393.

Croft H et al. "Effect on body weight of bupropion sustained-release in patients with major depression treated for 52 weeks." *Clinical Therapy.* April 2002; 24(4): 662–672.

Crook WG, Cass H. *The Yeast Connection and Women's Health.* Professional Books; 2003.

Crook WG. *The Yeast Connection: A Medical Breakthrough.* Vintage; 1986.

Csendes A et al. "Management of leaks after laparoscopic sleeve gastrectomy in patients with obesity." *Gastrointest Surg.* June 22, 2010.

Cummings DE et al. "Plasma ghrelin levels after diet-induced weight loss or gastric bypass surgery." *New England Journal of Medicine.* 2002; 346(21): 1,623–1,630.

Dargent J. "Laparoscopic adjustable gastric banding: lessons from the first 500 patients in a single institution." *Obesity Surgery.* 1999; 5: 446–452.

Degen L, Oesch S, Casanova M, Graf S, Ketterer S, Drewe J, Beglinger C. "Effect of PYY3-36 on food intake in humans." *Gastroenterology.* 2005; 129: 1,430.

Devière J et al. "Safety, feasibility and weight loss after transoral gastroplasty: First human multicenter study." *Surg Endosc.* March 2008; 22(3): 589–598. Epub November 1, 2007.

Diethylpropion. RXlist.com. www.rxlist.com/frame/display.cgi?drug=TENUATE.

Drezgic M et al. "Should we look for metabolic syndrome (MSy) in subclinical hypothyroidism?" *Endocrine Abstracts.* 2008; 16: 787.

Erasmus U. *Fats That Heal, Fats That Kill.* Alive Books; 1999.

European Agency for the Evaluation of Medicinal Products. [Press release.] September 9, 1999. www.emea.eu.int/pdfs/human/press/pr/232599en.pdf.

Ezrin C. *Your Fat Can Make You Thin.* Contemporary Books; 2001.

Fat cell hormone promotes type 2 diabetes. National Institutes of Health, National Institute of Diabetes and Digestive and Kidney Diseases. January 2001. www.niddk.nih.gov/welcome/releases/1-01.htm.

Fazylov R et al. "Laparoscopic Roux-en-Y gastric bypass surgery on morbidly obese patients with hypothyroidism." *Obes Surg.* June 2008; 18(6): 644–647.

Fen-Phen online information resource. James F. Early, LLC. 2001.

Fife B. *The Healing Miracles of Coconut Oil.* Piccadilly Books; 2003.

Forslund, H. et al. "Meal patterns and obesity in Swedish women." *European Journal of Clinical Nutrition.* 2002; 56: 740–747.

Fraser WD et al. "Are biochemical tests of thyroid function of any value in monitoring patients receiving thyroxine replacement?" *British Medical Journal.* September 27, 1986; 293(6550): 808–10.

Freudenrich CC. "How fat cells work." HowStuffWorks.com. home.howstuffworks.com/fat-cell.htm/printable.

Fung TT, Hu FB, Pereira MA, et al. "Whole-grain intake and the risk of type 2 diabetes: a prospective study in men." *American Journal of Clinical Nutrition.* 2002; 76: 535–540.

Fung TT et al. "Low-carbohydrate diets and all-cause and cause-specific mortality: two cohort studies." *Annals of Internal Medicine.* 2010; 153(5).

Gadde K. "Long-term study finds antidepressants effective for weight loss in women." DukeMed News Office. September 11, 2001.

Galletti P-M et al. "Effect of fluorine on the thyroidal iodine metabolism in hyperthyroidism." *Journal of Clinical Endocrinology.* 1958; 18: 1,102–1,110.

Gate Pharmaceuticals. Adipex-P (phentermine hydrochloride) product information. November 2000. www.gatepharma.com/Adipex-P/adipexscript.pdf.

Gittleman AL. *Eat Fat, Lose Weight.* Keats Publishing; 1999.

Gittleman AL. *The Fat Flush Plan.* McGraw-Hill; 2002.

Gittleman AL. *Guess What Came to Dinner? Parasites and Your Health.* Avery Penguin Putnam; 2001.

Gittleman AL. *Why Am I Always So Tired?* HarperSanFrancisco; 1999.

GlaxoSmithKline. Wellbutrin SR (bupropion hydrochloride), prescribing information. October 2002. us.gsk.com/products/assets/us_wellbutrinSR.pdf.

Glazer G. "Long-term pharmacotherapy of obesity 2000: a review of efficacy and safety." *Archives of Internal Medicine.* 2001; 161(15): 1,814–1,824.

Gobble RM et al. "Gastric banding as a salvage procedure for patients with weight loss failure after Roux-en-Y gastric bypass." *Surg Endosc.* April 2008; 22(4): 1019–1022.

Goglia PL. *Turn Up the Heat: Unlock the Fat-Burning Power of Your Metabolism.* Viking; 2002.

Goode E. "The heavy cost of chronic stress." *New York Times.* December 17, 2002.

Gortmaker S, Must LA, Perrin JM, et al. "Social and economic consequences of overweight in adolescence and young adulthood." *New England Journal of Medicine.* 1993; 329: 1,008.

Grayson CE, ed. insulin resistance syndrome. WebMD Health. November 2002.

Grout P. *Jumpstart Your Metabolism: How to Lose Weight by Changing the Way You Breathe.* Fireside; 1998.

Haines PS et al. "Weekend eating in the United States is linked with greater energy, fat, and alcohol intake." *Obesity Research.* 2003; 11: 945–949.

Halford JC et al. "Pharmacological management of appetite expression in obesity." *Nat Rev Endocrinol.* May 2010; 6(5): 255–269.

Hanks B, Rooney R. The Physique Transformation Program. www.physiquetrans formation.com.

Harrison L. *Master Your Metabolism.* Sourcebooks; 2003.

Hayashi T et al. "Ellagitannins from Lagerstroemia speciosa as activators of glucose transport in fat cells." *Planta Medica.* 2002; 68(2): 173–175.

Indications and side effects. Presentations at American Epilepsy Society 56th Annual Meeting. December 2002.

Insulin resistance and pre-diabetes. National Institutes of Health, National Institute of Diabetes and Digestive and Kidney Diseases, National Diabetes Information Clearinghouse. May 2003. www.idd.nih.gov/health/diabetes/pubs/insulinres /index.htm.

"Insulin resistance syndrome." American Academy of Family Physicians. *American Family Physician.* March 15, 2001.

Isidro ML et al. "Metformin reduces thyrotropin levels in obese, diabetic women with primary hypothyroidism on thyroxine replacement therapy." *Endocrine.* 2007; 32(1): 79–82. Epub October 2, 2007.

Jahnke, Roger O. "Oxygen metabolism." *HealthWorld.* www.healthy.net/asp/tem plates/article.asp?PageType=Article&ID=991.

Jonsson S, Hedblad B, Engstrom G et al. "Influence of obesity on cardiovascular risk: twenty-three-year follow-up of 22,025 men from an urban Swedish population." *International Journal of Obesity Related Metabolic Disorders*. 2002; 26: 1,046.

Judy WV et al. "Antidiabetic activity of a standardized extract (glucosol) from Lagerstroemia speciosa leaves in type II diabetics. A dose-dependence study." *Journal of Ethnopharmacology*. 2003; 87(1): 115–117.

Kakuda T, Sakane I, Takihara T, Ozaki Y, Takeuchi H, Kuroyanagi M. "Hypoglycemic effect of extracts from Lagerstroemia speciosa L. Leaves in genetically diabetic KK-AY mice." *Bioscience, Biotechnology and Biochemistry*. 1996; 60(2): 204–208.

Kalfarentzos F et al. "Weight loss following vertical banded gastroplasty: intermediate results of a prospective study." *Obesity Surgery*. 2001; 11(3): 265–270.

Kasza J et al. "Analysis of poor outcomes after laparoscopic adjustable gastric banding." *Surg Endosc*. June 30, 2010.

Kennett GA et al. "New approaches to the pharmacological treatment of obesity: Can they break through the efficacy barrier? " *Pharmacol Biochem Behav*. August 3, 2010.

Khan B et al. "Hypogylcemic activity of aqueous extract of some indigenous plants." *Pak J Pharm Sci*. 2005; 18(1): 62–64.

Khan MS et al. "Cinnamon improves glucose and lipids of people with type 2 diabetes." *Diabetes Care*. 2003; 26: 3,215–3,218.

Knudsen N et al. "Small differences in thyroid function may be important for body mass index and the occurrence of obesity in the population." *J Clin Endocrinol Metab*. May 3, 2005.

Kolata G. "The fat epidemic/new clues from the lab/how the body knows when to gain or lose." *New York Times*. October 17, 2000.

Krotkiewski M. "Thyroid hormones in the pathogenesis and treatment of obesity." *European Journal of Pharmacology*. 2002; 440(2–3): 85–98.

Lakka HM, Laaksonen DE, Lakka TA et al. "The metabolic syndrome and cardiovascular disease mortality in middle-aged men." *Journal of the American Medical Association*. 2002; 288: 2,709.

Lanc, James et al. "Caffeine affects cardiovascular and neuroendocrinology activation at work and home." *Psychosomatic Medicine* 2002; 64: 593–603.

Langer S, Scheer JF. *Solved: The Riddle of Illness.* Healing Arts Press; 1989.

Lanthaler M et al. "Long term results and complications following adjustable gastric banding." *Obes Surg.* May 23, 2010.

Layton, Julia. "How calories work." HowStuffWorks.com. home.howstuffworks .com/calorie.htm/printable.

Leeds AR. "Glycemic index and heart disease." *American Journal of Clinical Nutrition* 2002; 76: 286S–289S.

Lejeune M. "Additional protein intake limits weight gain after weight loss in humans. Abstract t4:02." Proceedings of the European Congress of Obesity. Helsinki, Finland. June 2003.

Linde, JA et. al. "Self weighing in weight gain prevention and weight loss trials." *Annals of Behavioral Medicine,* 2005. December; 30(3): 210–216.

Linquette A, Fossati P. "Hunger control with benzphetamine hydrochloride in the treatment of obesity." *Lille Medical.* 1971; 16(suppl 2): 620–624.

Liu F, Kim J, Li Y, Liu X, Li J, Chen X. "An extract of Lagerstroemia speciosa L. has insulin-like glucose uptake-stimulatory and adipocyte differentiation-inhibitory activities in 3T3-L1 cells." *Journal of Nutrition.* 2001; 131(9): 2,242–2,247.

Liu S, Willett WC, Stampfer MJ, Hu FB et al. "A prospective study of dietary glycemic load, carbohydrate intake, and risk of coronary heart disease in U.S. women." *American Journal of Clinical Nutrition.*" 2000; 71: 1,455–1,461.

MacGregor A, ed. "The story of surgery for obesity." American Society of Bariatric Surgeons (ASBS). 2002 Amendment.

Maeda H et al. "Fucoxanthin from edible seaweed, Undaria pinnatifida, shows anti-obesity effect through UCP1 expression in white adipose tissues." *Biochem Biophys Res Commun.* 2005; 332(2): 392–397.

Manson JE, Willett WC, Stampfer MJ, et al. "Body weight and mortality among women." *New England Journal of Medicine.* 1995; 333: 677.

Mason EE. "Vertical banded gastroplasty for obesity." *Archives of Surgery*. 1982; 117(5): 701–706.

Mason EE. "Why the operation I prefer is vertical banded gastroplasty." *Obesity Surgery*. 1991; 1(2): 181–183.

Mason EE et al. "Gastric bypass for obesity after ten years experience." *International Journal of Obesity*. 1978; v2(2): v197–206.

Mason EE, Ito C. "Gastric bypass in obesity." *Surgical Clinics of North America*. 1967; 47(6): 1,345–1,351.

Mazansky H. "A review of obesity and its management in 263 cases." *South African Medical Journal*. 1975; 49(47): 1,955–1,962.

"Medical encyclopedia: obesity." MEDLINEplus. May 17, 2002. www.nlm.nih.gov /medlineplus/ency/article/003101.htm#Definition.

Meigs JB. "The metabolic syndrome." *British Medical Journal*. 2003; 327: 61–62.

Mellin L. *The Solution: 6 Winning Ways to Permanent Weight Loss*. Regan Books; 1997.

Mercola J, Levy AR. *The No-Grain Diet: Conquer Carbohydrate Addiction and Stay Slim for Life*. E.P. Dutton; 2003.

Michaud E. "Healing with your sixth sense." *Prevention*. May 2003.

Miller PM. *The Hilton Head Metabolism Diet*. Warner Books; 1983.

Mogul H et al. "The endocrinopathy of obesity: correlate, consequence or cause?" [Abstract.] 84th annual meeting of the Endocrine Society. June 2002.

Mohos E et al. "Quality of life parameters, weight change and improvement of co-morbidities after laparoscopic Roux Y gastric bypass and laparoscopic gastric sleeve resection comparative study." *Obes Surg*. July 14, 2010.

Mokdad AH, Ford ES, Bowman BA, et al. "Prevalence of obesity, diabetes, and obesity-related health risk factors, 2001." *Journal of the American Medical Association*. 2003; 289: 76.

Moreno C et al. "Transoral gastroplasty is safe, feasible, and induces significant weight loss in morbidly obese patients: results of the second human pilot study." *Endoscopy.* 2008; 40(5): 406–413.

Moulin de Moraes CM et al. "Prevalence of subclinical hypothyroidism in a morbidly obese population and improvement after weight loss induced by Roux-en-Y gastric bypass." *Obes Surg.* 2005; 15(9): 1,287–1,291.

Muller FO et al. "Availability of phendimetrazine from sustained and non-sustained action formula." *South African Medical Journal.* 1975; 49(5): 135–139.

Murakami C, Myoga K, Kasai R, Ohtani K, Kurokawa T, Ishibashi S, Dayrit F, Padolina WG, Yamasaki K. "Screening of plant constituents for effect on glucose transport activity in ehrlich ascites tumour cells." *Chemical and Pharmaceutical Bulletin* (Tokyo). 1993; 41(12): 2,129–2,131.

Must A, Spadano J, Coakley EH. "The disease burden associated with overweight and obesity." *Journal of the American Medical Association.* 1999; 282: 1,523.

Nannipieri M et al. "Expression of thyrotropin and thyroid hormone receptors in adipose tissue of patients with morbid obesity and/or type 2 diabetes: effects of weight loss." *Int J Obes* (Lond). September 2009; 33(9): 1,001 6. Epub July 28, 2009.

Nannipieri M et al. "Expression of thyrotropin and thyroid hormone receptors in adipose tissue of patients with morbid obesity and/or type 2 diabetes: effects of weight loss." *Int J Obes* (Lond). September 2009; 33(9): 1,001–1,006.

Nathan PJ et al. "Neuropsychiatric adverse effects of centrally acting antiobesity drugs." *CNS Neurosci Ther.* July 7, 2010.

Ngondi Jet al. "IGOB131, a novel seed extract of the West African plant Irvingia gabonensis, significantly reduces body weight and improves metabolic parameters in overweight humans in a randomized double-blind placebo controlled investigation." *Lipids in Health and Disease.* 2009; 8: 7.

Nguyen NT et al. "The relationship between hospital volume and outcome in bariatric surgery at academic medical centers." *Ann Surg.* 2004; 240(4): 586–593, 594.

Nygaard B et al. "Effect of combination therapy with thyroxine (T4) and 3,5,3'-tri-iodothyronine versus T4 monotherapy in patients with hypothyroidism, a double-blind, randomised cross-over study." *European Journal of Endocrinology.* 2009; 161(6): 895–902.

O'Brien PE et al. "Prospective study of a laparoscopically placed, adjustablic gastric band in the treatment of morbid obesity." *British Journal of Surgery.* 1999; 86(1): 113–118.

"One-year prophylactic treatment of euthyroid Hashimoto's thyroiditis patients with levothyroxine: is there a benefit?" *Thyroid.* 2001; 11(3): 249–255.

Orlistat. RXList.com. www.rxlist.com/frame/display.cgi?drug=Xenical.

Osono Y, Hirose N, Nakajima K, Hata Y. "The effects of pantethine on fatty liver and fat distribution." *Journal of Atherosclerosis and Thrombosis.* 2000; 7(1): 55–58.

Overweight and obesity, defining overweight and obesity. Centers for Disease Control and Prevention, National Center for Chronic Disease Prevention and Health Promotion, Division of Nutrition and Physical Activity. April 22, 2003. www.cdc .gov/nccdphp/dnpa/obesity/defining.htm.

Palkhivala A. "New hormone might explain link between diabetes and obesity." *WebMD Health.* January 17, 2001.

Parsons WB. "Controlled-release diethylpropion hydrochloride used in a program for weight reduction." *Clinical Therapy.* 1981; 3(5): 329–335.

Patel SR, Malhotra A, White DP, Gottlieb DJ, Hu FB. "Association between reduced sleep and weight gain in women." *Am J Epidemiol.* November 15, 2006; 164(10): 947–954.

Patel S et al. "Reasons and outcomes of laparoscopic revisional surgery after lapa-roscopic adjustable gastric banding for morbid obesity." *Surg Obes Relat Dis.* 2010; 6(4): 391–398.

Peppard PE, Young T, Palta P, et al. "Longitudinal study of moderate weight change and sleep-disordered breathing." *Journal of the American Medical Association.* 2000; 284: 3,015.

Perrone, Tony. *Dr. Tony Perrone's Body Fat Breakthru.* Regan Books; 1999.

Pharmacia and Upjohn Company. Didrex (benzphetamine hydrochloride) product information. April 2002. www.pfizer.com/download/uspi_didrex.pdf.

Phendimetrazine information. Eon Labs. June 16, 1999. www.phendimetrazine .org/phendimetrazine-information.htm.

Phendimetrazine. RXlist.com. www.rxlist.com/frame/display.cgi?drug=BONTRIL.

Phentermine. RXlist.com. www.rxlist.com/frame/display.cgi?drug=ADIPEX.

Pi-Sunyer FX. "Medical hazards of obesity." *Annals of Internal Medicine.* 1993; 19: 655.

Pijl H et al. "Food choice in hyperthyroidism: potential influence of the autonomic nervous system and brain serotonin precursor availability." *Journal of Clinical Endocrinology and Metabolism.* 2001; 86(12): 5,848–5,853.

Plauchu M et al. "Trial of benzphetamine in treatment of obesity." *Lyon Medical.* 1969; 222(32): 317–321.

Polovina S et al. "The influence of low calorie–high dietary fibres diet on the change of parameters of the metabolic syndrome." *Endocrine Abstracts.* 2008; 16: 484.

Prachand VN et al. "Duodenal switch provides superior weight loss in the super obese (BMI [INSERT LESS THAN SIGN] or = 50 kg/m^2) compared with gastric bypass." *Ann Surg.* 2006; 244(4): 611–619.

Product review: weight loss, slimming, and diabetes-management supplements (chromium, cla, and pyruvate). ConsumerLab.com.

Purnell JQ. "What's new in medicine? *Obesity.*" Professional Publishing, 2003.

Rathi MS et al. "Weight gain during the treatment of thyrotoxicosis using conventional thyrostatic treatment." *J Endocrinol Invest.* 2008; 31(6): 505–508.

Report of the Dietary Guidelines Advisory Committee on the Dietary Guidelines for Americans, 2000.

Richards B. *Mastering Leptin.* Wellness Resources; 2003.

Rimm EB, Stampfer MF, Giovannucci E, et al. "Body size and fat distribution as predictors of coronary heart disease among middle-aged and older US men." *American Journal of Epidemiology.* 1995; 141: 1117.

Roos A et al. "Thyroid function is associated with components of the metabolic syndrome in euthyroid subjects." *Journal of Clinical Endocrinology and Metabolism.* doi:10.1210/jc.2006-1718.

Ross J. *The Diet Cure.* Viking Penguin; 1999.

Rubenstein R. "Laparoscopic adjustable gastric banding at a U.S. center with up to 3-year follow-up." *Obesity Surgery.* 2002; 12: 380–384.

Samaha F et al. "A low-carbohydrate as compared with a low-fat diet in severe obesity." *New England Journal of Medicine.* 2003; 348: 2,074–2,081.

Sanalkumar N et al. "Prevalence and potential implications of undetected thyroid abnormalities in a population of obese patients." [Abstract.] 84th annual meeting of the Endocrine Society. June 2002.

Sankar R. "Anticonvulsants: newest clinical trials focus on potential indications and side effects." *Medscape Neurology & Neurosurgery.* March 5, 2003. www.medscape .org/newarticle/450338.

Scopinaro N, et al. "Biliopancreatic diversion for obesity at eighteen years." *Surgery.* 1996; 119(3): 261–268.

Savard M. *How to Save Your Own Life: The Savard System for Managing—and Controlling—Your Health Care.* Warner Books; 2000.

Savard M. *The Savard Health Record: A Six-Step System for Managing Your Health Care.* Time Life; 2000.

Schmid S et al. "Sleep loss and metabolic response to breakfast." *Endocrine Abstracts.* 2008; 16: 524.

Seeley RR, Stephens TD, Tate P. *Anatomy and Physiology.* Time Mirror/Mosby College Publishing; 1989.

Shames R, Shames KH. *Thyroid Power: Ten Steps to Total Health.* Harper Resource; 2001.

Sibutramine. RXlist.com. www.rxlist.com/frame/display.cgi?drug=Meridia.

Simontacchi C. *Your Fat Is Not Your Fault*. Penguin Putnam; 1998.

Sjorstrom L et al. "Randomized placebo-controlled trial of orlistat for weight loss and prevention of weight gain in obese patients." *Lancet*. 1998; 352(9,123): 167–173.

Slotman GJ. "Non transectional open gastric bypass as the definitive bariatric procedure for 61 patients with BMI of 70 and higher." *Obes Surg*. 2010; 20(1): 7–12.

Smith S. "Pramlintide treatment reduces 24-hour caloric intake and meal sizes, and improves control of eating in obese subjects: a 6-week translational research study." *Am J Physiol Endocrinol Metab*. May 15, 2007.

Sohle J et al. "White tea extract induces lipolytic activity and inhibits adipogenesis in human subcutaneous (pre)-adipocytes." *Nutrition and Metabolism*. 2009; 6: 20.

Sonka J et al. "Effects of diet, exercise and anorexigenic drugs on serum thyroid hormones." *Endokrinologie*. 1980; 76(3): 351–356.

Spiegel K, Leproult R, Van Cauter E. "Impact of sleep debt on metabolic and endocrine function." *Lancet*. 1999; 354: 1,435–1,439.

St-Onge MP. "Physiological effects of medium-chain triglycerides: potential agents in the prevention of obesity." *Journal of Nutrition*. 2002; 132(3): 329–332.

Stein MR et al. "Ineffectiveness of human chorionic gonadotropin in weight reduction: a double-blind study." *American Journal of Clinical Nutrition*. 1976; 29: 940–948.

Strauss RS. "Childhood obesity and self-esteem." *Pediatrics*. 2000; 105: e15.

Suter M et al. "Band erosion after laparoscopic gastric banding: occurrence and results after conversion to Roux en Y gastric bypass." *Obes Surg*. 2004; 14(3): 381–386.

Suter M et al. "A 10 year experience with laparoscopic gastric banding for morbid obesity: high long term complication and failure rates." *Obes Surg*. 2006; 16(7): 829–835.

Suzuki Y, Unno T, Ushitani M, Hayashi K, Kakuda T. "Antiobesity activity of extracts from Lagerstroemia speciosa L. leaves on female KK-Ay mice." *Journal of Nutritional Science and Vitaminology* (Tokyo). 1999; 45(6): 791–795.

Swithers SE. "A role for sweet taste: calorie predictive relations in energy regulation by rats." *Behavioral Neuroscience*. 2008; 122(1): 161–173.

Taubes G. "What if it's all been a big fat lie?" *New York Times*. July 2, 2002.

Teitelbaum J. *From Fatigued to Fantastic*. Avery Penguin Putnam; 2001.

Telles S, Nagarathna R, Nagendra HR. "Breathing through a particular nostril can alter metabolism and autonomic activities." *Indian J Physiol Pharmacol*. 1994; 38(2): 133.

Tevaarwerk G. "Thyroid hormone replacement using a combination of levothyroxine plus slow-release liothyronine: beyond proof of principle." *Endocrine Abstracts*. 2008; 16: 771.

Tice JA et al. "Gastric banding or bypass? A systematic review comparing the two most popular bariatric procedures." *Am J Med*. 2008; 121(10): 885–893.

Triantafyllidis G et al. "Anatomy and complications following laparoscopic sleeve gastrectomy: radiological evaluation and imaging pitfalls." *Obes Surg*. July 24, 2010.

Tsesmeli N et al. "The future of bariatrics: endoscopy, endoluminal surgery, and natural orifice transluminal endoscopic surgery." *Endoscopy*. February 2010; 42(2): 155–162.

Val-Laillet D et al. "Chronic vagus nerve stimulation decreased weight gain, food consumption and sweet craving in adult obese minipigs." *Appetite*. June 19, 2010.

Valle-Jones JC et al. "A comparative study of phentermine and diethylpropion in the treatment of obese patients in general practices." *Pharmatherapeutica*. 1983; 3(5): 300–304.

Van Cauter E, Leproult R, Plat L. "Age-related changes in slow wave sleep and REM sleep and relationship with growth hormone and cortisol levels in healthy men." *Journal of the American Medical Association*. 2000; 284: 861–868.

Vigersky RA et al. "Thyrotropin suppression by metformin." *J Clin Endocrinol Metab*. 2006; 91(1): 225–227.

Volkova A et al. "Thyroid function is associated with insulin sensibility." *Endocrine Abstracts*. 2008; 16: 779.

Wadden TA et al. "Weight loss with naltrexone SR/bupropion SR combination therapy as an adjunct to behavior modification: the COR-BMOD Trial." *Obesity* (Silver Spring). June 17, 2010.

Weiner R et al. "Outcome after laparoscopic adjustable gastric banding 8 years experience." Frankfurt Center for Minimally Invasive Surgery, Section of Bariatric Surgery, Germany. rweiner@khs ffm.de.

Weintraub M et al. "A double-blind clinical trial in weight control: use of fenfluramine and phentermine alone and in combination." *Archives of Internal Medicine*. 1984; 144(6): 1,143–1,148.

Willett W, Manson J, Liu S. "Glycemic index, glycemic load, and risk of type 2 diabetes." *American Journal of Clinical Nutrition*. 2002; 76(suppl): 274S–280S.

Wittgrove AC, Clark GW. "Laparoscopic gastric bypass, Roux-en-Y–500 patients. Technique and results with 3–60 month follow-up." *Obesity Surgery*. 2000; 10: 233–239.

Wolcott WL, Fahey T. *The Metabolic Typing Diet: Customize Your Diet to Your Own Unique Body Chemistry*. Broadway Books; 2002.

Wolever TM, Mehling C. "High-carbohydrate-low-glycaemic index dietary advice improves glucose disposition index in subjects with impaired glucose tolerance." *British Journal of Nutrition*. 2002; 87: 477–487.

Wolf AM, Colditz GA. "Current estimates of the economic cost of obesity in the United States." *Obesity Research*. 1998; 6: 97.

Zieba R. "Obesity: a review of currently used antiobesity drugs and new compounds in clinical development." [Polish]. *Postepy Hig Med Dosw*. 2007; 61: 612–626.

Ziomber A et al. "Magnetically induced vagus nerve stimulation and feeding behavior in rats." *J Physiol Pharmacol*. September 2009; 60(3): 71–77.

INDEX

BOOKS BY MARY J. SHOMON

THE THYROID DIET REVOLUTION
Manage Your Master Gland of Metabolism for Lasting Weight Loss

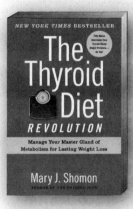

ISBN 978-0-06-198747-2 (paperback)

The expanded and updated edition of *The Thyroid Diet*—the groundbreaking guide for thyroid patients that revolutionized the conversation about thyroid conditions and weight loss.

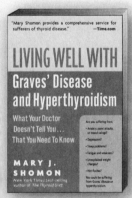

LIVING WELL WITH GRAVES' DISEASE AND HYPERTHYROIDISM
What Your Doctor Doesn't Tell You . . . That You Need to Know

ISBN 978-0-06-073019-2 (paperback)

A holistic roadmap for diagnosis, treatment, and recovery for the millions of people suffering from Graves' disease and hyperthyroidism.

LIVING WELL WITH HYPOTHYROIDISM
What Your Doctor Doesn't Tell You . . . That You Need to Know

ISBN 978-0-06-074095-5 (paperback)

This revised and updated edition incorporates up-to-the-minute diagnostic and treatment information, and features a broader range of alternative therapies.

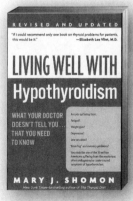